DOCTOR OF LOVE

James Graham and
His Celestial Bed

L Y D I A   S Y S O N

Dear Rosemary & Tom,

*hope you have an
mun fun with
this as I have...*

ll mu lov,

Lydia
x

ALMA BOOKS

ALMA BOOKS LTD
London House
243–253 Lower Mortlake Road
Richmond
Surrey TW9 2LL
United Kingdom
www.almabooks.com

First published by Alma Books Limited in 2008
Copyright © Lydia Syson, 2008

Lydia Syson asserts her moral right to be identified as the author of this work
in accordance with the Copyright, Designs and Patents Act 1988

Printed in England by TJ International, Padstow, Cornwall

ISBN: 978-1-84688-054-4

Contents

DOCTOR OF LOVE

Prologue

In 1780, James Graham was turning away carriages from his door on a nightly basis. He had London eating out of his hand, and images of the Doctor were everywhere – on stage, in the print shops, in the newspapers and on the streets. A Swedish visitor who sought him out said he kept the finest carriage and horses in the whole city, and seemed to see into the heart of every Englishman. "I am… not only a doctor of medicine, but a physician of the soul," claimed Graham. At the Temple of Health, overlooking the Thames, he ran the most exciting show in town. He had apparently succeeded in translating sexual knowledge into polite and rational entertainment.

Walking into the Temple was like entering the inner chambers of some enchanter's palace. Exotic perfumes and distant music seemed to seep as if without source into every room, and rainbow shards of light shining from one mysterious machine's prismatic pillar fractured in the spiralling glass columns of another. Glittering festoons of artificial flowers were mirrored in every shiny surface. A profusion of candles burning in silver-and-rhinestone candelabra added the scent of beeswax to an already heady atmosphere, designed to appeal to every sense. Meanwhile Graham had had a field day with a newly published guide to symbolism. Every crowing china cock, every rabbit, every mule, every fake stained-glass window pane radiated allegorical significance. Here was a bust of Hippocrates, here Cupid, here Galen – and there a salamander, a phoenix or a sphinx.

The vast and unmistakably phallic electrical conductor in the first room needed no interpretation though. This metal cylinder, eleven feet long and four in circumference, was suggestively described as ending in two semi-globes. It rested on six-foot-high pillars of intricately cut glass, reflecting and refracting all the coloured lamps and candles to dazzling effect. On metal shelves running its length glowed an enticing selection of the tools of Graham's trade: jars, vessels and phials filled with mysterious healing essences, supposedly impregnated with the electrical, magnetic and aerial forces which the Doctor claimed at his command.

On the other side of the room a six-foot sparkling golden drag-on appeared to fly, its wings outstretched, eyes ablaze and forked crimson tongue extended to receive the "lambent elementary fire". The electrical charge passed, visibly and loudly crackling, along the creature's scaly body and out through its tail. Connecting with the huge conductor, the charge continued along polished brass rods entwined with silken cords to activate a ten-foot-high throne, where crimson-flowered damask cushions could seat six or eight people for simultaneous treatment. Another five rooms displayed an equally eye-catching cornucopia. Everywhere, glass structures glittered and spiralled. The most stylish new techniques of the decorative arts did not just lend glamour to the latest inventions of natural philosophy. They were fundamental to the way Graham's Temple was constructed and construed. In the holy of holies, the Grand Apollo Chamber, the Doctor lectured an enthralled public.

Electricity was the most thrilling and visible of the scientific developments of the Enlightenment, "an Entertainment for Angels, rather than for Men". In a candlelit world, the drama of experiments involving showers of phosphorescent fire, liquids set alight and luminous bodies could hardly fail to bewitch the public. Extraordinary looking machinery generated static electrical "fire" by applying friction to hand-cranked spinning glass globes, cylinders and plates. The long tubes wielded by popular electrical demonstrators were uncannily like conjuror's wands, reinforcing the magical and miraculous air of this exciting new form of pyrotechnics. There was no escaping what else they resembled. Satirists and writers of erotica were quick to make the obvious associations, capitalizing delightedly on the newly familiar terminology of electrical "fluids" and "friction", the principles of attraction and repulsion, and the erections of human fibres.

James Graham took this several steps further, and he was perfectly serious. He firmly believed that "the venereal act itself, at all times, and under every circumstances, is in fact, no other than an electrical operation." It seemed to make every sense. Those "heart-piercing and irresistible glances" which shoot at critical times from soul to soul were "no other than electrical strokes or emanations!" Just as electricians had to charge up their capacitors, so the "animal electrical tube or cylinder" needed to be excited "for the accumulation, or mustering up of the balmy fire of life!... Then follows the discharging, or passage of that balmy, luminous, active principle, from the *plus* male to the *minus* female. These are all mere, plain, demonstrable, electrical processes." In Graham's mind and in the lectures with which he shocked and entranced an aristocratic

Georgian public, the fleshy-looking leather pad against which the glass of electrical machines rubbed as it rotated became a grotesque image of a woman's genitals. Both women and machinery were said to operate most effectively when pristine. Today cosmetic surgeons offer to rejuvenate women's sexual organs on the operating table. In the 1780s Graham promised that a combination of scrupulous hygiene and judiciously applied electrical "fire" could do much the same thing.

Putting the latest principles of natural philosophy to practical use in the act of procreation, the Doctor came up with his most extraordinary invention, the "medico, magnetico, musico, electrical" Celestial Bed. He opened a second Temple to house this astonishing piece of furniture-cum-medical apparatus. Marriages and families would no longer be ruined by infidelity and infertility. Britain could be populated with a race of superhumans, of the highest physical and mental calibre. In the Bed's final and most extraordinary incarnation, electricity, magnetism, mechanical musicians, fragrant airs, fresh flowers, seductive mirrors and miniature automata all came together to deliver sexual pleasures that were said to be sublime. By appointment only, couples could cough up £50 a night – a huge sum – to enjoy its prolonged delights. Officially, they had to be married, but discretion was assured.

Nobles, gentry and courtesans turned up in their hundreds to hear Graham lecture on the bed's wonders, even before it was unveiled. Alongside electricity and magnetism, Graham also harnessed the fashionable new discoveries of chemistry to his cause – mind-altering substances like ether and nitrous oxide. He pioneered music therapy, incorporating intriguing new instruments into his equipment and conjugal music-making into his love-making advice.

The adulterous, the barren and the prurient arrived in their silks and masks to enjoy the illuminated glories of Graham's regal decor, his glitzy gold-and-glass take on the most up-to-date scientific research. They left with discreet booklets that promised to put the sexual sublime into the lives of every married couple, even without the benefits of the famous bed.

Against the most stylish and splendid backdrop imaginable, the Doctor – tall, handsome and utterly charming – railed against the degeneracy of luxury. Later he ventriloquized sexual equality through Vestina, his Goddess of Health, and was equally outspoken in his objections to slavery in the Atlantic triangle and Britain's death-dealing part in the American War of Independence. Amidst scenes of decorative excess and between evocations of political liberty, he preached moderation and regulation: early hours, plenty of exercise, a vegetarian diet, open air and above all genital hygiene. Nothing was more important than cold-water washing.

It was all very confusing. While Graham came up with legal reforms for the horrors of prostitution, prostitutes themselves adopted his rejuvenating techniques with huge success. Miss Harriet Jones of Wapping, who could with lips and tongue "make a man of sixty young", and boasted a "beautiful *black fringe*" bordering her "*Venetian Mount*", was reported by a guidebook to pursue "the *Grahamitic* method". Whether this was "from a practical knowledge of its increase of pleasure, from motives of cleanliness, or as a certain preventative we will not pretend to say; but we well know it makes her the more desirable bed-fellow, and after every *stroke* gives fresh *tone and vigour* to the lately *distended parts*".

Graham's life reflected the rainbow colours of his times like one of the prismatic columns that supported his healing electro-magnetic structures. At the height of his success he trod a line every bit as precarious as that of the high-wire walkers who competed for audiences at Astley's amphitheatre over at Westminster Bridge, perilously poised between the sublime and the ridiculous. He used to argue that, like the wet nose of a dog, "a cold, glowing, full, liquid balmy firmness... of the genital parts" showed a state of "perfect health and strength!" Just as he touted the conditions of the genitals as "the true pulse, the infallible barometer" of a person's health, so the figure of Graham himself, endlessly rendered in caricature with phallic objects (whether the scroll of his famous lecture, or the prime conductor of his electrical apparatus), came to stand for the moral state of health of the nation. He quickly became an invaluably malleable image for satirists wanting to consider the ailments of the state. Gambling, riots, fashion, luxury, social climbing and public credulity were all anatomized through the figure of the electric empiric.

James Graham has long been regarded as one of the Enlightenment's best sideshows, good for a snigger, or an entertaining footnote to the stories of history's main players. As a one-off eccentric, he spawned no movement, gave rise to no lasting neologism, inspired no posthumous acolytes. But he was as typical of the eighteenth century as any of the great scientists, writers and philosophers. This, after all, was a period stuffed with little men trying to make it big in a vibrantly commercial world. Some, like Graham, briefly succeeded; others sank with no trace. In many ways the Doctor was an entrepreneur par excellence. He took up all the most exciting new developments of his era and remade them in compellingly original forms. But he was not a very realistic businessman.

Colourful though Graham's story was, it was also a tragic one. Even at the moment of his greatest success, the Doctor inevitably attracted notoriety. While half of London flocked in awe to his door, the other half denounced him as the King of Quacks, an impudent charlatan whose magnetic charms drew money from the pockets of gullible fools. It was a label that stuck, for two centuries and more, and one that has allowed history to misjudge him. For although Graham was a man who sometimes made himself ridiculous, he lived life with the best intentions. His spirited and humane take on the world's problems can hardly fail to strike a chord today. He was utterly convinced that he had been put on earth to improve the lot of humankind. But as his ever wilder ambitions exceeded his ability to pay for them, he found himself increasingly compromised and misunderstood.

In newspapers, handbills, health manuals and pamphlets, he poured "forth unreservedly his whole Soul!" His life was one self-consciously dramatized in his own publicity; he told his own tale, piecemeal, through florid advertisements and promotional literature that took hyperbole to new heights. In contrast to his prolific output in print, he left few manuscripts. What letters survive were written in a professional context to patients or patrons, and Graham tended to keep his family out of the limelight he loved. This lack of intimate evidence is inevitably a problem for a biographer. I have worried at times about being duped by my subject, fretted that I have simply fallen for the public persona of a contradictory individual. But what if Graham had written a full-length memoir, left a private journal, or preserved more personal correspondence? Would such documents be any more authentic, and should a biographer's wariness about them be any less acute? Is an individual necessarily any less self-deluding in manuscript than in print, in autobiography than in advertising? Print was where Graham made himself, and where he was destroyed, and he was born at a time when its possibilities were still being revealed. Brash, commercial and self-seeking, yet touchingly heartfelt, the Doctor's published remains are rich and colourful. They are the testimonials of an exceptional individual, a man entirely of his time. Here then, is a story in small ads.

"…though all the portals open stand
Of Health's own temple at her Graham's command
And the great high-priest baffling Death and Sin
Earth each immortal idiot to the chin,
Ask of these wretched beings worse than dead
If on the couch celestial gold can shed
The coarser blessings of a Peasant's bed."
       – Wordsworth, *Imitation of Juvenal*

1

The Beginning

> "From my earliest infancy, I loved
> the profession of medicine…"

At Edinburgh, an operation was a performance. It had been the same in Leiden, where most of the Scottish medical school's founders had learnt their trade. The surgeons usually scheduled their operations for Sunday afternoons – so as not to clash with lectures and church services – and advertised tickets beforehand on notices in the hospital's consulting room, alerting students and apprentices to the forthcoming drama. Like clinical lectures, autopsies and even religious services, surgery took place in the amphitheatre. It was the heart of Edinburgh's new Royal Infirmary, architecturally and philosophically, an airy room built over the hospital's generous central staircase, designed to allow plenty of space for patient-bearing sedan chairs. An elegant coved roof and glassed cupola let the light pour in from above, while steeply raked benches rising up on three sides of the theatre gave a fine view of the proceedings for several hundred observers. Others hung from galleries above.

Before scalpels were drawn, the surgeon would review the reasons for the operation under scrutiny, and discuss formally how it should be performed. What followed required strength of purpose for everyone present. "Und[a]unted firmness of resolution…" was essential for the operating surgeon, according to an eighteenth-century handbook on hospitals. He must be "staggered neither by tears, sighs, or groans, the sight of blood, or even death's pale image". Meanwhile the patient endured "unspeakable pain and torture". As the blood ran off the runnels of the operating table's oilskin cover, the surgeon, dressed in a frock coat stiff with the pus and human debris of previous operations, would kick a box of sawdust underneath to soak up the overflow. The fortifications surgeons needed for such scenes was not always exclusively mental: "I have seen several primed with a good dram of brandy just before they went to the theatre…" one Chair of Medicine revealed towards the end of the century, adding with heavy sarcasm, "I must do them justice to say that they drank their brandy most scientifically out of a cupping glass."

It wasn't encouraged, but the audience often passed audible judgement on the skill of different surgeons as though they were at a playhouse. One year the students' vocal criticism of one nervous operator attempting a delicate eye procedure with trembling hands provoked a serious reprimand. Others were occasionally expelled from the premises for clapping or hissing as an operation took place. From time to time, some left of their own accord, unable to stomach particularly gruesome scenes. An American student, James Rush, wrote home about a breast-cancer operation he had witnessed: "The mamma was taken off very expeditiously indeed, and I was about to give credit to the hand of the operator – But just as the ligatures had all been applied, and the dressings were about to be put on – It was discovered that the diseased part had not been entirely extracted… the barbarous handling and even *punching* of wounded flesh… which followed – was too shocking to look at."

The Royal Infirmary, where all this took place, had risen stone by stone on the far side of Edinburgh's Cowgate valley through James Graham's infancy, "reared by the hand of charity". It had been an exemplary municipal enterprise. The new landmark was a living, humming manifestation of the great age of improvement just dawning in Scotland. In the early 1750s, Edinburgh was a city consciously on the cusp of change. Scotland as a whole had only recently recovered from the economic devastation wrought by the 1707 Act of Union, destructive of the country's independent parliament and its self-confidence alike. Now Edinburgh's boom years were beginning. Politeness and civic virtues reigned as the economy surged.

Born in the middle of a cold wet June in 1745, Graham came into the world at the perfect moment to take advantage of Edinburgh's astonishing metamorphosis. The Grahams were a family of squarely middling means, that ever-growing band. His father, an "honest laborious" saddler, was a respectable burgess, his maternal grandfather a lawyer. The future Dr Graham may have had none of the advantages of a medical family, with its invaluable inheritance of knowledge, practice and professional networks, but neither was he brought up in rags and squalor.

At least, no more squalor than any other inhabitant of Edinburgh had to endure, rich or poor. Stinking "Auld Reekie", as Edinburgh is still affectionately known, then thoroughly deserved its nickname. The Old Town, with its memorably vile "morning smells", constituted the entire city at this point. The elegant New Town – which half a century later would earn the city an elegant new sobriquet, "the

Athens of the North" – was still unimagined. Most people lived in dark, cramped, multi-storey tenements: impossibly narrow buildings that clung defensively to the steep sides of the castle-topped, volcanic crag, or gripped the sweeping tail long ago left behind by retreating glaciers, now the backbone of the Royal Mile. Each floor housed several families, from all walks of life. William and Jean Graham moved from the outskirts of Edinburgh into its centre in 1751. Their new home in Veitch's Land was off the West Bow, leading up from the Grassmarket, and the tenement was shared with two coppersmiths, some merchants, an ale-seller, a glover and a blacksmith. It was near enough Cowgate – a thoroughfare with a less salubrious ring to it – to have been elided with it repeatedly in later accounts of James Graham's life.

The Grahams were not the kind of family who left much behind in the way of documentary evidence. When it comes to reconstructing the details of James Graham's childhood and early life, there is little more substantial on which to rely than the births, marriages and deaths recorded, with luck, in Old Parish Records. His earliest biographer was another Edinburgh resident called Charles Kirkpatrick Sharpe, whose brief handwritten account eventually found its way, undated, into the National Library of Scotland, tucked into a (probably pirated) edition of Graham's *Eccentric Lecture*. But Sharpe, an expert on matters antiquarian, a ballad-collector and a friend of Walter Scott, was barely a teenager when Graham died, so he must have collected his evidence from others. A respected scholar, he was also a man known for his taste for historical gossip and marital scandal. Though his version of Graham's life seems largely accurate, it's not completely reliable. The same is certainly true of a more detailed biographical sketch written in the late 1830s to accompany John Kay's 1786 portrait of Graham in a collection known as *Kay's Edinburgh Portraits*. It was probably written by a Scottish journalist called James Paterson, sixty years Graham's junior, who could never have known him personally. Errors in both these accounts have been unknowingly replicated in later writings about Graham.

From the *Edinburgh Portraits* sketch we learn that William and Jean Graham were "old-fashioned Presbyterian Whigs of the strictest kind". James grew up singing psalms every Sunday at Greyfriars church. In old age his parents would come to enjoy every attention from their most celebrated son, taking morning airings in his smart carriage, attended by gorgeously liveried servants and generally surrounded by the kind of "pomp and vanities" which Graham often found hard to resist. Mrs Graham was said to have helped out at the Temple in later life, selling medicines and pamphlets, but during James' childhood she must have been immured in domesticity, as one confinement followed another. She produced nine children in all, five of whom survived to adulthood. The eldest, Grizell, had been born in Falkirk, Stirlingshire, where William Graham had established himself as a saddler before his marriage. Elspeth, James, Robert, and Jean were all born at Crosscausey, then just outside the city. After the family's move to the heart of Edinburgh, twins were born, Rachell and Margaret, who survived at least a few weeks to be baptized on 13th January. They were followed by Ann, who, like Grizell and Elspeth, definitely grew up and married. But just a week before Ann's birth in October 1753, a child of a William Graham was buried in their parish. This was probably six-year-old Robert, since James later described his youngest sibling William as his "only" brother. The baby of the family, born in 1755 and named after his father, was said to be so like James that the brothers were sometimes mistaken for one another, despite the ten years between them. Like James, William began his medical training in his mid-teens. By his early twenties, he had inadvertently propelled his older brother into national fame.

The Graham family lived a stone's throw from the public execution site described by one of James Graham's future patients, Walter Scott:

> The fatal day was announced to the public, by the appearance of a huge black gallows-tree towards the eastern end of the Grass-market. This ill-omened apparition was of great height, with a scaffold surrounding it, and a double ladder placed against it, for the ascent of the unhappy criminal and the executioner. As this apparatus was always arranged before dawn, it seemed as if the gallows had grown out of the earth in the course of one night, like the production of some foul demon; and I well remember the fright with which the schoolboys, when I was one of their number, used to regard these ominous signs of deadly preparation.

Medical students took a different view of events, often their first introduction to people they would come to know at closer quarters. "Saw two men hanged for murder," one student, Sylas Neville, confided laconically to his journal in 1773. "I should not have gone if it had not been reported that they intended making some resistance.

Was afterwards at the College when the bodies were received for dissection. They bled on the jugular being opened but not at the arm." Corpses for anatomy classes were hard to come by, and tended to become familiar through long use.

The saddler's son embarked on his professional training probably only after a decent and inexpensive schooling at the nearby Royal High School, which was favoured by virtually every respectable Edinburgh citizen. There he would have had at least six years' education in Latin language and literature, instruction in Roman antiquities, comparative ancient and modern geography, and learnt a smattering of Greek. He would also have spent much of his boyhood on the far side of the high stone walls which surrounded the new Infirmary next door to the school, expressly built to repel invaders from the school yard.

Graham grew up witnessing a steady influx of aspiring medics arriving each autumn for the beginning of the Winter Session. They were a conspicuous city presence, swarming between lectures, and trooping in and out of the Infirmary. The students packed out Edinburgh's boarding houses and rented rooms, the richer young men frequenting the oyster bars and whorehouses, the poorer ones confined to an expensive daily grind of lectures and note-taking that left little leisure for debauchery. Edinburgh was still the only place in Britain to combine a university education with clinical instruction in medicine. (The kind of training available at London hospitals was usually seen as a practical addition to an academic degree rather than its substitute.) Graduates could walk away with the title of MD in just three years. Oxford and Cambridge medical degrees were no more prestigious but still demanded a seven- or eight-year investment, and were only open to Church of England men. Not surprisingly then, Edinburgh drew all sorts.

In the autumn of 1761, sixteen-year-old Graham joined a gathering of embryonic doctors to sign the Matriculation Album in the University Library. He must have stood out even then, if only thanks to his impressive height and undeniable good looks. But he was also clearly already blessed with that supreme self-confidence which would propel him through life in years to come. Sharpe noted retrospectively that his "impudence" at this age was said to have been "very conspicuous". This did not simply mean that he was impertinent, but rather suggests that Graham was marked by a kind of chutzpah, that brand of charming audacity that can slide so easily between self-assurance and arrogance.

Most newcomers were impressed by the cosmopolitan crowd of young men who assembled at the beginning of each academic year. A Danish physician who spent some months in the city as a student in 1765 remembered mixing with Americans and West Indians, Portuguese and Italians, Frenchmen and Englishmen, Irishmen and Dutchmen, Germans and Swiss, Russians and Danes. Edinburgh was internationally famous for its medical education: it "already rivals, if not surpasses, that of every other school of Physic in Europe", wrote a young American contemporary, one of the university's many Philadelphian graduates.

One self-satisfied English undergraduate, Walter Jones, divided the heterogeneous mass that assembled in the library on his first day into three "ranks or orders":

1st the Fine Gentlemen, or those who give no application to study, but spend the Revenues of Gentlemen of Independent Fortunes. 2ly. The Gentlemen, or Students of Medicine strictly speaking, these live genteely and at the same time apply themselves to study. 3ly. The vulgar, or those who, if they are not indolent, are entirely devoid of everything polite and agreeable. I believe you will not doubt for a moment with which of these orders I ought to associate.

Graham was not in a position to worry too much about the social status of his fellow students, nor did he need to write home to describe his new life. One new friend, Thomas Arnold, clearly relished the chance to broaden his horizons: "I need not tell you that Edinburgh is the place to my wish…" he enthused, when he arrived from the Midlands in 1762. Arnold had previously been apprenticed to Richard Pulteney, a non-conformist apothecary and botanist, and he went on to become a respected expert in lunacy, running an asylum in his home town of Leicester. In July 1766 Arnold married James's older sister Elspeth in Edinburgh. By this time she had refined her name to Elizabeth and he had added MD to his own. "A College Life is my Element," he wrote to his former master just after his first Christmas in the city. "I think it the most agreeable Life upon Earth: and at present my only Fear is lest it should be too short. And how can it be otherwise. When one is continually meeting with something new; daily, nay, hourly, Increasing our Stock of Ideas; and enlarging the petty Circle which had before Circumscribed our Knowledge; one cannot but receive Abundance of Pleasure, and wish that Pleasure may be long continued."

Arnold's friend Timothy Bentley had been another Pulteney apprentice, and he was just as taken with Edinburgh. "I am well happy and shall remember the Seat of the Muses with pleasure as long as I live," Bentley assured Pulteney, subsequently confessing, "I observe you allow me to think of the Girls now and then ... and tho' I keep them pretty much out of my sights I can't always keep them out of my mind."

Despite Graham's later claims to have been "regularly bred to Physic and Surgery", there was really no such thing as a typical Edinburgh student. Even aside from the divisions of social class, age and gentility which some young men were so quick to notice, there were quite a number of different routes to a medical education at the university. The gentlemen physicians could take their time over graduation, enjoying the benefits of membership of the official Medical Society as well as opportunities to hobnob with their professors after class. Many seemed to spend as much time in taverns, brothels and theatres as they did in lectures. For those who could afford it, the pleasures of attending the Assembly Hall and enjoying concerts and plays were not just distractions from study, but an indispensable part of a gentleman physician's grooming. He needed the skills to present himself as the social equal of his future patients as surely as he needed a knowledge of anatomy. Samuel Johnson had recently coined the word "clubbable": this was only one of the advantages for Sylas Neville and his friends of membership of the Beggar's Benison, an Edinburgh gentlemen's sex club which rejoiced in the motto: "May Prick nor Purse ne'er fail you".

In contrast to this, an apprentice's education was firmly directed by his surgeon or apothecary master. It was invariably dominated by shop-floor drudgery – sweeping up, rolling pills, washing bandages, making up bills and running errands. Note-taking in class must have come as light relief. An apprentice lived with his master's family, and was expected to avoid his daughters. According to Sharpe, Graham was apprenticed to a chemist and apothecary at this point. But no evidence remains of any such indenture, which, since it was taxable, should have been recorded officially at the time.

It's more likely that Graham was one of a third group of students, the largest and most elusive type, and a mixed bag in themselves. Until recently, very little has been known about the "occasional auditors" identified by an early nineteenth-century Royal Commission. What united these students was the fact that they attended classes when the opportunity arose, and left with no form of certification, sometimes not even a trace of their presence at the university. In commercial terms, auditors like Graham were the professors' bread and butter. They dominated the lecture halls, and often crammed as many lectures into the single year the vast majority of them spent at the university as a typical gentleman graduate might manage in three or four. These men studied alongside the "gentlemen physicians" (most of whom arrived with every intention to graduate) and the "industrious apprentices". Many were optimistic they would share the prestige of Edinburgh's graduates: "What should I have been…!" wrote one young auditor, grateful for his uncle's timely financial support for study in the city. "A mere ignorant country quack – and hereafter I can rank with the highest of them – Oh! delightful thought."

Many accounts of Graham's life written in the past century note snidely that although he studied at Edinburgh University, he never officially graduated. Nor, in fact, did the vast majority of his contemporaries. In the early 1760s, most Edinburgh medical students avoided the formal rigour of actually taking their degrees. Even to matriculate was optional. To graduate required a significant fee of £10, as well as writing and defending a thesis in Latin. (Thomas Arnold confessed himself "continually haunted with [his] Thesis, and public examination in that Language".) Lots of other reputable European universities had less onerous graduation requirements. Some demanded minimal attendance to obtain their medical degrees, and the Scottish ones of Aberdeen and St Andrews none at all. So chastising Graham for his lack of a degree is both anachronistic and meaningless. In 1763 just ten out of the three hundred students attending classes that year in Edinburgh took the trouble to go through the thesis ordeal, and those who did collect their degrees often had less clinical experience than the apothecary's apprentices they invariably disdained.

Doctoring was a business as much as a profession, and in time James Graham would take this fact to its logical extreme. Medical education was no less commercial, and in Edinburgh in 1761, how much you got depended almost entirely on what you could pay. Each newcomer simply had to glean what he could from friends, family and acquaintances about the merits of particular teachers and courses, and then tailor his programme of study according to income, ambition and available time. Nothing was obligatory for those not planning to graduate other than payment. Most students who have left letters or diaries refer repeatedly to class fees, which meant little to the gentlemen, but weighed heavily on students from poorer families. "When I consider the Money that it will cost me during my Stay at this place, it makes me confine myself too close to my Study; more so than is conducive to my Health," confessed Thomas Ismay, recording that courses cost three guineas apiece. Coughing up for a son's medical education was a serious investment, which did not always pay off. Ismay's concerns proved justified, for he died at the end of that academic year, "in the Bloom of Life", and was buried in Greyfriars' churchyard, his professors his pall-bearers.

On 7th October 1761 the annual announcement appeared in the Edinburgh newspapers:

The Professors of Medicine in the University of Edinburgh are to begin their Lectures on Wednesday the 28th October:
Anatomy and surgery by Drs. Monro sen. & jun.
Midwifery by Dr. Young.
Materia Medica by Dr. Hope.
Chemistry by Dr. Cullen.
Theory of Medicine by Dr. Whytt.
Practice of Medicine by Dr. Rutherford.

The list reads like a roll call of the luminaries of eighteenth-century medicine, the gods and heroes of a "golden age of physic". Graham was trained by men of global fame. These "ingenious countrymen", as Graham described them later, were "living ornaments", who could hardly have inspired more awe in the medical world.

"I think I would not fail of having heard [Dr Cullen's lectures] for ten thousand pounds. Illustrious Oracle of human Wisdom live – live for ever!" wrote Benjamin Rush of Philadelphia, a future Founding Father whose "Halcyon Days" were spent in Edinburgh. William Cullen, at this point responsible for chemistry instruction, later Professor of the Theory of Medicine, was both revered and adored. He was a towering figure of the Scottish Enlightenment and lionized as the "Scotch Hippocrates". Adam Smith was a close friend, and his philosophy seeped into Cullen's lectures. Thomas Arnold liked Cullen best of all his professors. Another student fell for him on his first day at lectures: "Dr Cullen the inimatable Cullen I say addressed his Class in the warmest manner that words could express. Sure a more warm affectionate and at the same time a more engaging instructive, extemporary Discourse I never hear'd from any before." Samuel Bard of New York also wrote home in awe after joining Cullen's course in chemistry in 1762: "it must certainly make him very happy… to see so many even from the Wilds of America crouding his Lectures, and listening to him with the greatest pleasure and attention—for he never speaks but you may see these emotions painted in the faces of allmost all his hearers & so universal a silence reigns that was a pin to drop it would be distinctly heard."

Of all these teachers, "the learned and sagacious Dr Whytt" was the most obviously influential on Graham. This professor of Medical Theory, like his colleague Dr Rutherford, had actually studied with an ageing Boerhaave at the University of Leiden. (The incomparably famous Dutch physician Herman Boerhaave (1668–1738) introduced the essential principle of academic clinical teaching on which Edinburgh medical school was founded.) Whytt's ideas about unconscious response were elaborated in a major work on nervous diseases published in 1764. In his view, the parts of the body operated in a particular kind of sympathy with the soul: illness came about when this relationship became distorted. This kind of thinking helped transform that vague complaint "the vapours", a term derived from the old-style humour-based understanding of pathology, by then on the decline, into the more fashionable "nervous disease". Whytt's controversial interpretation of the relationship between body and soul was at the heart of the mood-altering therapies Graham took up with such enthusiasm in the 1770s. Graham's prescriptive promotion of fresh air, exercise and simple nutrition would have been learnt from both Whytt and Cullen.

The charismatic Dr Alexander Monro *secundus* was the youngest of the Professors. Born into an impressive medical dynasty, he had inherited some of his father's anatomy classes in 1758 even before he'd graduated. In the mid-1760s he was lecturing without notes to nearly 200 students at a time on a daily basis. Arnold acknowledged him as "perfectly the Master of the Science he teaches; and… a very good Lecturer. But as to Affability, I think he seems to have very little. I don't find that he ever takes any Notice of the Students." His energy and eloquence were "like an electric shock" after his father's ponderous performances, according to another contemporary, while yet another pupil recalled the "copious stream of information – medical, surgical, physiological, and pathological – that flowed from him almost without art or effort."

Dr John Hope, "no Orator but a very Laboring Man", according to Bentley, taught his first session as Professor of Botany in 1761. He was one of the least experienced teachers in the medical school. Yet despite Hope's less than charismatic lecturing skills, Arnold wrote, "his Knowledge and Learning have gain'd my Esteem, and his good Nature and readiness to oblige my Affection. He seems to be desirous of doing every thing that may be of Benefit or Gratification to his Pupils."

The atmosphere of fermenting ideas at "the seat of the medical muses" comes across vividly in Arnold's letters. Teachers and students alike were excitedly advancing the boundaries of their knowledge, sometimes controversially. Arnold commented on a very public medical dispute raging between the anatomist William Hunter and Alexander Monro: "Such Clouds of dust are the combatants apt to raise, in these Engagements, that poor Truth is lost in the thick Obscure."

A student could expect to hear well over a hundred lectures from each of these "fine men" between November and May. On the first Wednesday of the Winter Session, students could sample each subject before making their choices. If the zeal and enthusiasm with which James Graham approached the rest of his life is anything to go by, he probably endured a similarly punishing student schedule to the one which finished off Ismay.

"I have also begun to attend the Hospital," wrote Neville in November 1772. "Walking the Infirmary" was not a leisurely break from lectures, nor the somewhat random exercise it often became in London institutions. From 1756, students who had a reasonable grounding in the principles of medical practice were encouraged to complement their theoretical education with formal clinical lectures. "I shall give you the history of the disease, enquire into the cause of it, give you my opinion as to how it will terminate, lay down the indications of cure which will arise, or if any new symptoms happen acquaint you of them that you may see how I vary my prescriptions," Dr Rutherford explained to his students. They made the rounds of the teaching wards in the company of clerks, physicians, surgeons and university professors. During Graham's time at the medical school, Alexander Monro *secundus*, William Cullen and Robert Whytt took responsibility for patient care and clinical lectures at the Infirmary on a rotating basis.

Of course, all this came at a price. Seven and a half guineas bought a year's worth of twice-weekly clinical lectures on current cases, as well as bedside instruction. Only the urban physician was able – indeed expected – to avoid physical contact with his patients, feeling only their pulses, and preferring to examine blood and urine to actual bodies. A provincial apothecary-surgeon was likely to spend more time lancing boils, draining pus, dressing abscesses or setting fractures than rolling up his sleeves to tackle the kind of "heroic" surgery admired in the Infirmary amphitheatre. So when it came to low-key technical skills like cupping and bloodletting, apprentices and auditors – students like Graham heading for medical practice in small country towns and villages – had rather more need than gentlemen would-be graduates to pay attention.

Bloodletting (technically called venesection or phlebotomy) had been used for centuries to correct excesses of "plethora", according to the humoral pathology which had dominated medical thinking until the early eighteenth century. But though the procedure was eventually proved useless and positively harmful, doctors promoting new mechanical and neuropathological theories remained enthusiastic about it, right through the century. (Bloodletting was only finally abandoned by the profession in the early twentieth century, *The Lancet*'s title a testimony to its endurance.) Phlebotomy was hard for physicians to give up because it provoked such impressive physiological responses. Four to eight ounces of blood, speedily removed, caused a patient's pulse rate and body temperature to fall, while sensations of pain seemed to melt away. Feelings of relaxation and faintness followed, and often then slumber and sweating. So although the justifying theory changed over time, the therapy altered little.

Doctors prescribed phlebotomy, but it was usually performed by surgeons or more often their clerks and dressers. First fastening a ligature around the chosen limb, they used a spear-pointed lancet, often with a spring mechanism, to plunge into a superficial vein in the arm, hand, leg, foot or even neck. Having little opportunity to try this in Edinburgh, Sylas Neville practised instead on his Norfolk servants, rather nervously, "knowing the dangerous and fatal consequences which have followed blood-letting in some cases." Leeches were also often ordered by the physicians, especially in the summer months. These lively tri-jawed bloodsuckers helpfully inject a natural anti-coagulant complete with a local anaesthetic as they attach themselves, making the process relatively painless. They were put on the temples for headaches, applied to the eyelids in cases of eye inflammations, and often attached to bodily cavities like the mouth, anus, urethra or vagina. When Timothy Bentley nearly lost his eye in an accident after overdosing on claret one night, he "sent for the best Surgeon in Town (for I did not care to send for any of the Apothecaries here who are a set of very bold adventurous Youths, and would not have made any hesitation in opening my temporal artery which I did not Care for) and he somewhat abated the Inflammation by 3 Leeches on my temple, and keeping me for 3 days on Barley Water and a Dose of Salts."

Cupping was another option. Again, the original idea was that "bad" blood could be usefully drawn away from vital organs. In "dry" cupping, a glass (rather like a miniature goldfish bowl) or sometimes a horn was attached to the skin with a partial vacuum. "Wet" cupping was more dramatic: the chosen site was scarified with a special instrument either before or after the procedure, and the blood collected in the cup. Dr Cullen was not averse to using bloodletting of all kinds to deter malingerers at the Infirmary.

Nearly a quarter of patients in the teaching wards also had to endure blistering. This was another long-established technique inspired by the theory of the humours, which continued, with elaborate "schedules", well into the late eighteenth century and beyond. The updated rationale was that the procedure stimulated the bodily system. A sticking plaster or dressing was covered with some horribly irritating substance, often a powder or ointment made of *cantharides*, or Spanish flies. No apothecary shop of the eighteenth century would have been complete without its jar of these Mediterranean beetles, in medical use since Roman times. Mustard flour, onions, leeks and sulphuric acid had similarly painful effects. Half a day or so after the plaster was put on a patient's shaved crown, neck, sternum or back, up would come the blister. A hospital underling would then pierce it and drain the clear fluid, before dressing the sore again. Infirmary patients who had been prescribed a heavy blistering schedule were sometimes known simply to pack their bags and walk.

The art of the physician, as succinctly defined by one Edinburgh professor, consisted in "exciting, promoting, restraining, and some-times irritating by art various operations of nature in the human body". Treatments were designed simply "to place the patient 'in the train', a vague phrase meaning a path that could lead to recovery".

Just as indispensable to standard practice as bleeding and blistering were various techniques for emptying the digestive canal, to "keep the system open". These evacuations also often harmed more than they helped, and their medical history was equally entrenched. The old humoral pathology saw the process in terms of cleansing the entire system so that any food or faeces left inside wouldn't unbalance the whole organism. Since vomiting, stomach pain and diarrhoea often spontaneously followed fever, it was reasoned that dosing with an appropriate preparation at the critical moment simply gave nature a helping hand. According to the neuropathology of Graham's mentor William Cullen, the digestive organs, particularly the stomach, were sympathetically linked to all other bodily systems. So whatever disease affected a patient, it was assumed that the contents of the stomach and intestines should be expelled as quickly as possible, whether by laxatives or emetics. It was little wonder that when Graham began to develop alternative treatments he laid such stress on their gentle friendliness.

Infirmary rules were strict. Students were forbidden "to stroll the wards, converse together, stand upon beds or benches, or do anything that may be disturbing to the physician, clerk or patients." The throngs of hangers-on accompanying staff on their rounds between twelve and one, talking to the patients, observing the dressers in their bandagings, cuppings and bloodlettings, copying from ward journals and ledgers, and chatting and joking amongst themselves, sometimes made it scarcely possible for normal hospital routines to continue.

Infirmary passes, presented to the porter on each visit, also allowed vital access to the record books. All lectures had to be written down laboriously by every student, and few found it an easy task. "I take notes at the Materium Medica and Chimical Classes," explained Bentley. "It's impossible to take all. I take as many as I can and such as I think worth writing down but cannot take all these, you are frequently interrupted by coughing and blowing noses..." The Professors were understandably proprietorial about their knowledge, and often reluctant to publish their lectures. They risked losing more than just class fees if their words of wisdom became too readily available. In this commercial world, trade secrets had to be maintained. Not surprisingly, there was a flourishing market in transcribed and borrowed notes, passing from student to student. Thomas Arnold got together with a friend called Fowler, one of "the Companions [he prized] the most", and two other students whom he fails to name (Graham may have been one of these) to form a small private medical society. "We meet every Saturday at 3 o'Clock in the Afternoon, and each o[f us] produce an Essay on any Medical Subject, and in what Language we [choose]. I have twice adventured to write in Latin."

When classes drew to an end in May, many students joined the rush to London. Some went just for the summer months, returning for the next Edinburgh winter session in October. Others used the private lectures and clinical experiences available in London to put the finishing touches to their Edinburgh education, taking the opportunity to acquire a certain medical finesse as well as to forge the vital connections that might secure a more rewarding career path. Few young doctors would have wanted to stay in Scotland, where country practice was notoriously poorly paid. Even in the north of England, medical fees tended to be much lower than in the south.

Opportunity above all determined a medical student's future. Degree or no degree, gentleman, apprentice or auditor, the first step in a medical career was rarely easy without a suitable sponsor. "Nothing is of greater service to Medical people, than the acquaintance and conversation of men distinguished in their profession," Sylas Neville wrote ingratiatingly to a well-established Norfolk physician, seeking letters of recommendation.

James Graham struck lucky with an Edinburgh connection, William Buchan, attracting his attention "by some chance unknown". Sharpe recorded that Buchan then "became his patron, and carried Graham with him into England". By the end of the eighteenth century, William Buchan would be a household name, his book *Domestic Medicine* well thumbed in family homes through Britain, Europe and America. A populist lay textbook, its mission was to help ordinary people take their health into their own hands. Buchan wanted to rescue medicine from the monopolizing grip of the "faculty", a theme Graham himself would echo in years to come. At this point though, Buchan was an unknown Yorkshire apothecary rather than a medical celebrity.

Perhaps Graham was introduced to Buchan when he returned to Edinburgh in 1761 to defend and publish his MD thesis. He had been the young student's predecessor in the classes of Rutherford, Whytt, the Monros and William Cullen. Perhaps they met through some Edinburgh family connection. Typically for a man of his status and wandering nature, Graham left little evidence of his movements during the 1760s – just enough to sketch an approximate plot for the early stages of his life story. He found his wife in the village of Ackworth where Buchan worked, so this supports Sharpe's account of his departure from Edinburgh. We also know for certain that by the time he married her, in the summer of 1764, Graham had set up his own apothecary practice fifteen miles away in Doncaster. The details of these years can only be surmised.

William Buchan was employed by a newly established found-ling hospital, one of six rural outposts of an institution dreamt up by sea captain Thomas Coram. It had been one of London's most fashionable charitable causes since the 1740s, a hospital in the hospitable rather than the medical sense, set up to take in the illegitimate offspring of first-time mothers. In London, it had the support of Georg Friedrich Handel and William Hogarth, as well as society painters like Sir Joshua Reynolds and Thomas Gainsborough. In Ackworth the prime mover was the local vicar, Dr Timothy Lee, "a gentleman who placed an intelligent and philanthropic mind almost entirely at the service of the young institution", and who designed an ingenious hammock to make the week-long "caravan" journey regularly undertaken by children and nurses from London to Yorkshire a little more bearable.

In this small West Riding village, Buchan ministered to hundreds of children. His basic salary was about £40 a year, though drugs charged separately could double this fee. When not on his rounds, he used his experience of working with the foundlings to write his MD thesis on the preservation of infant life, *De infantum vita conservanda*. (He was obviously quite successful at this task, since the orphanage administrators were fond of favourably comparing their own death rates with the public bills of mortality.) He also treated private patients, including the occasional hermaphrodite: "I was highly entertained today by a man who came to me for advice, and who firmly believed he was turned into a woman." From 1759 onwards, Buchan had written repeatedly to his friend William Smellie (who did eventually become a co-author and editor of *Domestic Medicine)* trying and failing to persuade him to give up printing in favour of medicine as a profession. He had a "scheme" that Smellie should come to Yorkshire, joining his existing assistant John Rutherford on much the same terms: "You shall be welcome to live with me until you learn pharmacy, and see as much practice as to be able to set up for yourself." This was generous. Usually an apprentice – or more often his parent – paid his master for an agreed term in advance; the going rate for an apothecary in Yorkshire then would have been about £60 for five years.

Smellie's biographer Kerr was churlishly convinced that Buchan simply wanted a "literary drudge" to help him edit an early version of *Domestic Medicine*. The portrait of Buchan drawn by his own Victorian biographer suggests on the contrary a man more convivial than conniving, whose sociable habits would have made him long for company as intelligent and stimulating as Smellie's. "Full of anecdote, of agreeable manners, benevolent and compassionate,

[Buchan] was unsuited to make or keep a fortune: a tale of woe always drew tears from his eyes and money from his pocket." Buchan's letters to Smellie reveal a man fired with enthusiasm for his medical research, his rooms filling up with bottled body parts, specimens, skeletons and textbooks. He was clearly frustrated that Rutherford (that "indolent rogue") didn't share his passionate urge to go beyond the borders of his scientific understanding: "he absolutely refuses to assist me in any one of my curious researches; and won't so much as touch a subject, or attend when I am opening a child, let the case be ever so curious, but wants always to sit and hang his head over a book... I am just now preparing a curious skeleton in the next room to where he sits; but he has never once deigned to give it a look, far less to give me any assistance, though I desired him in the most pressing manner. 'Who would be plagued with such nonsense?' is all his answer... Who, in his right wits, would not jump at such an opportunity?"

Smellie, for one. He continued to resist Buchan's entreaties, arguing that he was too "destitute of money and impudence" to try to make a living as a doctor. "Any booby with a little brass in his face and a doctoreal peruke, &c. would cut a much better figure either in town or country than your most humble servant," he wrote in the late summer of 1762. Graham was certainly a young man with brass in his face, if not a great deal in his pocket. And he was not the type to baulk at the ruses Smellie scorned – such as wearing a physician's distinctive long wig to improve his prospects. Buchan probably recognized that Graham combined just the opportunistic instincts and self-educating zeal that John Rutherford so sorely lacked, and offered him the chance of becoming his companion and assistant.

Buchan planned to leave Ackworth for Sheffield at the end of 1763. By this time, the Ackworth Hospital for the Maintenance and Education of Exposed and Deserted Young Children boasted a grand new building, with generous rooms for its medical officer just behind the hall of the central wing. Buchan's post was advertised several times in the *York Courant* through the month of October that year. "WANTED, A SURGEON AND APOTHECARY to attend the said Hospital, and visit the Children at Nurse in the Neighbourhood of Ackworth." This meant responsibility for the health not just of several hundred children living, working and learning in the Hospital premises, and even more babies and infants farmed out to local wet nurses in the surrounding villages, but also forty members of staff. Regular health reports on all of these charges were expected by

Dr Lee. The committee of local grandees – including the Marquis of Rockingham, yet to become completely immersed in Whig factionalizing – planned to make a decision on the appointment on 3rd November. A letter from the London committee suggests that it was a job worth moving for: Dr Watson, one of the metropolitan hospital's physicians, offered to "recommend a proper Person".

If Graham nursed any ambition to follow in Buchan's footsteps, he was unsuccessful. The position went instead to a very local man, a far more experienced apothecary called Mr Cope who lived a couple of miles away in Hemsworth. Fortunately though, there was no shortage of professional opportunities for a young medic in that part of Yorkshire. A few weeks after the Ackworth hospital appointment had been made, an advertisement appeared in the regional newspaper. Someone was looking for an apothecary with patients to spare. He proposed either taking over an existing business or going into partnership with an established practitioner. Meanwhile, another regular supplier of the foundling hospital, Mr Thomas Malin, a Doncaster apothecary, alderman and one-time Mayor, was in low circumstances and approaching retirement. Many of the town's other general practitioners and druggists were also getting on in years. A further advertisement in July 1764 sought "[a] JOURNEYMAN or two for Apothecaries and Surgeons in the Country".

But by this time Graham seems to have been in a position to strike out on his own. He was often described by contemporaries as something of a head-turner, and was clearly blessed with that kind of charismatic charm which amounts to more than the simple sum of good looks and pleasant manners. Before long it had attracted "a young girl with some beauty". Her name was Mary Pickering.

The Pickerings of Ackworth were not so rich or so influential as to offer their time to foundling hospital committee meetings. Neither were they so poor as to apply for foundling apprentices nor work as hospital staff. But like so many of their neighbours, they were involved with the institution. When the new buildings were going up in December 1761, Mr Pickering, along with quite a few local worthies, donated 200 bricks at two shillings apiece. The previous spring he had charged £1 6s for the hire of a cart and ten days' worth of labour. That winter seems to have been his last, and perhaps marked the point at which Mary's marriage prospects improved further, as wealth was added to beauty. Subsequent dealings recorded in the Hospital accounts are with a Mrs Sarah Pickering, presumably Mary's mother, who supplied the hospital over the course of the next few years with significant quantities of hay, beans and so on. So although there is nothing to substantiate Sharpe's claim that Mary was worth the precise sum of £1,600, she does seem to have been born into a successful farming family. Graham himself later recorded that she married him with "fifty five pounds a year… settled upon her out of her own fortune." According to Sharpe, this was the modest fortune which funded Graham's Doncaster apothecary shop.

Doncaster was halfway between Edinburgh and London, a popular stop on the main coaching route. As a local historian boasted in 1804, "the High-street, for length, width, and beauty, [was] generally allowed to be the best on the road betwixt the above capitals," and the town offered "fine promenades". It was a lively, bustling place, and enjoyed good roads, cheap coal and water, not to mention admirably "salubrious air". An efficient corporation levied modest local taxes, a rather splendid Mansion House was the scene of regular balls and assemblies, and new markets for meat and country produce had also recently been built. It was hardly industrial – attempts by would-be factory owners to capitalize on Doncaster's tradition of stocking-knitting never quite got off the ground, and the town's best-known product remained its famously fine asparagus – but a combination of passing trade and local gentry kept shopkeepers busy. It even had a Presbyterian Chapel, built in 1740, practising the same form of worship as that of the Church of Scotland, which may have appealed to Graham. In short, Doncaster could "vie with any town in the kingdom, as a most desirable residence, not only for the affluent, but more particularly for persons of small fortune". Since the city's historic ban on non-freemen joining the town's commercial community had been recently tacitly abandoned – it was simply impractical to enforce – there was nothing to stop a young Edinburgh-trained medic setting up in business as he pleased. In London and some other large towns, different professional bodies – physicians, surgeons, apothecaries – did their best to limit intruders through various systems of licensing and local guild regulations, but even in the capital their efforts were hardly successful. The provinces had temporarily become a commercial free-for-all for medical men.

The word "apothecary" still evokes a Shakespearean character "in tatter'd weeds, with overwhelming brows / Culling of simples", lurking in a shop hung about with stuffed alligators and tortoises. A 1783 print of Graham in his prime alluded to his past by showing a crocodilian creature suspended in the background above a pestle and mortar and a bust of Galen. Although some self-styled apothecaries in the mid-eighteenth century still confined themselves to trading, either as small-scale glorified grocers, or wholesale druggists with a regional network of clients, a great many had moved away from simply preparing and selling drugs. Straightforward shopkeeping was being left to chemists and druggists, and patent medicines were also available from booksellers. The apothecaries were inexorably heading for the more lucrative field of general medical practice. They were no longer simply expected to supply the drugs ordered by a visiting physician, but were increasingly being summoned to patients' bedsides to diagnose and prescribe themselves. A country doctor might call in his carriage to treat the family of a man of means, but his servants would be tended by the apothecary on his horse, riding round to the back door.

"This is a very genteel Business, and has been in great Vogue of late years," pronounced *A General Directory of Trades* in 1747, which also noted, without judgement, that many apothecaries had started to "officiate as *Physicians*, especially in the country, and often become Men of very large Practice, and eminent in their Way". The relative lack of start-up costs was certainly one incentive to take up the trade for anyone from a family of moderate means, like the Grahams of Veitch's Land. An anonymous pamphleteer arguing for greater regulation in the profession declared that "there is no business scarcely, that requires so little money, as that of an Apothecary. This is known to all, and this is the cause of such a number of mushrooms in that profession; it is no difficult matter for a druggist's porter to procure both credit for a few medicines and a sufficient assortment of gallipots, and bottles, and thus turn Apothecary." Graham was not in that category of medical impostor, but how much, exactly, would he have needed to get his business off the ground? A couple of hundred pounds would fit up a smart shop, according to the *General Directory*, though a little extra would be needed to keep a man going while he built up a good set of patients.

The apothecary's role in his local community rather depended on the gaps left by other medics. When Timothy Bentley was nosing around for a possible professional opening in the London area for Richard Pulteney, he came across an exhausted Epping apothecary whom he described as "knockt up by Midwifery". Most apothecaries regularly performed minor surgery of the ulcer-dressing, bleeding and blistering variety and gave other medical advice in their shops, crude precursors of modern family health centres.

Imagine then, a young James Graham busy in his shop – probably a rather beautiful place, with its impressive rows of matching jars all neatly labelled with their contents. Perhaps he is poring over a drugs manual, such as the *Pharmacopoeia Universalis; or, a new universal English dispensatory*, about to weigh out the active and inert ingredients for a one-to-ten mixture on his specially designed ratio scales. Perhaps he is transferring a snake of chalky dough from the marble slab where he has formed it to the corrugated brass runnels of a newly acquired pill-rolling machine. Maybe a heap of squirming leeches is waiting to be taken to a patient in a perforated china carrying case. The bell rings and in rushes a child whose father has fallen from a ladder. Ordering his shopboy to saddle his horse, Graham packs up a suitable poultice for the sprained ankle he suspects, snatching up some packages to deliver to some neighbouring houses on his way home – perhaps some sort of anti-scorbutic treatment for scurvy, or an all-purpose "cordial". He has managed to build up a practice of families all within about ten miles of Doncaster, but spends more time than he might wish on horseback, with loaded saddlebags. In his absence, some passing customers call in for plasters and salves, or maybe a mercury-based "Pox Lotion" for a distressing case of syphilis. Apothecaries had "no set Hours for Business", as the author of a directory of trades commented. They could expect to be summoned late into the night.

Pills and potions were adored by Georgians of all classes. Letters and diaries of the period display a nation obsessed with its own health, as ready to self-prescribe and recommend treatments for friends and family as they were to flock to the latest fashionable doctor. It seems to have been perfectly normal for a wealthy family to have almost daily deliveries of medicines, remedies for maladies real and imagined as well as preventative treatments and tonics. Making these up in individually charged packets and bottles boosted prices even more. Plenty of people still considered regular spring and autumn bloodletting essential to staying hale and hearty. As the market economy flourished and income levels rose, medicines and medical care increasingly became just another everyday expense. A culture of consumption and display was reflected in escalating numbers of ever more wealthy medical practitioners, swanning around in liveried carriages and happily claiming for themselves every social advantage their position could secure.

James Graham, "apothecary of Doncaster", married Mary Pickering on a Wednesday in high summer, on 22nd August 1764, at St Cuthbert's, Dr Lee's church in Ackworth. It stood by the village green, where the uniformed children from the foundling hospital used to play, boys in red-collared rough brown coats and leather breeches, girls in print dresses. The Pickerings' near complete absence from parish records suggests that they were a nonconformist family, but James and Mary were now obliged by law to marry according to the rites of the Church of England. Lord Hardwicke's "Act for the better preventing of Clandestine Marriages" had come into force in 1754 to protect both patriarchy and property – to the delight of the aristocratic fathers of potential runaway heiresses but to the dismay of many in dissenting communities. Quakers and Jews alone were exempt from the Act. Only marriages performed by an ordained Anglican clergyman in the premises of the Church of England after thrice-called banns or a licence bought from a bishop were now valid. At least one party had to be resident for at least three weeks in the parish where the marriage took place. Parental consent for those under twenty-one was supposedly strictly enforced.

James Graham was supported in his claim to be a twenty-one-year-old bachelor by a Doncaster grocer called Bethune Green, who presumably knew no better, and acted as his bondsman to the standard tune of £200. By avoiding the truth about his age, Graham avoided the need to seek permission from his parents. He was in fact only just nineteen, four years younger than his bride. Was he simply mistaken, or did he think his parents might not approve? Perhaps he could spare neither the time nor the money to return to Edinburgh. Certainly banns were not read, and the bond applied for bears the same date as the wedding, so it may have been a rushed affair. Then again, the couple might have chosen the more expensive route of buying a bishop's licence so they could celebrate more privately. For quite a while the gentry had tended to arrive and depart from their own weddings in anonymous closed carriages, stealing away to church "quietly as lambs" with just a few witnesses. If James and Mary were not regular St Cuthbert's churchgoers, they probably didn't want a reading of the banns to expose them to all the fun and games of a traditional Yorkshire country wedding, public rituals involving a variety of possible humiliations, like garter-chasing and having to leap a barrier to leave the churchyard.

Graham, the future lecturer on generation, soon became preoccupied with the idea of procreation, in theory as well as practice. In 1767 he subscribed to a work by a Scottish-born but Sheffield-based doctor called Thomas Short, *A Comparative History of the Increase and Decrease of MANKIND*. Short (who also supplied

Graham with a quantity of his proprietary mineral water) was one of a number of eighteenth-century individuals who, concerned at the lack of institutional interest in the counting of births and deaths in the national population, took the task upon themselves. Like many enthusiasts for quantification, Short was motivated by a generalized horror of depopulation. Rousseau had recently pronounced in *The Social Contract* (1762) that the multiplication of citizens was an indicator of good government. "Count, measure, compare!" he exhorted. Short tried to calculate the fertility and salubrity of over 160 different country parishes, factoring in topographical features such as elevation, type of soil and so on, as well as numbers of marriages and ratios of male and female children. The complicated tables he produced are pretty impenetrable. His message is not. There were, he believed, three challenges to be met in order to "make the Nation more populous, Cities and Towns more healthy, and Youth stronger and hardier". Firstly, marriage had to be encouraged. Secondly, vice should be suppressed and virtue promoted. Thirdly, it was necessary to "mend the Air".

In fact, it is now accepted that the population was firmly on the rise by the mid-eighteenth century. But from his provincial base, Short saw nothing less than a rural wasteland spreading before him, as he totted up the disproportion of buryings to christenings. He saw the countryside being drained not "of Children, or aged, weakly, infirm, decripid, lame, sick, maimed, or languishing Persons; but of the sprightly, robust, healthy, effective Youth in their Prime, the Flower of the Country of both Sexes." The consequences, he bewailed, were manifold: a weak Navy, press gangs, too few servants and the undercutting of British trade. Short's diatribes against luxury and debauchery, sexual incontinence and indiscretion, came down particularly hard on the young. He painted a picture of Britain's oversexed youth: "weak, feeble, and enervated, or emasculated, diseased, and useless, as well as pernicious to their puny, languishing Offspring, should they have any". Graham was clearly fired by these ideas. They were themes he took up and elaborated with vigour. Thirteen years later, they became the primary justification for his electrical-magnetic medical practice at the Temple of Health.

A poem that appeared in a two-shilling volume advertised in a Yorkshire newspaper in 1763 offered a more frivolous approach to improving the quality if not the quantity of legal offspring. "Advice to new-married person" was a translation of a work by a seventeenth-century French doctor, *Callipaedia: or the art of having pretty children*, and may have sown a seed which eventually germinated in the form of James Graham's notorious *Lecture on Generation*. Page after page of rhyming couplets instructs newly wed couples how "to propagate the manly breed". Quality semen was essential, and had to be saved up carefully. "HOLD, furious Youth", issues the poet's titillating command to the eager Groom:

> – Better thy Heat assuage,
> And moderate a while thy eager Rage;
> For if the Genial Sport you now compleat,
> Full of the Fumes of undigested Meat,
> A thin diluted Substance shalt thou place,
> Too weak in Basis for a Manly Grace,
> To rise in Figure just, and dignify thy Race.
> Advis'd, defer the Work, till Time produce
> A more mature, and well concocted Juice.
> Hard is the Rule, and Lovers oft complain;
> Tho' hard, yet proper for a vig'rous Strain.

Whether or not they followed this advice, Mary and James were fortunate in their fecundity, and must have conceived within weeks of their wedding. William Pickering Graham was born early the following summer, a hot and difficult season of high food prices and low wages. No baptism was registered at St Cuthbert's, or apparently in Doncaster. Probably the ceremony was performed in a non-conformist church whose records have not been preserved. No other births to the young couple were recorded in Yorkshire either, though at around this time they definitely produced their eldest daughter, Mary Ann, who lived to a ripe old age, and bore six children. But little William proved to be "a weakly Offspring", lacking in the vigour needed to dignify his race. Consumption carried him away before he was three and a half, and his death certificate remains the only evidence of his birth. Dated 11th October 1768, William's father, James Graham, druggist, was recorded in the document as "late of Doncaster". So it seems he was not there to mourn at the Ackworth graveyard where his first child was buried.

By his own account, Graham spent some time in the hospitals of London and Dublin during the 1760s. In 1768, he had probably already saved enough money to head for the metropolis, leaving his wife and family in Ackworth. The prestige of a period of London study would provide the perfect gilding to the broad practical experience he had already garnered in Yorkshire. England's capital offered plenty of opportunities for an aspiring practitioner anxious for a competitive advantage in his career. Hospitals and infirmaries tendered a broad choice of clinical experience and academic education. Fairly casual, cash-based agreements with individual surgeons or physicians at St Thomas's, Guy's, Bart's or the London Hospital bought the right to observe operations, walk the wards or attend classes, with little commitment on the part of the student other than to his own advancement.

The market in private medical lectures was also burgeoning. William Hunter's Great Windmill Street anatomy theatre was the biggest draw in a competitive field, and James Graham would have found Hunter's triumphant career as a self-made man particularly compelling. Here was a wealthy entrepreneur who shared Graham's unexceptional Scottish Presbyterian origins, whose first job had been as William Cullen's apprentice. Now he was lording it over his own establishment on the edge of London's West End. Significantly for a maverick like Graham, Hunter's awe-inspiring success was completely independent of the authority of any public institution. He had deliberately bypassed the College of Physicians and the Company of Surgeons. And though Hunter marketed guaranteed-hands-on-a-corpse anatomy lessons, he offered something else almost as alluring. When it came to social and material ambition, his lectures were as inspirational as his life story:

I firmly believe, that it is in your power not only to *chuse*, but to *have*, which rank you please in the world... Now, in our profession it seems incontestable, that the man of abilities and diligence always succeeds... and, surely the man who is really able in his profession, will have the best chance of being thought so. In my opinion, a young man cannot cultivate a more important truth than this, that merit is sure of its reward in this world.

2

The Spark

> "America… whose rising sun announced the great day of UNIVERSAL FREEDOM! And shone with intellectual light!"

While Graham was taking on the responsibilities of adulthood in Yorkshire, the American dream was in its infancy. Like him, it grew up quickly. With each passing season after Britain's ambiguous victories at the close of the Seven Years War in 1763, America became an ever more powerful magnet. Its British colonies were now loudly heralded as a place of refuge and hope for the dispossessed and persecuted, a land of opportunity for the discontented or ambitious. This was a time when "the spirit of emigration prevailed in North Britain", as another Scot later wrote, repeating a phrase that appeared over and again in newspapers, letters and journals. It was a time when Ireland and the Highlands seemed almost to be emptying themselves across the Atlantic. At Hebridean ceilidhs the Scottish exodus was exuberantly mimicked in a new dance, "America": a few lone dancers gradually drew in the entire assembled company until the whole room was on the move. And as fast as the real immigrant ships unloaded their human cargoes, families and lone adventurers already in the colonies were packing up carts, sledges, packhorses and wagons and heading into the unknown back countries.

On both sides of the Atlantic, men rushed shamelessly to make the most of what promised to be the greatest land boom in history. Meanwhile James Graham, apothecary, was confronted with the difficulties of making his way in England, little lubricated by influential family or connections. It would have been unthinkable for someone of his restless and opportunistic nature to have ignored the lure of America during those extraordinary years. Where better could anyone fashion his own choice of "rank" in the world?

"[I]t was the best country in the world for people of small fortunes… the best poor man's country… It takes a good while however, to get established on an agreeable footing," warned another Scot, Patrick M'Robert, in a series of letters supposedly written to a friend during a tour of Northern Provinces undertaken in 1774–75. They were published as a kind of travel guide for prospective emigrants, an ever more popular genre in succeeding decades. The difficulties to be faced were substantial. "Courage and resolution in the adventurer" were essential. Not so hard though for the young, as M'Robert observed, or for those escaping from hardships at home: "for men in this particular are like trees, they do not answer so well after a certain age for transplantation, nor do they do so well from a good soil as from a bad."

Graham was the perfect age to meet these challenges, turning twenty-four the year he sailed for Baltimore. He was not, in any case, a man given to putting down roots anywhere he found himself. He seems to have left with the intention of bettering himself so that he could return to his family with glory, reputation and (with luck) some capital. Charles Kirkpatrick Sharpe, ever alert for the whiff of scandal, claimed in his "biographical notice" of Graham that he quit Britain in some disgrace: "indulging in those extravagancies of fashion which impoverished him through life, he quickly got rid of his [wife's] sixteen hundred pounds and also of his wife, whom her parents very obligingly allowed to return home again." Given Sharpe's general vagueness about this period of Graham's life, and other discrepancies in his account, a more likely explanation is that the young apothecary was carried away by the tide of high expectations that swept so many across the Atlantic.

The kernel of this ambition may have been planted in his mind as early as 1761, when he studied alongside American-born medical students at Edinburgh. It was certainly well watered by Thomas Short's book on population trends: Short had enthusiastically reprinted the notes to a sermon preached in Rhode Island in 1760 by the Revd Mr Ezra Stiles – president-to-be of Yale University. Stiles used Bible-derived calculations to make optimistic estimates of the growth rate of America's British colonies, and called for "every Encouragement" to be given to the Settlers by "Great Britain" to "extend their Commerce, and thereby increase both their Property, their Produce and their Numbers." This was an enticing prospect.

Part of James Graham's motivation may have been political. He might simply have become intoxicated with the rhetoric of liberty associated with America. The young apothecary was perhaps already mixing in the kind of republican circles which quickly became his milieu on returning from the colonies. This was a time when many English republicans still celebrated the execution of Charles I by symbolically dining on calf's head every 30th of January. Battling against the perceived tyrannies of George III, they were generally convinced that liberty seemed "to be flying from this country & making a desirable progress there".

We know nothing of Graham's crossing. Perhaps it was as uneventful as M'Robert's agreeable "tho' tedious" passage. In the category of "nothing material" this traveller blithely recorded a little girl of about nine falling overboard and drowning, and the death of another sickly child. On a happier note, "to make amends for that loss" a third infant was born on board. And after an initial three weeks of debilitating sickness, M'Robert found his sea legs and kept his health very well, enjoyably diverted on the journey by the flying fish, swordfish and large tuna following the boat. Steering for the southern latitudes to catch the trade winds these voyagers met with such intense heat that passengers could not lay a finger on any metal on deck without burning their hands.

Graham may have avoided that danger by courting others. He would have made a considerable financial saving by travelling crammed into steerage. Here indentured servants and shackled convicts were trapped together below decks, sometimes as many as a hundred men, women and children in a low, dark, airless space. The hatches were often kept firmly battened down to prevent flooding from rain and breaking waves. At times it was barely possible to breathe. During ocean storms, hatches were bolted shut against the elements. Soaking-wet emigrants had to keep standing, or sitting upright, holding tight to their children for days on end to stop them drowning in the deep pools of water that sloshed around in the hold. On days like these, the only light came from the cracks in the decking above. There was certainly no chance of cooking the inadequate allowances of oatmeal, peas or potatoes that bulked up bread or ship's biscuit, supplemented on a good voyage by molasses and scraps of meat and cheese.

Perhaps Graham stretched his finances to pay for a cabin and a slightly more generous share of what were still often mouldy rations and brackish water. But if he had to endure severe weather on the way over, survival would have felt precarious wherever he found himself on ship. A "Lady of Quality" and fellow Scot, Janet Schaw, who endured a particularly violent Atlantic tempest at around this time, wrote afterwards of waves running "mountains high". They crashed into the cabins, filling them to the upper berths, while Miss Schaw and her maid clung on to whatever they could. Water, live poultry, cooking equipment and barrels of pickled meats all came loose from their fastenings and were swept off the decks. The crew could neither control the helm nor keep hold of the wet ropes which tore their hands to pieces and snapped in the gales, throwing the ship and all its contents from side to side.

Sailing up Chesapeake Bay and finally tying up at a Baltimore wharf was not the end of the ordeal for many passengers. Arriving in the late summer of 1769, Graham would have doubtless witnessed a scene of the kind that unfolded repeatedly through the 1760s and early 1770s in ports and riverside villages up and down the colonial shoreline south of New England. From stinking holds emerged the men and women who had come to be sold on the American labour market, separated by sex once on deck. Frequently sickly and mal-nourished, the survivors by this stage were often dressed in little more than disintegrating rags. Yet they had to do their best to look faintly respectable to make a decent sale and secure the chance of a half-decent future.

Local merchants, planters, farmers, shopkeepers and labour-marketeers boarded the ships to scrutinize the newly arrived wares, inspecting and picking out people as they might livestock, watchful above all for signs of fever or disease. "They sell the servants here as they do their horses," a shocked British officer stationed in Philadelphia wrote home, "and advertise them as they do their beef and oatmeal." These auction sales for indentured servants were little different from the sales of black slaves, as other English letter-writers made clear: "They might as well fall into the hands of the Turks, they are subject nearly to the same laws as the Negroes and have the same coarse food and clothing." One James Cheston, who marketed both convicts and these servants listed them in his ledgers without distinction, and referred to them all as his "children".

Graham may originally have been drawn to Maryland by the strong presence of Scottish tobacco merchants and their agents in the region; the Chesapeake and the Clyde had long been linked. On his arrival, it did not take him long to see this was hardly the ideal community in which to make his mark. Looking at the people around him, it would have been hard for an aspiring medical entrepreneur like Graham to pick out significant numbers of potential patients. Half the population of the Chesapeake area were black slaves. A sizeable number of the rest were white convicts or indentured servants who only received bed and board for their labour. At the other end of the social spectrum, the pseudo-aristocratic "First Families of Chesapeake" were a haughty lot, little given to intellectual improvement or straying far from their rural properties. The outward magnificence of their mansions often belied the depths to which their owners were sunk in debt. A London vicar who had toured the middle settlements about a decade earlier sketched the characters of rich white Marylanders and Virginians with equal disdain: "they seldom show any spirit of enterprise, or expose themselves willingly to fatigue. Their authority over their slaves renders them vain and imperious... they scarcely consider [Indians and Negroes] as of the human species."

In January 1770 Graham was advertising London origins as he touted for an audience for a "Lecture on the Eye", to be performed in the modest Maryland capital of Annapolis, "a small neat town... [with] the finest water-prospect imaginable". It can hardly have been oversubscribed, since it was not repeated there. By the time the heat of August had arrived, the young doctor had moved to New York – a journey as likely to have been made by sea as by land in those days. In this city, half Dutch, half English in appearance, he took rooms at Mrs French's in Maiden Lane. Running between Broadway and the eastern waterfront of the southerly tip of Manhattan, the street had once been a lovers' walk.

A burst of Cicero at the head of his first New York newspaper advertisement was a pompous signal of Graham's learned status: *Homines ad deos nulla re proprius accedunt quam salutem hominibus dando.* Those who actually understood Latin might have wondered at his lack of modesty: "in nothing do men more nearly approach the gods as in doing good to men". Doctor Graham, "Physician and Surgeon from London", announced his availability for consultation at his apartments in Maiden Lane, and listed his specialities. He boasted of his education "at the justly celebrated University of Edinburgh" and the hospitals of London and Dublin, not to mention lectures "of the most eminent professors in several parts of Europe".

This made Graham one of the best-qualified doctors around. Even in America, an Edinburgh training was becoming a near-essential claim for any truly reputable medic. By today's standards, Graham's self-congratulatory small ad was hardly sophisticated. But by the standards of his own time, his debonair and expansive advertising style shows how quickly the young doctor had grasped the possibilities offered by the explosion in the printed word. The number of newspapers now available in America was still not vast. These four-page rag-paper weeklies typically averaged a print run of about 1,500 for each issue. But subscribers invariably passed on or posted their copies to friends and family members, and every coffeehouse or tavern had newspapers laid out for free perusal and animated discussion.

> 'Tis truth (with deference to the College)
> News-papers are the spring of knowledge,
> The general source throughout the nation,
> Of every modern conversation.
> What could this mighty people do,
> If there, alas! were nothing new?

Graham was a self-made man, and the newspapers were where he began to create himself. In print, conviction could be converted into fact. A significant investment in column inches and some carefully chosen phrases allowed Graham to introduce himself to New York as a cosmopolitan and experienced medic, rather than the provincial apothecary who had left British shores just over a year previously. Away from the stricter professional demarcations of London, in New York he described himself as a physician and surgeon. Like many medical newcomers, he promoted his "tenderness and moderation, to even the poorest individual", as well as his particular expertise in diseases of the eyes and ears: "He has resided in Maryland, about Twelve Months, and in that Time he hath happily restored great Numbers to their Sight and Hearing, who had been deemed incurable by other Practitioners."

This third-person claim to cure the incurable was a favourite one of quacks and nostrum vendors, specialists in last-resort solutions. So in terms of public image, it was a risky strategy. Clearly aware of what this implied, Graham concluded his lengthy advertisement with the pious hope that he might stand "recommended to some Share of the Favour of the candid and respectable Inhabitants of these Parts of British America, who can readily distinguish Merit from pretended Knowledge".

It was an astute appeal, which, like the fact of his Edinburgh training, Graham repeated in marketing material for most of his life. It conjures a world in which a medical training was probably easier to counterfeit than many others. In late August 1771 he would have been particularly keen to set himself apart from the newly arrived Dr Anthony Yeldall. Like many medical charlatans of previous centuries, Yeldall promoted himself with a wire-walking acrobat and a performing clown and sold cure-alls from a portable stage.

He owned a medicine warehouse on Front Street in Philadelphia and toured the middle colonies like a medieval mountebank. At "Brucklyn, on Long-Island" he attracted enormous crowds "by his harangues, the odd tricks of his Merry-Andrew, and the surprising feats of activity of his little boy". It was reported that several thousand New Yorkers "flock'd to see and hear him every day of his exhibition" – so many one Monday that they capsized the ferry boat on their crossing.

Graham formed part of a modest invasion of oculists, aurists and dentists crossing the Atlantic to hawk their expertise. These medics joined a wave of itinerant European culture-mongers offering instruction and entertainment of every variety: dancing teachers, fencing masters, portrait painters and musicians all promoted themselves in newspaper advertisements or sold their services door-to-door. Yeldall was certainly more colourful than most newcomers, but he had some dramatic competition. Ezra Stiles witnessed a well-dressed alcoholic from London, Dr Isaac Calcott, lick the eyes of a six-year-old boy and instantly restore his sight. Calcott promoted himself as the seventh son of a seventh son.

"Few physicians among us are eminent for their skill," wrote a pre-revolutionary historian of New York: "Quacks abound like locusts in Egypt" As the numbers of medical graduates increased, the better-qualified expressed their frustration at the impossibility of distinguishing themselves from "all those who by the courtesy of America" were "promiscuously" styled doctors. Both New Jersey and New York attempted to bring in licensing legislation at around this time, but it was hardly enforceable. And at this still relatively primitive stage of medical history, the quacks probably had a success rate just as good, if not better, than orthodox physicians.

New York kept Graham busy and wealthy enough to run his advertisement nearly every week till the end of November, sometimes in several different newspapers at once. The heavy flurry of self-publicity on his arrival seems to have paid off, and Graham stayed for the best part of another year. By M'Robert's account, it was a fine city at the time, New Yorkers "in general brisk and lively, kind to strangers, [and dressing] very gay". M'Robert found it remarkable that even the five hundred prostitutes living incongruously close to the "Holy Ground" around St Paul's lived more harmoniously together than those in Britain or Ireland, but noted that it "rather hurts an Europian eye to see so many negro slaves upon the streets, tho' they are said to deminish yearly here".

James Graham's advertisements – the only paper trail he left in America – promised to attend to "letters and messages from the country" as well as to New Yorkers. They record occasional forays into nearby New Jersey. Here he picked up or invented useful testimonials from patients relieved of the eye problems in which he specialized: failure of the optic nerve (now known as amaurosis) and ulcerated tear ducts. Graham himself naturally referred to these by their Latin medical names: *gutta serena* and *fistula lacrymalis*. He highlighted cancers, old sores and an unpleasant scurvy-related skin condition among his other cures: "obstinate" (and eye-catchingly capitalized) "SCORBUTIC ULCERS", as well as "FEMALE COMPLAINTS in general".

The bustle of New York certainly beat Baltimore and Annapolis. But Graham was always alert to new possibilities and opportunities, and there was an even more tempting prospect luring him on again. The colonies as a whole boasted an active and dedicated community of individuals interested in Enlightenment progress. They were in close touch with European circles by private letters and print, and always anxious to extol America's independent achievements in the sciences. "The means of conveying knowledge… are now become easy," wrote Charles Thomson, when the American Society for Promoting Useful Knowledge was reinvigorated in 1768, referring to widespread printing houses and postal services: "…in this country almost every man is fond of reading, and seems to have a thirst for knowledge." Nowhere in America was this thirst more evident nor more easily slaked than in Philadelphia, a city which offered enlightenment like no other.

The recently launched "flying machine", a stagecoach from New York, allowed passengers to alight at the Indian Queen Tavern in Fourth Street, Philadelphia, a mere two days later. Travellers arrived in a city which promised more people in one place than anywhere else on the continent, their numbers growing faster than ever or elsewhere. It was the fourth biggest in the British Empire – only London, Bristol and Dublin were larger – and new shiploads of immigrants disembarked at the three-mile long waterfront daily. The unfamiliar prospect of broad, clean, paved, well-lit streets and a municipal night watch were further enticement to a man who would later make a business of hygiene and order. As for the brotherly love for which the city was named, Dr Graham claimed it as his motivating force, referring to himself in years to come simply as "a Lover of his Species".

Philadelphians adored lectures. By the time Graham arrived in town in October 1771, opportunities for self-improvement for visitors and townsfolk offered themselves in a huge variety of forms. Since 1762 a rudimentary medical education had been available through lectures on anatomy and dissection classes given by Dr William Shippen, a disciple of the Hunter school. (He also made use of anatomical drawings and plaster casts donated by the English doctor, John Fothergill, who was soon to transform Ackworth Foundling hospital into the Quaker boarding school it remains to this day.) Shippen had been joined by a fellow Edinburgh graduate, John Morgan, in 1765 to inaugurate America's first medical school in embryo. Genteel competition was promoted at the "Anatomical museum" in Vidal's Alley by the elderly English Tory Dr Abraham Chovet, who had practised in Philadelphia since 1770. Shippen's rival taught his specialism using "elegant Anatomical Wax-Work Figures" to spare his pupils "the disagreeable sights or smells of recent disease and putrid carcasses, which often disgust even the students in Physick, as well as the curious". (Memories of Shippen's dismembered corpses of criminals lingered well into the early nineteenth century, when small boys continued to frighten themselves with tales of body-snatching and boiling flesh as they dashed past what they took to be his dissecting theatre.)

In 1767 the Provost, William Smith, had widened the audience for his lectures on natural philosophy at the city's College (now the University of Pennsylvania) to admit any "gentleman" who had attended the institution in the past. Less high-brow courses on natural and experimental philosophy by Revd John Ewing and Dr Hugh Williamson at the Masonic Hall in Lodge Alley were so well attended that all tickets had to be booked in advance, except by "Strangers to the City". In 1770, Provost Smith had arranged a particularly ambitious public-lecture series, including three on chemistry by Dr Benjamin Rush, which were positively lapped up. Admission fees went to a fund to buy for the College an exquisite orrery made by a local hero in philosophical circles, David Rittenhouse. Bowing to "the prevailing taste", this self-educated astronomer had contrived the clock part of the instrument to play music. Select groups came to admire it, and receive instruction on the movements of the planets from Rittenhouse himself: "There wond'ring crouds with raptur'd eye behold / The spangled Heav'ns their mystic maze unfold." Philadelphians were naturally delighted that their orrery rivalled any in Europe. The mechanical planetarium became an icon of American enlightenment.

Shippen's brother John had returned from studying in France in 1770 to join the growing throng of lecturers with an illustrated series on the theory and history of fossils for those "who are daily making Collections". A year later the Irish "engineer and architect" Christopher Colles opened an evening school, teaching "hydraulics, hydrostatics, pneumatic, optics, perspective architecture, and fortification". This was useful knowledge indeed. It could be applied to the building of waterways, docks, bridges, aqueducts and other vital structures. The following year Colles added geography and natural philosophy to his curriculum.

So in Philadelphia Graham was quite spoilt for choice. In later years, responding "[t]o those Gentlemen who enquire from what sources I have drawn my Medical Knowledge – improvements – and superior skill", he described habits of learning both voracious and opportunistic:

> After a regular classical and medical education at the celebrated University of Edinburgh, I diligently consulted the literary monuments of the most illustrious and most *excentrick* dead, by ransacking and culling from every book ancient and modern I could meet with, and even from manuscripts written before printing was invented;—I courted too, information and instruction from the most eminent among the living; and after collecting what I could in every part of the Islands of *Great Britain* and *Ireland* I travelled for further intelligence and improvements in many foreign nations.

Graham's account suggests he made the most of Philadelphia's well-stocked libraries. Some were highly specialized: the Loganian Library, for example, had few but dedicated readers, "obscure mechanicks who have a turn for mathematics". More usefully for an information-hungry doctor, Pennsylvania Hospital was beginning to boast an outstanding medical library; borrowing had yet to be restricted to the institution's managers, physicians and their students. But nothing better represents the city's autodidactic and democratic intellectual spirit than that long-standing institution, the Library Company.

It was founded by Benjamin Franklin, who argued in 1771 that the colonies' libraries had "made the common Tradesmen and Farmers as intelligent as most Gentlemen from other Countries". The Library Company's ever-expanding collection was beginning to overflow from the shelves of its State House premises by 1772. That year it was frequented by twenty tradesmen for each "person of distinction and fortune". As a self-consciously civic institution, it opened its doors to "any civil person" who showed no evidence of fleas and did not have to be woken up more than once in a session. Users who kept their eyes open could make the most of one of the best collections of English literature in the colonies, as well as the latest British periodicals and an ever-growing cabinet of curiosities – an eclectic museum which included some unusual fossils and a complete electrical apparatus donated by Thomas Penn, Pennsylvania's colonial proprietor.

Performing his *Lecture on Generation* years later in London, Graham would drop references to Benjamin Franklin as though he had been his personal tutor. By that time the American's international reputation as an electrician was well established. "[T]he great prince of philosophers... the venerable prince of politicians!" eulogized the Doctor, irredeemably prone to sycophancy. In his *Travels and Voyages* (1783), Graham even claims that one of the reasons he had embarked for America in the first place was his conviction, from reading "the writings of an American, one of the greatest Philosophers in the world, that in *Philadelphia* Electricity had been more improved, was better understood, and more generally cultivated than in any other part of the world." (This doesn't explain why it took Graham two years to reach the city after his arrival in the colonies, but it gives a good sense of the currency of Franklin's name, even when only implied.) The ambitious doctor recorded his two years' residence in Philadelphia as ones spent "attending the public Exhibitions and Lectures on Electricity in that College, as well as applying closely to private experiments and to general practice". In fact during all the years Graham was in America, Franklin himself was away in Britain. He was officially in London as the agent of the Philadelphia Assembly, making a political mark only possible because of his already well-established reputation as an innovative and rigorous natural philosopher.

The windswept, red-cloaked sage gathering electricity from the string of a kite helpfully flown by angels in Benjamin West's well-known portrait, Fragonard's majestic figure sitting in the clouds with wise Minerva, or even the sterner face glaring from the back of every hundred-dollar bill today, represent the Benjamin Franklin of mythology, the lone genius inventing unheard-of things in a savage wilderness. The reality was actually very different. The inexhaustible polymath who dominates historical memory of this time may have led the way, but he was far from alone. Already a successful businessman-printer and innovatory newspaper editor with leisure and wealth to spare, Franklin is thought to have begun tinkering with static electricity in 1746, after he was sent an irresistible package by a well-connected English friend, the Quaker botanist Peter Collinson. The American unwrapped a simple glass tube and directions how to use it, now lost. "As this may I think very justly be stiled an age of wonders, it may not perhaps be disagreeable to just hint them to you... now the vertuosi of Europe are taken up in electrical experiments," Collinson wrote at around the same time to another friend in New York. Franklin found further inspiration in an intriguing account of some German philosophers' recent experiments with the new science, generally assumed to be an influential article in the *Gentleman's Magazine*, to which the Library Company subscribed:

[P]rinces were willing to see this new fire which a man produced from himself, which did not descend from heaven. Could one believe that a lady's finger, that her whalebone petticoat, should send forth flashes of true lightning, and that such charming lips could set on fire a house? The ladies were sensible of this new privilege of kindling fires without any poetical figure, or hyperbole, and resorted from all parts to the publick lectures of natural philosophy, which by that means became brilliant assemblies.

The writer of this article (probably William Watson, a fellow of London's Royal Society) conveys not just the overwhelming wonderment such experiments provoked, but gives a usefully precise description of the physical sensation of electrification in those early days:

It is neither a burning nor contusion, but a dry and quick impression of an agitated matter, which pierces to the very bone, and most affects the person not electrified... [The fire]... is brighter than any artificial fire, and when it proceeds from the skin its flame is bluish, with a red point, but whiter when produced from silver, and is of different colours according to the bodies from whence it is emitted, or some other circumstances.

Franklin began to introduce a wide circle of friends to these unusual excitements, and quickly came up with ever more novel ways of using his new-found knowledge. During those exhilarating early months his house "was continually full for some time, with people who came to see these new wonders". To share the burden of attention he ordered tubes to be made at the local glasshouse, and encouraged his friends to perform too. One, a Transylvanian called Samuel Dömjén, had kept going from Philadelphia to Charleston giving lectures based on these new skills, much to his mentor's delight.

> ...he had lived eight hundred miles upon Electricity, it had been meat, drink, and cloathing to him. His last letter to me was, I think, from Jamaica, desiring me to send... [more electrical] tubes... to meet him, at the Havanah, from whence he expected to get a passage to La Vera Cruz; designed travelling over land through Mexico to Acapulco; thence to get a passage to Manilla, and so through China, India, Persia and Turkey, home to his own country; proposing to support himself chiefly by electricity. A strange project!

But Franklin's most successful fellow performer was "an ingenious Neighbour" called Ebenezer Kinnersley. Kinnersley took up Franklin's electrical baton and ran with it alongside him for over twenty years, becoming the best commercial lecturer on the subject in the colonies and the principal popularizer of Franklin's ideas in America. He did this job so effectively that his own contributions to early electrical research have now been largely sidelined. James Graham's post-hoc claims to have profited from Franklin's labours were economical with the truth, but did have some substance, since he seems to have done so indirectly through the work of Kinnersley.

Ebenezer Kinnersley, a Baptist minister without a congregation, was out of a job at this point for the very reasons that made him the perfect candidate to take up this emerging profession. He had found himself in trouble after preaching vehemently but rationally against the emotional manipulations of the likes of George Whitefield, leader of a widespread and intense religious revival movement of the 1740s known as the Great Awakening. Disgusted at the fear and passions aroused at mass salvation meetings sweeping the American colonies, Kinnersley declared in a letter published by Franklin in his newspaper, the *Pennsylvania Gazette*: "What Spirit Such Enthusiastick Ravings proceed from, I shall not attempt to determine; but this I am very sure of, that they proceed not from the Spirit of God, for our God is a God of Order, and not of such confusion."

In contrast, Kinnersley clearly had a gift for rational sensationalism. A month after he started his first lecture programme in May 1749, the *Maryland Gazette* reported a magnificently exciting and public piece of self-promotion. Setting up his electrical generating machine on the south side of a local creek, Kinnersley placed a small vessel of spirits of wine on the northern bank. Through 200 yards of water, he sent an electrical spark to set the spirits ablaze in an instant. The spectators were thrilled; even more so when he then used his apparatus to fire "a battery of eleven guns". This was an utterly persuasive demonstration of several of the scientific points made in his new lecture syllabus: that electricity "does not, like common Matter, take up any perceptible time in passing thro' great Portions of Space", and also that "it will live in Water, a River not being sufficient to quench the smallest Spark of it". It is hard to imagine a more striking way to draw in audiences to the colonial lecture halls that were the usual venues of *A Course of Experiments on the Newly Discover'd Electrical Fire* in Kinnersley's early days.

In these lectures, each experiment was carefully devised to develop the principles of the one before. They were designed to appeal to colonial pride as much as simple scientific curiosity, promoted as "…containing not only those that have been made and published in Europe, but a number of new ones lately made in Philadelphia…"

By the early 1770s, Kinnersley was a familiar figure in the College of Philadelphia, where his official post was Professor of English and Oratory. (His wife took care of the students' laundry.) One contemporary admired him as a "master of words", who was "truly respectable" – anything but some transient bandwagoner. By popular demand, alongside his other duties Kinnersley carried on performing ever more inventive versions of the lectures on electricity which had already sustained him for several decades. His intriguing advertisements for these continued to appear in the Pennsylvanian newspapers – whose distribution went far beyond the boundaries of that colony. In 1772 alone, Kinnersley lectured on electricity at the College at least nine times, making him far and away the most likely source of Graham's electrical inspiration and education.

In October 1771, Graham set up practice in Arch Street, a couple of blocks back from the waterfront. Within a few months he had his first chance to see one of Kinnersley's performances. Electricity is now so fundamental to everyday life in the developed world that it is almost impossible to picture the impact of a lecturer like Kinnersley on an ignorant audience. As likely as not, Graham had already encountered some of the surprising effects of static electricity – perhaps after a dinner, or performed by a roving experimenter in the Dömjén mould. Francis Hauksbee, chief experimentalist of the Royal Society in London, had built the first hand-cranked light-up electrical machine, using an evacuated glass globe, in the early years of the century. In the 1730s, a pensioner in London's Charterhouse, Stephen Gray, had spent his last years assembling apparatuses (including living children suspended by silken ropes) to demonstrate how electricity could be communicated from one object to another, inventing many of the technologies that would become staples for electrical experimenters for decades to come. The Leyden jar, the first ever method devised for storing electrical charge, had been invented the year James Graham was born in 1745.

But in Britain, public demonstrations of the wonders and enchantments of "electrical fire" were relatively few and far between by the time Graham was of an age and income to appreciate them. Electricity had become domesticated to a certain extent. Modest versions of once truly spectacular scientific shows were widespread as parlour games. An entertainment like Kinnersley's "artificial spider, animated by electrical fire acting like a live one, and endeavouring to catch a fly" was just one display of attraction and repulsion quite easily replicated with tabletop equipment in any well-to-do home. Natural philosophers on both sides of the ocean continued to experiment, but they concentrated on communicating their work through international networks of "learned societies" rather than public displays.

Without the support of the academies enjoyed in continental Europe, the 1760s were depressed times for British physics lecturers. Public attention, ever fickle, was increasingly turning to political controversy, local celebrities and the Seven Years War. An electrician who inspired ridicule for experiments involving his own black-and-white sparking silk stockings commented acidly to a friend, "Some Notice may be taken abroad, of what is new and ingenious in Matters of Natural Philosophy; but here we think of nothing but Politicks, Money and Pleasure."

So until Graham sat down in the apparatus room at the College in Philadelphia before Ebenezer Kinnersley, the Doctor was unlikely ever to have grasped either the principles or the potential of the new physics with quite such startling clarity. Kinnersley began his performances with a simple, striking image. He held up a golden chunk of amber. Rubbing it for some time with a scrap of woollen cloth, Kinnersley showed how the ancient Greeks first noticed that it could then be used to attract "any light Matter", drawing to it feathers, straw and so on.

Then he brought out his next exhibit: a simple glass tube, about two and a half feet long, an inch and a half across. This too he rubbed with some leather or cloth. Adding an iron rod suspended by silken strings, the simplest of "prime conductors", Kinnersley showed how the same power of attraction could be passed to one end of this rod simply by holding the glass tube near the other end.

The next step was to show the difference between conductors and insulators, first recognized (though not named as such) by Stephen Gray, who discovered that wax, pitch, silk and several other things, would stop "the Electric Virtue from running off, or dissipating in the Common Mass of Matter". So supporting the prime conductor on wax allowed it to retain its "virtue", but holding the rod in the hand or laying it on a table (earthing it) led to its escape. Kinnersley conveyed wonderfully the sense of excitement such a "seemingly small experiment" generated, and how this knowledge became the cornerstone for electrical research. He explained how, through the 1730s and 40s, "electricians", as these experimenters were called, gradually learnt how best to retain and then increase the quantity of "the Electric Matter" until it became a tangible thing, to be felt, heard and seen in strange sensations, snaps, cracks and flames. They had "this subtle, flying fluid" in their power, and began to investigate its nature in ever more ingenious trials. The preacher-turned-orator's audience learnt of electrical developments in France, Germany and Holland, then England and finally Philadelphia.

By the time Graham began to boast of his American experiences, the "Philadelphian experiments" were world famous. Until Franklin, natural philosophers (the word "scientist" had yet to be coined) had understood electricity not as a force but either as a kind of fluid, imagining it in terms of vapours, ethers, airs and effluvia, or as a type of fire. Kinnersley used the word "fluid" in the context of electricity not because he thought it was one, but as a way of suggesting that it sometimes behaved like one. He actually followed Franklin in maintaining that electricity was in fact a special type of matter, a real element as old as the creation, but "newly taken notice of". In 1733, a French savant called Charles du Fay, a close friend of Stephen Gray, had identified two different varieties of electricity – vitreous (or positive), which comes from rubbed glass, and resinous (or negative), acquired by resins such as amber or gum copal. He then formulated the law which became a core principle of electrical science: that objects with the same kind of charge repel, while those with opposite charges attract. Franklin and Kinnersley's great shared insight was to use the discovery of the Leyden jar, which eventually put paid to all effluvial theories, to test their hypothesis that "vitreous" and "resinous" electricity were actually one and the same. They simply behaved differently under different pressures. The collaborators were the first to label them as positive and negative, and Franklin is often also considered to have been the first to understand the principle of how charge could be stored.

Kinnersley's emphasis on careful distinctions and rational explanation made him unique among popular lecturers, and set him apart from the kind of society entertainers who had been doing the rounds in Europe up to this point. Many demonstrators were still only too happy to manipulate their audiences with the apparently magical effects of their electrical kit: though increasingly sophisticated machines were on the market, some preferred to use old-style hand-rubbed devices to convey the impression that their own bodies were the source of this mysterious power. The vast majority were simply crowd-pleasers, who diverted onlookers with a succession of tricks, more or less dramatic, and some downright exploitative.

Kinnersley understood perfectly how best to draw on the public's desire for choreographed fear and amazement, yet never made undue mystery of the processes. Shock and suspense were literalized in his capable hands, but always explained. His training in the pulpit had given him a keen sense of the requirements of an audience and, although he rejected the aims of the Great Awakening, Kinnersley recognized the compelling power of the revivalists' dramatic public oratory. He was also happy to adapt that kind of theatricality to his own presentations. After all, no congregation would sit happily through the same sermon ad infinitum. Over the twenty-five years in which he lectured on electricity, Kinnersley not only kept track of the latest advances in the field, but was responsible for quite a number of them. As new ideas and experiments were incorporated into his performances, the sense of wonder and marvel which attracted the earliest audiences was never lost, but neither was the seriousness of his intentions.

So the artificial spider mentioned earlier (usually regarded as a Franklinian device), and the "Shower of Sand, which rises again as fast as it falls", both demonstrated the continual powers of attraction and repulsion. "A Leaf of the most weighty of Metals suspended in the Air, as is said of *Mahomet's* Tomb" showed the equal powers of attraction and repulsion while "An Appearance like Fishes swimming in the Air" demonstrated the different effects of sharp and smoother points in transmitting the "Fire". Before moving on to high theatre, Kinnersley had to explain the workings of what he described as "Mr Muschenbrock's wonderful Bottle", the Leyden jar. Its discovery, according to the Dutch Newtonian physicist credited with its invention, Pieter van Musschenbroek, felt like "a clap of thunder" and struck him "such a violent blow he thought his life was at an end". A Leyden jar is a kind of condenser or capacitor – an instrument for accumulating electric charge in which two conductors are separated by an insulator. Kinnersley would have shown the assembly a wide glass bottle partly coated in metal foil. Water inside was connected by a wire or chain to a metal rod and knob set in a cork in the bottle's neck. When this knob approached or contacted the "prime conductor" of an electrical machine while the outer metal was temporarily grounded (for example through its contact with the demonstrator's body) the jar could be "charged". There the static electricity could be stored until someone connected its two conductors (the knob and the foil) with a wire or their hand.

Once this had been made clear, all kinds of different wonders emerged like genies from the bottle. Each effect seemed more marvellous than the last, although the bulk of any electrical demonstrator's repertoire actually tended to illustrate the same few principles over and over again in different ways. The "circle shock" could be experienced by everyone in the room if they all held hands and connected themselves to a Leyden jar. Electric mines were sprung, coins were electrified to repel any would-be thieves in the audience, and an impressive electric hole punch neatly pierced through a quire of paper before the onlookers' astonished gaze. Another experiment set alight a glass of alcohol using "Fire darting from a Lady's Eyes (without a Metaphor)". Small animals were even electrified to death.

Some way into the first lecture of a series, an intrepid volunteer would be called up from the audience. Once electrified, his finger would acquire the amazing power to kindle a flame in a glass of spirits. This was an experiment first carried out by a poetically inclined German professor, Georg Mathias Bose, in 1744. (Oil of turpentine was initially a favourite substance, for it "rises into bubbles at the approach of the electrified finger".) Kinnersley's interpretation of this piece of performance art must have delighted

Graham. Underscoring the theological underpinnings of his views on natural philosophy, he would remind his audiences that "a few years since, this firing of spirits by a finger might have passed for a miracle, and an impostor might have used it among the ignorant to establish a false doctrine and overthrow a true one."

Another experiment, towards the end of the first lecture, showed the "mutual Repulsion of electrified Bodies" using seven suspended cork balls representing the planets. (Uranus and Pluto had yet to be discovered.) It was the ideal illustration for a hypothesis – inaccurate, as it happens – about the workings of the solar system. Kinnersley strikingly imagined the "Creator" bowling planets through the "unresisting Aether" from his "form-finishing hand", with the electrified sun at the centre. Kinnersley's ideas about the forces of nature operating through the will of an orderly, loving deity would later emerge in Graham's works, with very different emphasis.

As he travelled through the colonies, Graham could not have helped noticing one obvious sign of Philadelphia's scientific revolution. Lightning conductors, Franklin's best-known invention, were now widespread. Their rods proudly pointed to the heavens on buildings throughout the well-cultivated Pennsylvanian countryside, in ostentatious defiance of the frequent summer thunderstorms to which people and property previously regularly fell victim. Foreign visitors often remarked upon the fact that most ordinary houses boasted "a spike of iron fixed upon the highest part of the building, and carried down along the side of the wall till it enter the ground." They were as efficient as they were ubiquitous, wrote the traveller Revd Andrew Burnaby a decade earlier, and "seem to be means put into our hands by Providence, for our safety and protection".

This endorsement was progressive thinking from a vicar in an era when attitudes towards lightning conductors tended to be suspicious, and often downright superstitious. For centuries it had been traditional in Europe to ward off the supposed wrath of God in the form of punitive lightning strikes by ritualistic bell-ringing. Succinct inscriptions often appeared on the actual bells: "*Deum laudo, vivos voco, / mortuos plango, fulgura frango.*" (I glorify God, call the living, / mourn the dead, break the thunder.) Ironically, of course, not only were church spires the very buildings most likely to be struck in a storm, since they were usually the highest point in a particular area, but bell-ringing in such weather was a potentially fatal activity in itself. In the event of a lightning strike, electricity would be all the more likely to be conducted down the ropes to strike the ringers themselves. Enlightened thinkers around the world had been left wringing their hands in despair at the stupidity of rebuilding St Bride's steeple in London with no conductor after it had been already been destroyed by lightning twice in fewer than fifteen years.

Even in America, it had not been easy to overcome deeply ingrained superstitions about the evils of interfering with divine design. "Atheistical presumption" was a charge levelled at experimenters with lightning conductors. The educated but pious (among whom Graham tended to number himself) concluded eventually that thunder and lightning were actually no more instruments of Divine Vengeance than any other elements. If lightning rods were "presumptuous", so too were sun hats, house roofs and umbrellas.

By the early 1770s, reports on lightning damage and destruction in American newspapers were often accompanied by warnings as to the advisability of guarding buildings "with pointed Iron Rods, for their Preservation", particularly hay and grain barns. Ebenezer Kinnersley had been pioneering a far more visceral version of these scare stories even before Franklin's theories about lightning had been formally published. Within twenty years experiments like his were being replicated by electricity lecturers from America to Europe. The most dramatic of these anticipated cartoon explosions in Tom-and-Jerry style using enchanting wooden model buildings known as "thunder houses" or "powder houses". These had hinged walls and roofs, and were topped with a little chimney complete with a diminutive polished lightning rod. The more elaborate versions were suitably decorated with moss and painted stonework. A small panel on the façade of the house allowed a section of the rod to be slid away, so that the conductor was no longer earthed. Inside the house a spark-gap arrangement was set in a small brass cylinder containing some gunpowder. Lightning was replicated in miniature using electrical apparatus. Finally, downy feathers suspended nearby expanded theatrically like thunderclouds when charged. When the lightning rod was properly earthed, the house remained safe and sound. If not, with a spark from a Leyden jar or prime conductor, the little building would fly apart with a loud bang.

Kinnersley's intentions were always serious, but he leavened his more prophetic pronouncements with theatrical grace. In an intriguing, even titillating experiment, innocent members of the audience were invited to come and kiss a woman standing on an insulated stool, or a cake of resin or pitch. Little did they know that she was charged, her entire body turned into a kind of electric chastity belt. Its original inventor, the poetic Bose, described the trick as the "Venus electrificata". Suitors were painfully repelled as they approached the woman's lips. Following the electric kiss, a Leyden jar was made to ring "a Number of small Bells", and the performance was rounded off in high style with an explosion from an electrical cannon, fired with a spark from someone's finger.

When Graham arrived in Philadelphia Ebenezer Kinnersley was introducing a topic which would transform the oculist's life. In an advertisement in late December 1770, he promised that "...as Electricity is now become a considerable article in the Materia Medica, directions will be given for the proper application thereof". Newspaper reports of seemingly miraculous electrical cures in Italy and Germany in the late 1750s had been enough for desperate paralytics from around Pennsylvania and beyond to throw themselves as guinea pigs on Benjamin Franklin, who remained sceptical about electricity's medical benefits. But Kinnersley's announcement quoted approvingly from Joseph Priestley's influential history of electricity:

Antonius de Haen, one of the most eminent physicians of the present age, after six years uninterrupted use of it, reckons it among the most valuable assistances of the medical art; and expressly says, though it has often been applied in vain, it has often afforded relief where no other application would have been effectual.

Another seed was sown. At the Temple of Health in London, Graham would later put to medical and theatrical use in vastly magnified forms many of the impressive effects he probably first witnessed in Philadelphia. Perhaps he was present on the November night in 1772 when Kinnersley was performing for Kayashuta, an Iroquois chief. Having been entertained by philosophical experiments on a previous visit, he gravely asked to see "Thunder and Lightning produced by human Art". This seems to have been one of Kinnersley's specialities, and certainly one which Graham took up with enthusiasm: he would subsequently claim, with Franklinian reverberations, to be able to "draw down into the room... the lightning from the clouds of heaven."

"A bright Flash of real Lightning darting from a Cloud in a painted Thunderstorm" was repeated a number of times during the course of Kinnersley's lectures. It was in fact a very simple effect achieved by touching a Leyden jar to a rain cloud painted onto a decorated backdrop. On the reverse of the painted scene a wire connected it to the other side of the jar. When he first started doing this part of the performance in the early years of electrical experimentation, it must have been on a fairly small scale. A glass rod alone could produce a lightning-like spark only an inch long. The flash doubled in size with the use of a globe electrical machine and a Leyden jar. During the early 1770s electricians around the world set themselves the task of creating ever larger and more powerful machines. One particularly large machine made for the Grand Duke of Tuscany in 1773 by the London instrument-maker Edward Nairne using a huge glass cylinder could generate sparks a foot long.

Kinnersley was clearly working along similar lines. At the end of that same year he announced "some considerable addition to his Electrical Apparatus" in the form of "an elegant case of seventy bottles, each lined and coated with tinfoil". This extra battery power would have hugely increased the drama of uncomfortable experiments such as one in which a "Flash of Lightning" was made to strike a small house, and "dart towards a little Lady sitting on a Chair, who will, notwithstanding, be preserved from being hurt, whilst the Image of a Negro standing by, and seeming to be further out of Danger, will be remarkably affected by it". (Both "Lady" and "Negro" took the form of small models.) Another of Kinnersley's novelties that year was a representation of part of the starry heavens, exhibiting a variety of beautiful electric stars. The earliest surviving announcement of this innovation was in late December 1773, by which time Graham was almost certainly on a boat returning to England. Seven years later though, the Doctor described in remarkably similar terms an effect which took place during the performance at the Temple of Health. After a burst of song, he would plunge his audience into darkness. Then the apartment would be "illuminated, in a Moment, with many Thousands of Electrical Stars, and Meteors of celestial Brilliance".

Graham was always a great recycler, of his own as well as other people's ideas. Eyeing up the medical competition in America, Graham must have noticed the success of a group of medics known as "Indian doctors", white colonists who specialized in the root and herbal cures used by native Americans. Their treatments were not taken very seriously by most orthodox physicians. "We have no discoveries in the *materia medica* to hope for from the Indians of North America," declared Benjamin Rush arrogantly in 1774 (by which time the Native Americans of the eastern seaboard had been more or less wiped out by colonial infectious diseases to which they had no immunity). The vast majority of immigrant doctors and American-born practitioners trained in Europe confined themselves to the European materia medica in which they had been educated, relying on familiar imported medicines, which would certainly have had more kudos in their patients' eyes.

But there were exceptions to these attitudes. In 1752, Dr Richard Brooke of Maryland sent notes about some Indian cures he was using in his practice to the Royal Society in London. A few plants had already been naturalized into the English Pharmacopoeia, such as snakeroot (*polygala senega*) and ginseng (*panax trifolium*), while imports to England of the root-beer-scented tree sassafras, a favourite treatment for rheumatism and venereal disease, reached 77 tons in 1770. Native American methods of curing these particular complaints were singled out for attention by Graham, who claimed in the course of his "tour of all the principal Colonies" to have spent time associating with and even bribing "Indians" whom he met, in order to discover their medical secrets.

He is reticent about the nature of these bribes. A colonial career criminal and professional chancer, Henry Tufts, found ten gallons of rum the most useful means of extracting such information. Tufts originally sought out a renowned healer, Molly Occut of the Western Abenakis, in 1772, for treatment to help him recover from a deep and festering jackknife wound in his thigh. After the success of this encounter, he lived for three years in the borderless wilderness between what was then "lower Canada" and "New England", trading furs for rum and that "fatally intoxicating potion" for medical knowledge.

"Gadding about quack-like" was at the more honest end of the spectrum of work Tufts found in the course of a life otherwise spent variously as a burglar, counterfeiter, army deserter, bigamist, farm-worker, fortune-teller and itinerant Evangelical preacher. (The bones he set were sometimes those of the man he had wrestled to the ground for prize money moments previously.) Like Tufts, Graham must have been planning to store away his knowledge of Native American medical practice for future use. While he was actually working in the colonies, Graham was probably anxious to dissociate himself from medical fly-by-nights in the Tufts mould, and certainly made no mention of Indian cures in any promotional material.

It was at this point that Graham's investigative attentions took him in a more original direction, one which would come to define his life. Separated all this time from his wife, his mind returned to the themes which had preoccupied him in Doncaster. The more he learnt about electrical therapy, the more obvious the parallels between electrical fluids and sexual fluids appeared. He was "suddenly struck with the thought, that the pleasure of the venereal act might be exalted or rendered more intense, if performed under the glowing, accelerating, and most genial influences of that heaven-born, all-animating element or principle, the electrical or concocted fire".

He was hardly alone in speculating about a connection between sexual and electrical energies. Barely had research into animal electricity been published, than it found its way into contemporary erotica. John Cleland, writing as Fanny Hill, mentioned "that principle of electricity which scarce ever fails of producing fire, when the sexes meet". Others were even more graphic. *The Electrical Eel*, one of a number of parodies of scientific articles along the lines of those published by the Royal Society, could not resist the unmissable visual associations between this remarkable fish and male anatomy: "let one of the nicest Ladies take a Male-Root into her Hand, and she becomes instantly electrical, and you may observe the quick and sudden Flashes of Electrical Fire dart from her Eyes." Female desire, like electrical effluvia, was imagined to emerge tangibly from a woman's organs of sight.

In Paris in 1772, a professor of surgery, Joseph-Aignan Sigaud de la Fond, was directing an electrical performance for the Duke of Chartres. Sigaud de la Fond was a successful disciple of Franklin's chief European rival, Abbé Nollet. His display was not as extravagant as Nollet's famous circuits using 180 shocked jumping guardsmen, or a kilometre and a half of Carthusian monks, but it was no less suggestive. Only twenty men formed this electrical chain, but crucially they numbered among them three castrati. The idea was to test whether the electrical conductivity of the human body was dependent on the presence of sperm. Of course, the experiment disproved the hypothesis. It had been initiated by an earlier failure in one of these human chain spectacles. When the experiment broke down, it was immediately surmised that it had done so at the moment the electrical "fire" had reached a man who was not a man. In fact, the accused participants were merely standing on a patch of damp ground.

Being "young, enterprising, impatient, and eccentric", as Graham described himself in retrospect, he decided to take his theories about electrical sex to their logical practical conclusion. He converted an ordinary bedstead by replacing its legs with strong glass pillars to insulate it from the ground and set up in the next room a fairly sophisticated electrical machine. Certainly, he refers in the plural to its "great globes". Graham was aware how old-fashioned even multiple globes must have sounded to an audience in the 1780s, when he first made these experiments public. By this time people were used to far more modern electrical apparatuses, in which cylinders or large glass plates had replaced globes.

One electrical machine designed by Joseph Priestley in 1768 looked something like a cross between a small three-legged mahogany table, a spinning wheel and a large crystal ball. Turning the handle rotated a leather pad at the bottom of the glass globe. The friction from this rubbing ensured that the glass built up a positive charge, while the pad developed a negative one, which could then be conducted away from the brass back plate of the pad and, in this particular experiment, sent along glass-enclosed iron rods through the wall and into the frame of the bed next door.

For his new purposes, Graham needed to generate more electrical charge than something like this could produce. He probably constructed a version of the more elaborate compound machines devised by German professors in their own quests for higher power. One of Bose's machines had three glass globes, up to one and a half feet across, which all rotated simultaneously, producing a charge capable of bruising with its shocks. Johann Winkler took a slightly different approach, connecting together the collecting devices of no fewer than eight glass cylinders, each with its own friction cushion. Although these sorts of multi-globed electric machines were largely superseded by the invention of the Leyden jar, some natural philosophers, like Priestley, believed that such machines could charge large Leyden batteries to a higher intensity, and he wrote about this idea in 1767. This would explain why Graham and Kinnersley were both intrigued by experimenting with magnitude at this period. Kinnersley, Franklin and at this point, surely, Graham, were all able to benefit from the expertise of the glassblowers at the nearby Wistarburgh Glassworks in New Jersey, which had a profitable line in making "electerising globes and tubes" for local experimenters.

The first patient to try out Graham's electric bed was a stout Dutch woman from Lancaster, sixty miles away, still childless after seven years or so of marriage to a "strong likely man". Now she had become partially paralysed, and incapable of speech. To make matters even worse, her periods had completely stopped. Her mother and husband brought her to see Graham in the hope that he could cure her "palsy". (Graham blamed her paralysis on the very strong coffee she drank every morning and her bizarre and unvarying evening diet of old tea leaves with salt and vinegar.) Every night she slept ("sometimes alone, sometimes with her husband") in the charged-up bed. Morning and night she plunged into an icy bath scented with herbs and flowers, followed by a firm massage "with the whole strength of her worthy husband". As soon as she could, she took up open-air exercise – "walking, running and rolling". Within two months she was on her way back to Lancaster, "in perfect health, in high-spirits, and happily pregnant".

After a result as spectacular as this, how could Graham resist recommending a session on "this *then* whimsical bed" to his "medical, philosophical, and gay friends"? These trials are reported in Graham's uniquely decorous yet explicit tone. Not surprisingly, the participants remain frustratingly anonymous. Viagra, today's answer to erectile dysfunction, only delays orgasm, but Graham claimed his bed also magnified the sensations of sexual climax. "They all found... that the pleasure was... rendered not only infinitely more intense, but at the same time, infinitely more durable!" This was the case for men, at least, whose anecdotes provide our only clues to the experience. These were hardly gathered with the rigour of a clinical trial – the concept was barely in existence at the time: "[A]fter a few months, when they were merry over a glass, and when it had circulated so freely as to make them forget themselves, and depart from that delicacy and reservedness which ought ever to be observed in these matters, they talked not as other men might have done, of the happy minute, or of the critical *moment*, – no!—They talked comparatively of the critical HOUR! ! !"

The account of the German experiments in the *Gentleman's Magazine* recorded the vast increase in power of multiple-globe apparatuses. These apparently caused a pain "insupportable to the philosophers themselves, [which] makes them cry out", a pain which increased "when you approach metal to the part where the bones are least cover'd with flesh". Graham must have designed his inventive apparatus in such a way as to avoid any danger of couples making direct contact with the metal conveying electricity to the bed. Users of the bed would have imagined themselves as "bathing" in a kind of pervasive electrical atmosphere. Its force would probably have been capable of agitating gold leaf to a distance of four or five feet around the bed, to judge from the *Gentleman's Magazine* article, but was not intended to shock. Graham quite likely set up special devices in the chamber to demonstrate this fact, perhaps using silk or feathers. Lovers doubtless found their hair floating upwards.

This electrical atmosphere was widely perceived as a nebulous vapour, possessing an almost mystical vital force. "I call it an atmosphere, because it really is so, as appears by the smell, which naturalists have compared to that of oil of vitriol." (In other words, sulphuric acid.) Other observers thought the smell more like phosphorus, and described electrified iron, and even jewels, "when impregnated with an electric virtue" as emitting an "acid smell". Hardly an atmosphere conducive to love-making. Little wonder that Graham chose to conceal this off-putting side effect when the bed became "celestial" by the strategic use of highly scented fumigators throughout the Temple of Health. He makes no mention of what kind of mattress was used in the original "whimsical bed".

Of course an element of exhibitionism may well have magnified any genuine therapeutic effects of this new invention. The fantasy of being observed in the act of sex could come close to being fulfilled for any lover using the electrical bed: to operate it, the Doctor himself must have been fairly audible as he cranked or treadled away behind the partition which divided the two rooms, quite possibly with the help of an assistant or two. The perceptible presence of even merely the aural equivalent of a potential voyeur is likely to have enhanced the sexual pleasure of a proportion of "patients". Such titillating partitions litter the erotic literature of the eighteenth century – Fanny Hill spends almost as much time secreted in a state of arousal behind screens and hidden in closets observing others in the act of sex as she does in bed herself in John Cleland's *Memoirs of a Woman of Pleasure* (1748). In the pornographic *Rambler's Magazine* of the 1780s, the serialized "Adventures of Kitty Pry" featured a sequence of erotic encounters through suitable holes in boudoir doors, written to appeal to voyeur and exhibitionist alike. Probably the most socially acceptable face of eighteenth-century erotica were the newspaper and magazine reports of civil adultery trials known as "crim. con." (short for "criminal conversation"). More or less overtly salacious according to the periodical in which they were reported, these could be hard to distinguish from the fictional versions which also appeared. Not surprisingly, witnesses to such cases were often servants. A particular kind of "knowing" concealment became a recurrent sexual motif. The frequency of the scenario in both genuine reports and parodies suggest readers found the idea particularly arousing.

The play of the imagination in sexual arousal – a theme he elaborated vividly in his "eccentric" lectures at the Temple of Health in the early 1780s – seems to have fascinated Graham, even in these early days. It was a logical train of thought probably derived from a developing medical interest in the workings of the nervous system. Stimulate the body, and you stimulate the mind, Graham later explained: "the influence of the electrical fire… warms and invigorates the whole system! – expanding the imagination, and every faculty of body and soul! – exciting and exalting the amorous ideas of both sexes – stimulating them to the enjoyment of love; and greatly heightening and prolonging its sweet pleasures!" Increase the intensity of pleasure, and, Graham quickly came to believe, you increase the likelihood of pregnancy. The Celestial Bed itself was promoted as a means of conception, but increasing fertility was initially an unforeseen side effect of electrifying sex: the Bed's Philadelphian prototype was clearly developed with pleasure rather than conception in mind. "Wonderful, oftentimes, are the effects of holding venereal congress in situations where the passions are very highly excited," wrote Graham in retrospect, adding diplomatically, "or where the hopes of progeny are very strongly impressed on the mind. To these strong mental impressions I formerly attributed, in some measure the unexpected conceptions which took place in the infancy of my celestial bed!" Like most sex therapists ever since, the Doctor always advocated diversity as the secret of a successful sex life, recommending celebrating the "rites of Venus… in a variety of ways and places, and on singular occasions". What could be more singular than a glass-legged electrical bed, in the consulting rooms of a handsome and charming Scottish doctor, who spoke so persuasively about such novel and inspiring ideas? Graham's guinea pigs were thrilled.

Graham later referred to Philadelphia as "that wise and all-tolerating city", perhaps an oblique reference to the apparent ease with which he found experimental subjects to test this bed. As his equipment expanded, so too did the space he needed to house his extraordinary apparatus. During his two years in Philadelphia, Graham changed his address with regularity. He had initially taken apartments "at a Mrs Dugdale's in Arch Street, between Second and Third streets, where he [gave] advice in all the diseases of the eye or its appendages; and in every species of deafness, hardness of hearing, ulceration, noise in the ears, &c." His advertisements at this point were becoming ever longer and more florid, Latin tags multiplying. The most extravagant were vaingloriously addressed "To the Inhabitants of *British* America", and contained a detailed third-person career sketch, panegyrics from satisfied patients and Graham's self-congratulatory reflections on his own profession:

> How noble, therefore, how deserving of the nicest attention and cultivation must that art be that can restore sight to the blind, hearing to the deaf, speech to the dumb, and keep in order the springs of those master pieces of Creative Wisdom! That art must needs be divine, because, thus assisted, our minds are inspired with the grandest apprehensions of Almighty God!

In March 1772, he advertised for an apprentice for the first time. He clearly hoped to earn both a reputation for being magnanimous and a decent fee for it. The usual habit of so-called oculists and aurists in Europe was, according to Graham, to protect their trade by keeping their methods and knowledge secret. Graham explained that his "concerns in England" – presumably his wife and children, and possibly already some debts – prevented him from remaining long in America, and he wanted to leave behind him someone trained in his methods.

By July that year he was doing well enough to move out of his latest lodgings with Mrs Rivers, also in Arch Street (where he had set up shop in March) and into his own house, much closer to the College, on "the Corner of *fifth* and *Market Streets*". The "greene Country Town" envisaged by its original proprietor William Penn in 1681, "which will never be burnt, and allways be wholsome", was rapidly disappearing, the squares of its generous grid filling up, typically with shingle-roofed brick residences. The 1760s had seen about two hundred built every year. In 1774 a medical student at the College, Solomon Downe, commented on the racket that came through his window on Second Street, complaining that "the thundering of Coaches, Chariots, Chaises, Wagons, Drays, and the whole Fraternity of Noise almost continuously assaill our Ears."

Not long after Graham had moved uptown, his advertisements began to include a favourite device for drumming up trade. He announced that he was proposing to stay in Philadelphia only until the beginning of May 1773. "Those, therefore, who have occasion for his assistance, are desired to apply as soon as possible." He also published his personal performance indicators, complete with a gruesome breakdown of the commonest complaints:

Since his arrival in this city in November 1771, upwards of four hundred patients have been cured or relieved of the following disorders, many of which had been of very long standing, and deemed altogether incurable by other practitioners, *viz.* Total, partial and periodical blindness; weakness and dimness of sight; squinting; pain, swelling, and inflammation of the eyes; spots, specks, and films, occasioned by the small-pox, colds, blows and extraneous substances; falling off of the hairs of the eye-lashes, weak, watery, red, spongy, and ulcerated eye-lids, involuntary weeping of the tears; tumours and excressances; *fistul lachchrym.* – Total and periodical deafness; thickness of hearing; pain and inflammations, cracking, itching, continual and unremitting noises and sounds in the ears; offensive runnings, occasioned by colds, swelling, swimming, picking and improper applications, long and severe sickness; ulcerations with caries of the bones; *polypi, etc.*, and several persons born deaf and dumb, who have made very considerable advances in speaking and hearing; insomuch that perfect cures will probably be effected.

Autumn 1772 found the Doctor making a brief circuit of outlying towns such as Lancaster, York and Reading. As well as his routine treatments, he was now offering to replace perished eyes with artificial ones, "so curiously fixed and adapted to the orbis, as to have (in appearance) the beauties, motion, &c. of the natural eye in its healthy state". Setting out his stall in copious newspaper advertisements, (including in the German-language press) Graham became repetitively lyrical about his expertise.

When Dr Graham left Philadelphia for a further New York tour in the summer of 1773, he went with a flourish. The young oculist who had begun his spell in the city as an eager member of the lecture-circuit audience had now thoroughly reinvented himself as a professional lecturer. His "Rational and Pleasing Entertainment", a development of his less successful effort back in Maryland, seems to have had its first airing in early October 1772. It was decisively aimed at "the Gentlemen of the Learned Professions, particularly those of the *Faculty*, and the respectable and intelligent Inhabitants of [the] City in general" as well as "the Ladies". It was repeated in early November. On Tuesday 23rd March 1773, he gave, supposedly for "one night only", a three-part "Lecture on the Eye" in the State House Assembly Room (still then the scene of regular subscription balls, though three years later it would host the debate, drafting and signing of the United States Constitution). A fortnight later, on 7th April, he was advertising the same lecture "by particular desire" at Philadelphia College Hall, a splendid finale indeed. He was apparently expecting quite a crowd since the gallery was open for half a dollar a ticket, while admittance to the hall cost twice that.

Following Kinnersley's lead on such matters, Graham published his syllabus in lengthy detail, taking up an entire column of the newspaper. Even when merely summarizing his lecture's content, Graham's rhetorical exuberance characteristically ran away with him. Still greater heights of grandiloquence were no doubt reached in performance. Sight was hymned as the most "refined or spiritual" of all the senses, that "most nearly approaching to those Pleasures that are purely Intellectual". Whereas the gratification of the other senses can apparently exhaust the spirits, "the Pleasures of the Eye restore the Mind and act as a Physician to the Soul". Ultimately, beholding beauty was lauded as an exalted religious experience: "the extensive Group of glorious Objects spread out on the wide Earth, and through the blue Expanse of Heaven, finding a Passage through the Eye, expand the Heart with the most lively Emotions of Sublimity and Grandeur, and transport the Mind to the Deity while it overflows with Admiration, Gratitude, and Love!"

His lecture began practically enough, with illustrations of the "anatomical and mechanical structure of the Eye" and its associated parts, probably using a Russian-doll-like model of the eye made out of wood, glass and ivory. These had been available since the previous century and could be dismantled layer by layer to reveal the eyelid, the sclerotic coat, the choroid tunic, the aqueous humour, the crystalline lens and so on. This first section of the lecture ended with an ingratiating apostrophe to the College of Philadelphia.

The principal eye diseases and their cures were the theme of the second part, which covered everything from cataracts and glaucoma to blindness, myopia and squinting. Just as he was applying his scientific research to the field of sexuality, so too did he eroticize his lecture on the eye. At this point Graham began to rehearse a theme which he pursued to its logical conclusion at the Temple of Health. The Doctor launched into an "Address to the Ladies on the Art of managing the eye". Essentially this was a coy guide to successful flirtation. The eye was described as "opening a direct Avenue to the female Heart", while the language of the eye was said to be one employed by Nature and understood by all. He pronounced (less helpfully) on the most pleasing colour for eyes, waxed lyrical on the

"Tender social Emotions how inspired by the Eye", gave advice on eyebrow-shaping, and explained "in what Manner the Eye of a fine Woman returns the more lovely after having rested on large green or black Objects". (It is worth bearing in mind that a 1743 book on "the Art of correcting and preventing deformities in children" listed in great detail no fewer than fourteen different malformations of the eyebrows alone.)

In his deliberate blurring of the medical and the erotic, Graham drew on long-established associations between sight and desire. There was an intense physicality about ancient theories of sight. The pattern of thought which regarded lovers' eyes as a very literal conduit of sexual passion went back to Plato. Vision was thought to come about when a stream of particles flowing from an object or person actually impinged on the onlooker's eye. So the meeting gaze of two lovers came close to a kind of copulation.

A well-developed body language is explicitly referred to in a popular piece of erotica of 1741. *A New Description of Merryland* describes the people of that country as having little use for words, "for they have the Art of communicating their Sentiments very plainly by their *Eyes and Actions*". Stimulated by the success of his experiments with the electrical bed, Graham began to perceive as electrical even those vital interactions between the sexes which were without physical contact. He was beginning to develop the theory that "those bewitching, those heart-piercing and irresistible glances, which shoot from the female eye to the male heart, and indeed reciprocally from soul to soul, at certain critical times, are no other than electrical strokes or emanations!"

In the third part of Graham's lecture, after a "Digressive Inquiry" into the dignity of physic and the illustrious history of the medical lecture, he launched into what he described as a "Eulogy on the Eye". This seems also to have been the point at which he introduced an early and undoubtedly more discreetly dressed incarnation of the Rosy Goddesses who would later controversially grace his lectures on generation at the Temple of Health. Perhaps inspired by the popularity of the female assistants who used to demonstrate "the Electric Kiss" or "*Venus Electrificata*" in the lectures of Kinnersley, Bose and other professional electricians, Graham illustrated his "Eulogy" with a description of "a young Female Quaker, in whose eyes are expressed such gentle and amiable Qualities of the Mind, as correspond with the Softness and sweet Simplicity of her outward Form and Dress".

This strongly suggests that Graham had begun to enjoy the advantages of sharing the stage with a pretty young woman in his public performances well before his Temple days. Her physical presence could gratify the gaze of an intrigued audience and yet still represent an irrefutably high-minded argument about beauty, simplicity and religion.

Kinnersley's lectures were usually scheduled for late morning or early afternoon, to avoid the damp evening air which could jeopardize the success of electrical experiments. Graham opened the doors at 4 p.m. for a performance that began, like a theatrical event, at seven o'clock. Between each part of the lecture the audience were entertained with a musical concert. Graham's gift for stagecraft was already revealing itself. It must have been quite a night.

3

The Treatment

"…and may excentric medical geniuses arise!…"

When James Graham finally made his way south down the eastern seaboard of America in late September 1773, he had left Philadelphia for the last time. For an expedition of rather greater international significance was simultaneously taking place: seven ships laden with tea setting sail across the Atlantic from the London warehouses of the near-bankrupt East India Company. Their cargo would affect the lives of millions. With the sanction of the British Parliament, some 600,000 pounds of tea from the Company's vast unsold "mountain" were heading for Boston, New York, Philadelphia and Charleston, due to be sold at a bargain price. But the tea tax, resented and despised by the American colonists since its imposition alongside a slew of other import duties six years previously, was still provocatively in place.

By the time the first vessel docked in Boston in late November, Graham had set up his practice in Baltimore. His arrival in America nearly four years previously had coincided with a brief period of stability in colonial relations. After the lifting of most of the harshest tax laws imposed in 1767 to recoup the costs of war, even patriotic Americans were once again enjoying the luxuries of imported British goods. It had been a relief, for the time being at least, to abandon homespun clothing and experimental herbal brews. By that autumn though, it was clear that the status quo was about to shift again dramatically. The British Parliament's insidious offer of cheap but duted tea was seen as a plot to tempt colonists into accepting taxation without representation. Mass meetings began to gather up and down the east coast to decide how to meet this latest threat to liberty.

In late November Philadelphia's "Committee of Tarring and Feathering" declared ominously "that Matters ripen fast here". The Committee wrote threateningly to Captain Ayres of the tea ship *Polly*, warning him that "the *Pennsylvanians* are, *to a* Man, passionately fond of Freedom; the Birthright of Americans". He was advised to fly "without Hesitation – without the Formality of a Protest" if he wanted to avoid a halter round his neck and the feathers of "a dozen wild Geese" laid over "ten Gallons of liquid Tar decanted on [his] Pate". Ayres hesitated on the Delaware. Way down the coast in Charleston, planters and merchants spent much of December debating what to do with tea impounded in a dockside warehouse, which eventually rotted where it lay. Up in Massachusetts there was a more portentous collision between the "Sons of Liberty" and the Governor. In the late evening of 16th December, barely disguised rebels, some with blackened faces and tauntingly dressed in Mohawk costumes, were sweeping the Boston tea ships' decks of their last stray leaves. The rest lay heaped unevenly in the low waters of a dark harbour. 342 crates had been emptied at the end of the famously silent riot that constituted the Boston Tea Party.

Though it would be another month before London learnt of these events, the news spread quickly through the agitated colonies. Never a man content to stay too long in one place, Graham decided it was time to go. The political turmoil was hardly conducive to business. More important matters would soon squeeze the comings and goings of a travelling physician out of the newspaper columns on which he depended. The troubles looked unlikely to blow over in a hurry and the threatening war risked separating him from his family in England permanently. "I returned to England at the commencement of the eternal downfall of European power in America! Yes, at the great aera!" he later declared, "when British and other European children, forced reluctant from their native homes, had attained to the age of majority, and were taking formal possession of that glorious and immense country! Which the luxury, the folly, and the infatuation of their parents had forced them over tremendous oceans to seek for."

When James Graham came back he was still, relatively speaking, a nobody. But in his absence he had transformed himself. No longer a run-of-the-mill apothecary, Graham was now an experienced doctor with some unusual specialisms and a sheaf of testimonials to his name. His peregrinations in the colonies had introduced him to a whole new approach to medicine – most significantly the exciting therapeutic possibilities offered by electricity. They had also transformed him into a master of self-promotion. These new skills would be vital in his solitary campaign to achieve celebrity status in Britain. Within seven years he would take London by storm with his Temple of Health. But long before the Temple was unveiled, newspapers, satirists and letter-writers were referring to Graham as "the advertising doctor", "the aërial doctor", or "the electrical empiric", confident that their readers would identify him with no difficulty.

Celebrity culture may seem a uniquely modern phenomenon. In fact it was very much an invention of the eighteenth century. Britain was a country which then revelled in a free press, personal libel laws so weak they might as well not have existed, and a brash delight in consumption that had grown up hand-in-hand with the explosion of print – newspapers, magazines, advertising bills, novels, cartoons and all the rest. They reported on a monarchy no longer divine, but with feet clearly of clay. The King was often referred to in the press simply by his initials, and soon everyone knew that his son and heir was more likely to be found gambling or whoring the night away at a drinking club than studying affairs of state. By 1770, sixty newspapers were printed in London alone every week, many of these dailies, and their gossip was reprinted in hundreds of provincial papers across the nation and as far away as the American colonies. Conditions were ripe for the public to embrace new kinds of national figures, individuals whose private lives quickly became commercial commodities. Fame had acquired more transient, earthly qualities. Candidates for celebrity could not hope for immortality, but novelty and sensation could win them a temporary share of the nation's applause.

James Graham did not just want to make a good living. He craved the limelight. In years to come he would rise from his box at the theatre to confront the actors impersonating his servants on stage, and then read about the event a few days later in the London press. At this point in his life, since he was neither thespian, politician nor courtesan and obviously lacked the more usual trappings of breeding or beauty, he had to create his own route to celebrity. The first step was to garner a share of glory from an already established public personality.

Graham got his helping hand into the public arena from one of its stars. It did not happen overnight, but it was well worth waiting for. In 1774 Catharine Macaulay was a woman already secure in her celebrity, all the more astonishing since it was neither for her looks, her sexual alliances nor through a stage career, but for her intellectual performance. She had become a national idol with the publication in 1763 of the first volume of her monumental *History of England*. "She is one of the sights that all foreigners are carried to see," attested a visiting French aristocrat. Like so many of those erudite eighteenth-century women known as "bluestockings", her reputation today does scant justice to the enormous reverence with which she was regarded in her lifetime. When Mary Wollstonecraft was a writer beginning to achieve renown, and Macaulay close to the end of her life, Wollstonecraft wrote to her heroine and declared her profound respect for a woman who "contends for laurels whilst most of her sex only seek for flowers..." Through the 1760s and 1770s this "very prodigy" had appeared in every possible medium. In porcelain, wax and marble, in oil paintings, prints, and on stage her figure and character were widely reproduced, usually in muse-like attitudes. Macaulay's wit and intelligence, her grace and amiability were almost universally admired. But she was a contradictory figure. Her princessly airs also attracted attention, particularly alongside her egalitarian political views, and both were cruelly mocked by Samuel Johnson and others.

Graham had particular reason to pursue a potential patient like Macaulay. Celebrity endorsement was as important to the uninhibited consumerism of the eighteenth century as it has been ever since. Medicine was very much part of that culture, and patients had to pick and choose their cures, nostrums and practitioners with little way of determining the validity of any particular treatments other than the recommendations of satisfied customers. Without Macaulay, Graham would have struggled to rise from the advertising columns of the provincial press. For most of his life, he proudly acknowledged her as the person to whom he owed his earliest success.

Barely had Graham disembarked in Bristol than one friend of Macaulay seems to have referred to him sourly as "the dapper doctor". The Revd Augustus Toplady wrote a warning letter to the republican historian on 18th February 1774 from his parish in Broad Hembury, Devon: "Above all, beware of being seen with him in public... He would derive lustre from you, but, like a piece of black cloth, he would absorb the rays, without reflecting any of them back."

It has been previously assumed that Toplady (whose own lasting legacy was the rousing hymn 'Rock of Ages') was cautioning her against a different doctor, a recently widowed and somewhat grasping minister called Thomas Wilson. Dr Wilson became very publicly and rather ridiculously infatuated with Macaulay at around this time. Widowed herself with a young daughter, and in a fragile state of health after working feverishly to finish five of the eight volumes of her *History* in less than a decade, Macaulay was certainly vulnerable to the blandishments of either man. Of the two, Graham was indisputably the more dapper, and shared Macaulay's own taste for extravagant sartorial display. A Swedish astronomer later commented on the fine lace on his velvet suit and the exceptionally large curls of his hair, while the novelist Sir Walter Scott remembered him turning up at Greyfriars in a white and silver outfit, a folding hat under his arm and "his hair most marvellously draped into a sort of double toupée, which divided upon his head like the two tops of Parnassus". Macaulay and probably Graham were both in the West Country in early spring. Few people in England were following events across the Atlantic more closely than the "female historian". The previous April, John Adams (the United States' future president) had written to Macaulay of "a System of Tyranny gaining ground upon us every day". Macaulay would undoubtedly have been anxious in these times to meet newly arrived and sympathetic witnesses of the progress of liberty in America.

When the Doctor dedicated a medical book to "the female historian" in 1778, he confessed it had "acquired not a little of its importance from the renowned name of MACAULAY". But the story of Graham's involvement with Macaulay turned out to be a great deal more complicated than a straightforward seal of approval from a recognizable "name". And in fulfilment of Toplady's prediction, as far as reputation was concerned, Dr Graham benefited rather more than she did from their curious association.

Whichever predatory doctor Toplady intended to steer her clear of, Macaulay chose to ignore his advice. On Christmas Day 1776, Dr Graham and Dr Wilson were both sitting down to dinner with Mrs Macaulay in Bath. This was recorded in the diary of fellow diner John Wilkes, that hideous and charming champion of liberty and libertarianism, who began to keep a watchful eye on events in the Macaulay household. But unlike the course of light (to borrow one of Graham's favourite metaphors), the Doctor's path to triumph and scandal in Bath was a little tortuous.

His exact movements in the early months of 1774 are mysterious, but he probably sailed from Baltimore into Bristol, where he established a practice in Queen's Square. Bristol was the perfect spot for Graham at this point. Its deep involvement in the Atlantic economy meant close links with America, and the possibility of recommendations from previous patients. Meanwhile Hotwells, in the nearby suburb of Clifton, was still enjoying a brief spell of glory as a fashionable spa resort. (Its later reputation as a last resort for the incurable was still a decade or so away.) What has now been reduced to a plume of steam emerging from under the Clifton suspension bridge was in the 1770s the focus of an economic boom offering rich pickings for land speculators, builders and rival physicians. May, the month Graham began to advertise in the Bristol local press, was the beginning of the holiday season for Hotwells. Graham must have planned to attract the more affluent aristocratic invalids who often moved on to Bristol as the Bath season drew to a close. He traded on the specialization in sight and hearing which he had developed in America.

In typically flamboyant style, Graham opened for business in the city's most elegant square: close to the harbour, Queen's Square was also the site of the Custom House. Its grand townhouses were home to many of Bristol's wealthiest slave and sugar merchants. The *Bristol Gazette* announced Graham's presence on 5th May with an advertisement thinly disguised as an item of news, a classic eighteenth-century "puff", reporting the Doctor's determination to settle in a few months in London.

In fact, Graham stuck it out in Bristol until the end of the year, further expanding his business in the autumn by delivering public lectures at the new Assembly Room in Prince's Street, close to Queen's Square. These talks covered much the same ground as his American lecture series. The following year Graham published his first small book, *Thoughts on the Present State of the Practice in Disorders of the Eye and Ear* (1775). His exuberant style bursts out of this slim volume, as it must have done in the lecture hall. Fired with enlightened ideals absorbed both in Philadelphia and Edinburgh, he clearly also believed that his Godlike purpose – making the blind see, the deaf hear – endowed him with Godlike powers. Was he not, after all, restoring the function of those most noble of human senses, "so far superior... as to approach to the faculty of *spirit* itself"? Graham almost swooned with self-importance and painted a pathetic picture of the lonely path he trod in his pioneering office as oculist and aurist. "What, alas! can be expected!" in the way of progress from general practitioners, who, unlike him, refused "to step out of the regular trammels" or leave "the old narrow track" of medicine "to mount on the shoulders of modern improvements", he bemoaned. His sentences characteristically pile up into striking and elaborate images. Distinguishing itinerant mountebanks who hawked a medical living from town to town from progressive specialists like himself, he compared the destructive powers of lightning with the illuminating properties of light itself:

May ignorant and unprincipled wretches, who puffing and posting *like lightning* from place to place, pretend to give light and sound, but who like lightning too, blast and destroy wherever they pass, and whoever they touch; may the number of such be small!... But may the number of liberal men, who shall confine their studies and practice to diseases of the same class, or of a single part, fast encrease! and may excentric medical geniuses arise, who *like light* shall with velocity proceed in *one* straight direction – like light too, chearing and illuminating the dark and gloomy regions and habitations of science and men!

This was rousing if convoluted stuff. Tradespeople perhaps did indeed "croud for relief" as Graham puts it – some coming from as far as Monmouthshire. But, to judge from the grateful letters in *Thoughts* economically recycled from the Bristol papers, bar the odd vicar, the visiting and local gentry were content merely to send their servants. Eighteenth-century medics usually operated a sliding scale of payment. The fees that could be charged to treat the ear infection of a cooper's son, the near blindness of a publican or a milliner's deafness were not going to amount to enough to support Graham's business plans. The rent on an apartment in Queen's Square was hardly cheap, and the kind of equipment Graham needed to develop required substantial investment.

The Doctor made it clear he was looking to reap a more rewarding "pecuniary harvest". Having met with only qualified success in one spa town, perhaps he wanted to test the commercial waters of another while it was convenient. So he spent January 1775 in Bath, whose season was then in full swing. More significantly, Catharine Macaulay had settled there the previous year, in the hope of improving her failing health. The Doctor had a joyous gift for fanfare. Graham's arrival and lodgings were instantly announced in the local papers, one of which reported that he had been expected for the past two months. Third-person puffs declared that he rejoiced in the applause of the world, exulted in the approbation of his own conscience, but that since London was his favourite place, he would shortly be heading for "that great metropolis".

In London, Graham's hopes of success seem to have been frustrated once more. Even after nearly a year in the capital, he still seemed to be struggling to attract the kind of upmarket patients he must have imagined an address in Pall Mall ("nearly opposite the King's Palace") would impress. The pages of *An Address to the Inhabitants of Great Britain* (1775), appended to *Thoughts on the Present State*, are crowded only with letter-writers from the middling to lower ranks of society. Vivid pictures of the psychological damage wrought by sensory deprivation touched the hearts of sentimental readers in affecting scenarios: an East End schoolmistress almost too deaf to go on working, a hard-of-hearing Smithfield butcher, a servant blinded by "an itinerant London operator", or the (particularly touching) case of Mrs Agnes Renwick – "so exceedingly deaf as not to hear the rattle of carriages when close upon her, and sometimes not even thunder, or the loudest church-bells;... trumpets in her case were useless. In this lonely – this dismal and truly pitiable condition she mopp'd on gloomy and dejected, till accidentally she came under Dr. Graham's care". Graham's instinctive understanding of the emotional condition of his prospective patients was always one of his strengths.

He implied the existence of more "noble personages" seeking his attention by declaring in tones of loud moral integrity that he "NEVER PRESUMES TO MENTION ANY OF HIS PATIENTS NAMES OR RESIDENCE without they desire it, or give him their intire consent". So he may have enjoyed the patronage of more illustrious patients than he could reveal. The writer, politician and Gothic revivalist Horace Walpole has only been exposed as one of these since the twentieth-century publication of his lengthy correspondence. In the mid-1770s he was still a close friend of Catharine Macaulay. Tormented by gout for the previous twenty years, Walpole sought help from Graham in April 1776, describing him as an "apothecary".

Though this period in London did not launch Graham in society quite as successfully as he had hoped, it was a time of frenzied activity which eventually bore fruit. During these months, the Doctor seems to have been peculiarly receptive to new ideas, and open to all kinds of different experiments. One night in February 1776, he went to an oboe concert given by the composer Johann Christian Fischer, recently settled in London and a member of Queen Charlotte's band at court. Fischer was a virtuoso player, and the novelist Fanny Burney, daughter of a musicologist and a young woman rarely given to superfluous praise, admired the "sweet-flowing, melting, celestial notes" of his oboe. Fischer bored Mozart, who found his concertos excessively long and repetitive, but they had a very different effect on Graham. He rushed home, inspired by the "inimitable sweetness" of Fischer's "*long-winded* variations on some fine old tunes" to attempt a similar effect in "literary composition". Graham went to bed and sat up all night writing a wild and passionate riff on the Lord's Prayer.

The result, *The Christian's Universal Prayer*, now reads as a distinctly hysterical piece of writing. It clearly shows the theological direction in which the Doctor was already heading. The third edition of the *Prayer* was confidently introduced with the hope that "the humble pious Heart of every Denomination... [might] feel the Warm Sparkling – the Delightful Elevation – the Holy Enthusiasm of true Devotion, – and may it give New Wings as it were to the Soul, in its onward Flight, till it FEELS itself in the blissful Circle of Divine Attraction – melting at last in the Immensity of Divine Love!"

Some eighteenth-century Christians believed in a rational religion, in which experience and the physical world gave order to faith; others, spiritually inspired by scripture, sought a personal, fervent relationship with their deity. Through the 1770s the divide was growing. With this publication Graham firmly rebuffed the scepticism of natural theology, and put himself on the side of revelation. Kinnersley would not have approved. Graham gave full vent to his instincts for hyperbole, swooping from crescendo to crescendo in an outpouring of faith modulated by the familiar phrases of the Lord's Prayer:

OUR FATHER – our good and gracious Father! – thou permittest, nay teachest us, to address thee by that affectionate – that endearing appellation. – How great the privilege! – How comfortable the condescension! – With humble confidence, therefore, and with cordial affection, we look up to Thee, and grasping, with the arms of kindness and compassion, not only our kindred and our kind, but the whole Universe, we address thee jointly and in their behalf, not as MINE only, but, as thou hast taught us, as OUR Father – WHICH ART IN HEAVEN... How sublime!...

In 1780, reprinting the prayer as an appendix to his first description of the Adelphi Temple of Health, he backtracked. Graham confessed: "On publishing this prayer, in order to give as little offence to the world as possible, and to please as many of the little bitter persecuting churches and sects as I can, I have used some phrases, and expressions, which are not very philosophical, and what is still worse, which I do not very well understand." All his life Graham tended to be carried away by rhetorical excess, but this was one of the few moments he revealed any awareness of the trait.

Rejecting dogma in the fields of both religion and medicine, Graham replaced it with a curious conflation of independent thought and emotional appeal. But he went on reading furiously in scientific fields, keeping himself abreast of new discoveries and publications so that he could incorporate the most up-to-date ideas into his medical practice. He travelled to Germany to pursue his research. There he learnt of "a person in Russia, who had devoted almost his whole life to the study of magnetism". With extraordinary enterprise, the Doctor set off on a round trip of nearly four thousand miles, to St Petersburg, where Catherine the Great was expanding her empire and establishing herself as the Enlightenment's most extravagant patron of the arts and sciences. When Graham's life became entangled with that of Catharine Macaulay, he was fond of comparing the two great Kates. At times he even implied that he had treated the Russian monarch as well as the British historian. Graham's account of these European travels first appeared in his third publication, a promotional pamphlet called *A Short Inquiry into the Present State of Medical Practice* (1776).

He is frustratingly brief about his mission to meet a man whom he does not name, but who must have been Franz Aepinus. A former director of the Berlin Observatory, Aepinus was by then a luminary of the St Petersburg Academy of Science, and its first Newtonian physicist. Graham could hardly have approached a more rigorous mentor. The fact that he sought him out shows how seriously he was pursuing this train of thought. Aepinus was the first of a new breed of mathematical physicists, spearheading a revolution in modern science with his developments of Benjamin Franklin's not entirely conclusive theories about electricity. His book was discussed in the popular *Gentleman's Magazine* the moment it was published, but its algebraic intricacies prevented most English electricians from hailing it immediately as a masterpiece. Whether because all this was beyond his own understanding (quite likely), or that of his intended audience (almost certainly), Graham offered no details about what he may have learnt from Aepinus, nor much information about the rest of his Russian expedition. Even in a later hurried rewriting of earlier works he fashionably entitled *Travels and Voyages* (1783), he preferred to dwell sentimentally on an encounter with a particularly generous and devout "Tartar peasant" with whom he shared a boat ride and a meal on the way from St Petersburg to Kronshtadt in the Gulf of Finland.

But the Doctor certainly felt he had made some spectacular improvements to his apparatus after this trip. His infectious zeal for novelty sings out of *A Short Inquiry*, reflecting the general excitement being stirred up around the globe by progress in natural philosophy as much as his own delight in the results of his new discoveries. Every day, he said, his astonishing cures afforded him "the highest and most exalted pleasure that the human mind is perhaps capable of enjoying". Graham must also have enjoyed some exalted pleasure at the realization that he could now go back to Bath with something truly original to offer prospective patients. For while he was refining his therapeutic practices, he was also refining his understanding of his market.

Bath was Britain's most thriving health resort, and its visitors were drawn to the city as much by the social whirl as for medicinal reasons. Of course the afflictions which Graham had previously made his speciality were, as he so vividly described, also the very ones most likely to prevent the sufferers from participating fully in society. Even more to the point, restoring sight or hearing may have been dramatic, but it was a one-off affair. Problems with the nerves, digestion or the "constitution" could run and run. So Graham extended the field of his advertised treatments, widening his appeal to the very type of invalid most likely to come to Bath – typically those of a hypochondriac disposition, suffering from vague, grumbling, non-specific complaints. Now his specialisms included "Consumptions, Asthmas, Gout in the Head or Stomach, spasmodic or paralytic Affections of the Nerves" and – what must surely have caught Catharine Macaulay's eye when she read it – "every species of nervous Weakness".

His next commercial move was to shift the promotional spotlight from particular disorders to his unique treatments. "My method of cure," he wrote, "consists chiefly in a variety of Effluvia, Vapours, and Applications ætherial, magnetic, or electric, adapted to the nature of each case, conveyed with certain curious machines into the lungs, stomach, or other parts… and so applied to the parts affected, as to act immediately, and powerfully, on the cause of the disease… they are of so extraordinary, active, penetrating, and salutary a nature, as not only to correct, in many cases, the *materies morbi* – the immediate case of the disease – but also to supply a vivifying spirit – a *pabulum vitæ*, to the injured or decayed constitution…" It sounded thrillingly modern, but pleasantly vague, and a lot more fun than the purging and bloodletting regimens prescribed by the mainstream medical faculty. Perfectly adapted, in short, to the seekers of revived health and respite from life's tedium who flocked to Bath. "When the silver cords are loosed, and the balmy juices dried up – when all the vital functions languish, – then the golden fountain of life runs low, – and pleasure charms no more, – then these ætherial, vivifying medicines refresh, restore, and reanimate, acting INSTANTLY and powerfully, as a Divine restorative!" Soon he was confidently referring to the rather vague vaporous substances he employed in his treatments as "effluvia" which were "strictly speaking, celestial".

Georgian Bath was another boom town, its appearance and inhabitants in perpetual flux. New vistas in golden, glowing stonework were materializing and new visitors arriving to occupy and admire them all the time. "Elegancies daily seem to spring up here by enchantment," commented one late-eighteenth-century newcomer to the resort. Bath's glamour and glory had been carefully invented in the first half of the century by a triumvirate composed of a professional gambler, an entrepreneur in postal services and a visionary architect with an ambition to rebuild Rome in Britain's West Country. Between 1700 and 1800 a market town with two or three thousand inhabitants became an international metropolis, its population increasing tenfold. Richard "Beau" Nash, Ralph Allen and John Wood were all dead by the time James Graham moved to Bath, but the transformation which they had begun was still in full swing. Critical of its follies, Graham was ready to reap its benefits.

Bath social life was highly structured, even ritualized, and yet unusually permeable. It was largely organized in communal meeting places, such as the Assembly Rooms, the Pump Room and the actual Baths themselves. The King's Bath was "a huge cistern, where you see the patients up to their necks in hot water". They were tended by professional guides, stained orange from long immersion in the mineral waters. By "their Scorbutick carcasses, and Lacker'd Hides, you would think [they] had lain pickling a Century of Years in the Stygian Lake". Bath's rigid rules of propriety were explained to the last detail in regularly updated guidebooks. Provided a visitor had enough money and had "registered" with the black-wigged Master of Ceremonies (a role invented by Nash and replicated in resorts from Tunbridge Wells to Buxton), anyone from virtually any rank in life could join in. This was fundamental to architect John Wood's uniquely egalitarian design for Bath. In 1742, he wrote that "when proper walks were made for exercise, and a house built for assembling in, rank began to be laid aside, and all degrees of people, from the private gentleman upwards, were soon united in society with one another".

The results of this kind of social experimentation are described with autobiographical clarity in *The Expedition of Humphry Clinker*. Tobias Smollett portrays the very milieu in which Graham had come to mingle, with some exemplary snapshots of the peculiarities of Bath's "entertainment". His principal character, the grouchy valetudinarian Matthew Bramble, despairs that Wood's vision has resulted only in "a monstrous jumble of heterogeneous principles; a vile mob of noise and impertinence, without decency or subordination". He is merciless about Bath's migratory visitors: "Knowing no other criterion of greatness, but the ostentation of wealth, they discharge their affluence without taste or conduct, through every channel of the most absurd extravagance; and all of them hurry to Bath, because here, without any further qualification, they can mingle with the princes and nobles of the land." His nephew Melford finds himself "...extremely diverted... to see the Master of the Ceremonies, leading, with great solemnity, to the upper end of the room, an antiquated Abigail, dressed in her lady's cast-clothes whom he (I suppose) mistook for some countess just arrived at the Bath... These follies, that move my uncle's spleen, excite my laughter."

It's clear why this city offered a doctor like Graham opportunities for "casual rencounter" far superior to those of London. "Taking the waters" either internally or externally was rarely a private affair. Bath social life was structured and often ruined by its visitors' tedious preoccupation with the details of their own health. When Graham turned up, conversation at Bath's public meeting places had probably not improved since the bluestocking queen Elizabeth Montagu had acidly described it to the Duchess of Portland some thirty years earlier:

The morning after I arrived I went to the Ladies' Coffee House, where I heard of nothing but the rheumatism in the shoulder, the sciatica in the hip, and the gout in the toe. I began to fancy myself in the hospital or infirmary, I never saw such an assembly of disorders... there is no place where one stands in greater need of something to enliven the brain and inspire the imagination. I hear every day of people's pumping their arms or legs for the rheumatism, but the pumping for wit is one of the hardest and most fruitless labours in the world. I should be glad to send you some news, but all the news of the place would be like the bills of mortality, palsy, four; gout, six; fever, one &c. We hear nothing

but Mr. such-a-one is not abroad today. Oh! no, says another, poor
gentleman, he died to-day… my party was made for quadrille to-
night, but one of the gentlemen has had a second stroke of the
palsy, and cannot come out; there is no depending upon people, no
body minds engagements.

As Smollett and Graham both observed, even those who arrived
at "that giddy vortex" in fine fettle were unlikely to remain so for
long. Quaffing in the pump room the scrofulous "scourings" of
other bathers, or inhaling at an assembly the mingled odours arising
from "putrid gums, imposthumated lungs, sour flatulencies, rank
armpits, sweating feet, running sores… hungary water, spirit of
lavender… and sal volatile" must have been testing for the strongest
of constitutions.

It is a melancholy assertion, but I believe a true one, that as many
persons who come here well, go away in a bad state of health, as
there are of diseased who receive a cure. The former is owing, in
[Graham's] opinion, to the constant racket of amusements and
dissipation; – to the crowds that are crammed up for many hours
every night, in over-heated rooms both public and private; – and
above all, to frequent and fatiguing dancing in that poisoned air.
Need I mention, moreover, the fatal effects of Tea, hot water,
&c. the ridiculous tight lacing of the women of the *Ton*; and the
enervating… exhausting indulgencies of both men and women of
fashion!

Showing the flair for inventive engineering that would later come into
play so spectacularly at the Temple of Health, Graham came up with
a novel proposal to deal with the foul air trapped in Bath's hot and
crowded ballrooms: "They ought to have had if possible, machinery
to have raised the roof and ceiling a dozen feet from the tops of the
walls…" He also threw himself provocatively into a controversy in
swing for some decades about the actual content of the city's spa
water. Graham fearlessly mocked "the ridiculous Manner of using
the celebrated and very salubrious Waters of Bath", taking issue with
the false "air of science" assumed by doctors devoted to laborious
bathing routines.

There were two obvious stars in the city's social firmament in the
mid-1770s, and Graham courted both with success. Opposite the new
Upper Assembly Rooms (a second "temple of sociability" which had

opened in 1771), Catharine Macaulay now presided over the equally recently built Alfred House. It remains the most elaborate façade in the terrace, its front door still marked by the bust of King Alfred – one of the heroes of eighteenth-century republicanism. Dr Thomas Wilson had moved to Alfred House on his retirement to Bath in 1772, the year his wife died. In October 1776, the same month that Graham himself returned to the city, Mrs Macaulay and her daughter moved in with Dr Wilson, to make use of both his library and his wealth.

Catharine Macaulay was no more short of like-minded admirers in Bath than she had been in London, though her republican views were always too controversial to exempt her from criticism in some quarters. She was said to have "made herself the centre of a little circle of politicians to whom she was accustomed to give lessons on general politics and English constitutional history". Alongside these tutorials, she held stylish private dinner parties where she enjoyed the adulation of Bath's more Whiggish inhabitants and visitors, Graham included.

Bath's other female celebrity could hardly have been more different from Macaulay, in either politics or abilities. Mrs Miller of Batheaston was an ambitious social climber with literary pretensions, who managed to accumulate a quite astonishing coterie in a very short time. Her talents were for partying rather than poetry. Mrs Miller and her husband had built an ostentatious new villa just outside Bath, shortly after their marriage in 1765. They then had to offset the extravagance of Batheaston with an extended and mind-expanding continental tour – travelling abroad was more economical than entertaining at home.

"Alas!" sighed Horace Walpole with heavy sarcasm when they came back in 1775, "Mrs Miller is returned a beauty, a genius, a Sappho, a tenth Muse…" Mrs Miller's ingenious plan to launch herself into tasteful society with a distinction money alone could never have achieved was a huge success. In London it provoked much ridicule. Into Bath's complex social programme she introduced a morning assembly which centred around an Olympian-style poetry contest. One element of this, the *bouts-rimés* (highly artificial six-line poems with preordained rhyme endings) was a society craze imported from seventeenth-century France. At Batheaston, verses on a set theme were dropped into an antique Roman urn recently dug up in Italy, the Millers' prize purchase during their grand tour. The poems were judged by the guests, and laurels awarded by "Mrs Calliope Miller", as Walpole renamed her.

The Vase poems, which were published from time to time as *Poetical Amusements from a Villa near Bath*, ostensibly to raise money for charity, frequently featured ingratiating portrayals of Mrs Miller, who appears endlessly as the "sprightly Laura" of "polish'd mind", "fair among the fair", with "taste refin'd, and classic sway". The novelist Fanny Burney, who visited Bath in 1780, declared herself "a faithful historian" and wrote in contrast: "Lady Miller is a round, plump, coarse-looking dame of about forty, and while all her aim is to appear an elegant woman of fashion, all her success is to seem an ordinary woman in very common life, with fine clothes on. Her manners are bustling, her air is mock-important, and her manners very inelegant."

But anyone able to attract "above fifty carriages drawn up in a line… and… four duchesses" at a single assembly was a worthwhile patient for James Graham. Within a month of beginning to practise at Bath, he elicited an approving letter from Anna Miller. Unfortunately it was about the vastly improved health of Mrs Miller's French maid, now back to fulfilling the "duties of her place", rather than the Queen of Batheaston herself. She only made use of Graham's medicines, and her ailments were hardly severe enough for their cure to be impressive.

From Mrs Macaulay Graham extracted a far more persuasive testimonial. It secured her role as chief patron of his social and professional ascent. Though an exceptional woman in most other ways, Macaulay was a typical Bath invalid. Throughout her life, letters arrived from her friends and family littered with anxious inquiries about her health, a preoccupation which she evidently shared. She regarded herself as having been born "with a very delicate constitution, and a weak system of nerves". Less typically, she had embarked on a strenuous writing project in "this very weak state of health", and ventured that this may have contributed to her symptoms: "I do not know whether it is not impertinent to add, that seven years severe application, reduced an originally tender frame to a state of insupportable weakness and debility; continual pains in the stomach, indigestion, trembling of the nerves, shivering fits, repeated pains in the ears and throat, kept my mind and body in continual agitation: and marked, those which would otherwise have been the brightest of my days, with sorrow and despair."

She was in one such fit of despair, Macaulay publicly informed Graham, when his pamphlet came to her hands.

Its contents awakened my curiosity; I sent for you; you undertook my cure with alacrity, and gave me the pleasing hope of a restoration of health, or rather a new state of constitution; and I have the happiness to declare, that a great part of my disease immediately gave way to your balsamic essences, and to your aerial, aetherial, magnetic and electric applications and influences; the pains in my ears and throat subsided, the fevers and irritations of my nerves left me, and my spirits were sufficiently invigorated to break from a confinement of six weeks, and to exercise in the open air.

Macaulay's letter was incorporated so quickly into a new edition of *A Short Inquiry* that it is impossible not to suspect collusion. An advertisement appeared announcing its inclusion in the book even before the date the letter was supposed to have been written. Like so many earlier newspaper plaudits, the testimonial echoes much of Graham's own phraseology. It seems remarkable from the pen of a professional writer, and particularly a woman who knew her own mind as well as Macaulay clearly did. This wholesale adoption of Graham's doctrines and forms of expression by such an independent thinker as Macaulay is very revealing. The "advertising doctor" clearly had an enormous talent for empathy, and a persuasive and sympathetic charm. He seems to have performed a role in patients' lives similar to that of some modern health gurus and complementary therapists. A large part of the power he exercised over his patients' bodies seemed to involve power over their minds.

He had certainly made himself indispensable to Macaulay and her circle. In January, her "friend" Dr Wilson found himself "cured" of troublesome and dangerous complaints – he had feared consumption – a cure which he made public a year later. Another highly respectable member of this social group, also recently settled in Bath, was Edmund Rack, a founder member of the city's Agricultural and Philosophical Societies. He was delighted with Graham's treatments, addressed his letter to his "good friend" and described Wilson as "a living monument of [the physician's] skill and success". Less than six months after Graham's arrival, instead of leaving Bath, as he had originally intended, he exchanged his lodgings near the Cross Bath for larger apartments in an elegant new terrace close to the popular Spring Gardens. Here he expanded his practice and apparatus so that "a much greater number of patients [might] partake of the inestimable blessings of his new discoveries and peculiar art".

What exactly did this mean? When he opened the Temple of Health in London, Graham's extraordinarily elaborate apparatus became the focus of the spectacle into which his medical practice had developed. Equally elaborate written descriptions of every aspect of his equipment's appearance also made him money. At this point though, he seemed wary of giving too much away. He tended to play up his own role in administering his treatments. In the wrong hands, he claimed, his methods might be useless or dangerous. So he revealed very few details of what it actually involved, preferring simply to repeat enticing adjectives such as "rational", "speedy", "elegant" and "certain".

But for all the evasiveness in his publicity, it is not too difficult to build up a picture of what went on in the South Parade consulting room. Over the previous decades, electrotherapists throughout Europe and the American colonies had been gradually standardizing many of their techniques. When he eventually installed his American-built "curious machine" in the Temple of Health, Graham wrote that it was "for throwing by the force of electricity, aetherial essences, vivifying air, and the magnetic effluvium through the whole body or into any particular part of it – especially the glands, limbs, joints, &c we would wish to confine their action upon".

The contraptions of Edward Nairne give a good sense of the scope and scale of this kind of apparatus. Nairne was a distinguished instrument-maker who collaborated with the likes of Benjamin Franklin, Joseph Priestley and Henry Cavendish. As well as taking on individual commissions, he had been steadily increasing the size, power and functions of commercially available electricity apparatus. Dismembered limbs float eerily on the pages of Nairne's illustrations of these patented machines – here a waving hand, beautifully laced at the cuff, there a neatly stockinged calf with buckled shoe – clasped by spidery robotic arms in a lightning-fingered embrace. He designed accessories which could draw visible sparks from a particular part of the body, giving the sensation of an "electric wind" at the afflicted area. Multiply jointed metal sticks leading from the spinning cylindrical machine ended in small copper balls, which could be directed with great accuracy to any particular spot using long glass handles. Two of these used at once passed a "current of electric fluid" through the entire body. The machine Graham had designed for himself in America operated similarly, and took the form of a cross. "The prime conductor which is wreathed with gold and silver upon a metallic surface of tin foil, lies horizontally on a pillar of clear flint glass, and is perforated with openings, and furnished with hooks for attaching and fixing chains, tubes, conic electrical brushes, and other instruments for conveying and confining this action of the above mentioned powerful agents to the weak, obstructed, or diseased parts."

The Doctor seems to have also been submitting a system known as the "electric bath" to ever more sophisticated redesigns. This was a particularly popular treatment for "female" disorders, as well as what Graham termed "spasmodic, or paralytic affections of the nerves, fits, and lethargic complaints". "Electric bath" is perhaps a misleading term – though it must have seemed exquisitely appropriate when practised at a Spa town. No actual immersion took place. Instead the patient was insulated from the ground by specially designed furniture with glass legs, and then connected (usually by a wire or chain leading directly to their body) to a prime conductor, charged by the hand-cranking of the therapist or an assistant. In other words, this was a less risqué version of the electric bed with which Graham had been experimenting in Philadelphia.

The so-called "electric bath" generally provided fairly painless treatments, during which invalids experienced only the mildest electric shock if their doctor connected them to the electrical machine before charge had accumulated on the conductor. They probably felt some warmth, a subtle skin-crawling sensation, and sweated a bit more. Most visibly, their hair would usually stand thrillingly on end – an indisputable sign that *something* significant was happening. "It is well known to every one who knows any thing at all about electricity," wrote Graham in 1783, "that when a person is insulated, that is placed on a stool, chair, or platform, suspended by silk, or supported by glass, and the machine excited, all the solid fibres of the body are braced, and even every hair of his head that is not tied down or heavily plastered with pomatum, becomes in a moment erected, like the quill of a porcupine, or the bristle of a boar."

The Doctor was constantly looking for new ways to heighten the psychological effect of his treatments. Where most electrotherapists sat their patients down on a mere stool, Graham's were invited to ascend an electric throne. This stately piece of furniture was probably also equipped with artificial magnets (commercially available since the 1740s) which would have contributed little to the patients' sensations but added much to the glamour and drama of the treatment. It was around this time that Graham also began to consider the therapeutic possibilities of music. "What may not the divinely harmonious musical modulations and influences – with a lively imagination, perform?" This was an adventurous proposal in a period when most musical experiences demanded the presence of live musicians, but one he would develop further at the Temple of Health.

Graham's hints about treatments "ethereal" and "celestial" suggest a new direction. After his success with electricity and magnetism, he seems to have been at this moment mid-leap onto the bandwagon of another groundbreaking science, pneumatic chemistry. The new doctor in town had clearly come under the influence of Joseph Priestley's exciting discoveries about the composition of air. Earlier that century, the "flat-earth" theory of phlogiston had been devised, mistakenly thought to explain how things burn. When Priestley isolated oxygen in 1775, he called it "dephlogisticated air" because it allowed candles to burn in bell jars and mice to survive. Graham must have been inspired by Priestley's prescient comment: "Who can tell but that in time this pure air may become a fashionable article in luxury." Up to that point only the scientist himself and two rodents had "had the privilege of breathing it". Why not fill entire rooms with this "pure air", he suggested, or construct a laboratory which could generate it, pumping it into a room as fast as it could be produced? Priestley had felt his own breathing become "peculiarly light and easy": perhaps this air might even be able to extend life itself?

Ignoring Priestley's warnings that, just as a candle burned faster in oxygen, so might a human being, and neglecting the moralist's position that "the air which nature has provided for us is as good as we deserve", Dr Graham got to work. In Bath he became the precursor of those twentieth-century entrepreneurs whose portable scented oxygen bars started popping up in the 1990s in shopping malls, music festivals and nightclubs all over the developed world, charging for breathing by the minute. Their claims to reduce stress, increase alertness and help hangovers often read remarkably like Graham's own advertisements.

The Doctor was also making use of another recent innovation. He claimed credit for pioneering the healing properties of a volatile liquid then known as "vitriolic aether", now called diethyl ether. In the nineteenth century it launched an anaesthetic revolution. One pioneer from that later period, a Massachusetts doctor called Henry Bigelow who self-tested numerous potential anaesthetics, reported that inhaling relatively small doses of ether produced effects almost as exhilarating as nitrous oxide (laughing gas) or "the Egyptian haschish". It was small wonder then that Graham's patients were reporting "immediate relief" from their sufferings, and enjoying cures described as "memorable".

Graham must have had a lot more physical contact with his patients than the average physician of his day. Milk baths and "dry friction" (a kind of massage) were also part of his regimen. Like many natural philosophers, he probably believed that the electric "fluid" in the body was brought into a continual motion by the movements of the body. "Animal heat" was thought to be produced by blood rubbing against the walls of the blood vessels as it circulated, setting free "elementary fire" in the process. There were also theories that the amount of electricity contained within a human body was affected by exercise, and that electric fluid was produced by the friction of the limbs against particles of air.

Like his manner, Graham's procedures were intended to be soothing and relaxing. He always emphasized the gentleness of his methods: "genial" was a favourite adjective. Of course they were a welcome alternative to the agonies that accompanied most orthodox treatments. "My neck is now broiling and smarting with blisters, and literally speaking I have my part in the lake that burns with fires and brimstones," wrote an American woman in the early nineteenth century after having been blistered with cantharides. But, as later case notes make clear, Graham did not entirely depart from the central tenets of blistering, bloodletting and purging in which he had been trained: it would have been a brave move, which many patients would probably have resisted, so indoctrinated were they about the necessity for such treatments by the conventional wisdom of contemporary medical practice.

As well as making constant improvements to his equipment, and inviting consultations for ten hours a day, the indefatigable doctor somehow found time to compose poetry. Who but Graham himself could have penned the verses which appeared in the *Bath Chronicle* of 27th March, 'On reading Mrs Macaulay's Letter to Dr. Graham'? Who but Graham would have risked such a combination of sycophancy and self-congratulation? The poem, which Graham reprinted with great regularity in later publications, opens with an image of the Greek muse of History begging for help from the god Apollo. The muse is in inadvertently comic despair about the imminent death of her favourite on earth, Catharine Macaulay. No need to worry, replies the "indulgent God": Apollo has trained Graham to save the day:

Dear maid, let all thy tears be dry'd,
Cath'rine shall yet be thine;
Her hand shall reassume the quill
And bid the faithful record still
Along thy pages shine.
To stop the ravage of the foe,
My GRAHAM instantly shall go,
And set thy fav'rite free;
No more let sorrow fill thine eye,
On GRAHAM's skill secure rely,
For he was taught by me.

Essentially a vigorous promotion of both Graham and his esteemed patient, the poem also exposes the rivalry between the two doctors in Macaulay's life. To the fury of the parishioners, Wilson had recently made plans to put up a marble statue of Macaulay "in the character of history" in the London church of which he was the absent rector. He had even ordered a vault for her remains. (His wife's were already entombed there.) These, say the Muse, have provoked her fears about Macaulay's health:

Behold in yonder fane,
The marble tomb arise:
Alas! the monumental bust,
And tribute to her fame, though just,
Are horror to mine eyes!

But, as the poem smugly concludes, though Wilson might anticipate with pride his role as chief mourner, only Graham has the power to step in and whisk their shared idol from death's jaws.

Wilson had already made himself and Macaulay ridiculous by his fawning treatment of the historian. With a competitive eye on Batheaston, he had begun to refer to Alfred House as "our little Tusculum which is honoured with the visits of all the Literary Persons who frequent this place…" Wilson's reputation as an "obsequious courtier" had been established in his youth, thanks to his relentless "pursuit of preferment". George III was said to have sent a message to the minister after one of his more grossly flattering sermons to say that "he came to church to hear God praised, not himself". He never did reach the longed-for status of bishop, hence Walpole's reference to Wilson as "that dirty disappointed hunter of a mitre".

But Graham's aptitude for servility easily equalled Wilson's. Together they planned a party at Alfred House for Mrs Macaulay's forty-sixth birthday that would have disastrous consequences. The two doctors seem to have egged each other on to ever greater excess. To judge from the flair for showmanship which Graham was displaying a few years later, he would have been only too pleased to make the most of this occasion. Six gentlemen from a "numerous and brilliant company" delivered six ingratiating poems to their hostess, who was seated in "a conspicuous, elevated situation". Published the following month as *Six Odes, presented to That justly-celebrated Historian, Mrs. Catharine Macaulay* (1777), these poems present an occasion in itself so absurd that its straight-faced description has been mistakenly catalogued in the British Library as a satire.

On 2nd April, Wilson and Graham vied ostentatiously for attention. The *Bath Chronicle*, published by one of Wilson's cronies, eagerly provided a to-the-moment report: "The morning was ushered in by ringing the Abbey bells" (an honour it was well known anyone could pay for) "and we hear, a very elegant collation is prepared for the entertainment of many of the genteelest company in Bath this evening, who (we are just informed) are now met there, to wish the Lady many happy returns of this happy day, and health to carry on and complete her History… to the present times". Macaulay's twentieth-century biographer was so appalled by the folly of this occasion that she could barely bring herself to describe it. The disgust, mockery and dismay the birthday celebrations provoked in observers at the time was even greater. When news of it reached him in Devon, Toplady, one of Macaulay's oldest allies, referred to her "contemptible vanity". The scholarly polymath Elizabeth Carter wrote to Mrs Montagu, "Surely nothing ever equalled that farcical parade of foolery with which she suffered herself to be flattered, and almost worshipped by that poor wrong-headed firebrand of party." Satirists had a field day.

It was the kind of self-important behaviour the world could forgive and forget of a Mrs Miller, but not someone with the former prestige of Mrs Macaulay. The irony of this revered republican receiving her honours from what was in effect a throne was not lost. Neither did the mirroring of Macaulay's majestic position in her treatments on Graham's electromagnetic throne need underscoring. Punning humour was derived from Macaulay's twin obsessions – her own constitution, and that of her country – and Graham's extravagant claims regarding his own powers to affect the former.

After "the pious, learned, and patriotic Dr. WILSON" had advanced to bestow a "large and curious Gold Medal" on the historian, Graham himself presented her with a copy of the latest edition of his book, *The General State of Medical and Chirurgical Practice*, apparently "with great modesty and diffidence" now dedicated to Macaulay. He took the opportunity to remind the world (already "pouring out Thanks to him from every Quarter") of "the valuable Discoveries and Improvements which he has made in the Cure of Diseases". Attending Macaulay, he declared at the party and in the preface, was "the happiest and most honourable incident" of his life. Two of the six odes were almost as flattering to Graham as they were to Macaulay. One was the poem already published in the *Bath Chronicle*. The other, 'A Vision', was written by someone very familiar with Graham's prose and practices (the italics and footnote are the poet's):

Yet let not Graham unnotic'd pass away,
Who, in her health, adds lustre to the day;
Who, to the noon of aeth'ral knowledge run
Its influence pours, diffusive like the sun
To *all* its *subtle*, *genial* heat displays,
Within the circle of its *fluid* rays;*

[*A philosophical, tho' figurative, disquisition of the qualities of Æther.]

But this extraordinary evening did not end there. "They then dispersed into different elegantly furnished apartments, which were finely illuminated on the occasion, and entertained themselves with dancing, cards, and conversation, 'till nine o'clock; when the doors of another apartment were thrown open, in which side-boards were ranged round, and covered in a sumptuous manner, with syllabubs, jellies, creams, ices, wines, cakes, and a variety of dry and fresh fruits, particularly grapes and pine-apples."

"The pleasures of Bath indeed!" one of the partygoers, Richard Graves, had written four years earlier in his comic novel, *The Spiritual Quixote*. "…It is a tedious circle of unmeaning hurry, anxiety and fatigue: of fancied enjoyments and real chagrins: today one is in vogue, and Lord knows why; tomorrow deserted, and equally without reason." Within days of the birthday celebrations, Graham's therapeutic claims came under attack in a letter in the *Bath Journal* of 7th April. Though this letter hasn't survived, Graham's extended response to it was published in a rival paper. His detractor is most likely to have been Matthew Turner, the Liverpool-based author of a practical sixteen-page pamphlet entitled *An Account of the Extraordinary Medicinal Fluid, called Aether* (1761).

Matthew Turner had reason to be angry with Graham. Turner had experimented carefully before starting to manufacture and sell the first commercially available solvent of ether for medical purposes over a decade previously. The Scottish doctor's boasts about his own originality must have been infuriating. It may even have been Turner's vivid descriptions of ether that had attracted Graham's attention to its potential in the first place: "It is the most light, most volatile, and most inflammable, of all known Liquids: It swims upon the highest rectified Spirit of Wine as Oil does upon Water, and flies away so quickly as hardly to wet a Hand it is dropped upon; from which Properties it probably has obtained it's Name. It is so readily inflammable, as to take Fire at the approach of a Candle, before the Flame touches it. Any Electrified Body will also produce the same Effect." Unlike Graham's publications, crammed with obscure references to "chemical essences" and "Aerial [and] *Aetherial... Vapours* and *Applications*", Turner's little book on ether was distinguished by unselfconscious clarity and modesty. Its instructions on exactly how the solvent could be used in different medical circumstances were helpfully detailed:

> To apply it Externally, you must procure a Bit of Linen Rag, of such a Dimension as to be conveniently covered by the Palm of the Hand; moisten this Rag with a little of the AETHER as it lies upon your Palm, and instantly apply it to the Part affected, pressing it very close, so as to prevent the Escape of its Fumes, for two or three Minutes, in which Time the Rag will be found dry, and may be taken away.

Ether was also open to abuse:

> This is the Secret of a present famous Practitioner, who having a Method sometimes of concealing his Application, is said to cure the Head-ach, fixed Rheumatic Pains, &c. by the Touch of his Hand.

Graham was obviously not this practitioner. In any case, he preferred the mystique of the natural philosopher to that of the faith healer.

But Turner's attack on Graham would undoubtedly have been clear and well argued. An experimental chemist and surgeon, Turner was also a dissenting theologian known for the rigour of his thought. (It was his lecture-demonstrations in Warrington which had provoked Joseph Priestley's initial interest in chemistry.) Two of his close friends were in Bath at around this time, either of whom could have alerted Turner to Graham's advertising activities. The innovative industrial potter Josiah Wedgwood had recently opened a West Country showroom there, while the artist Joseph Wright of Derby was attempting to emulate Gainsborough's success as a society portraitist in the city.

It took Graham a little while to muster his arguments against Matthew Turner's assault on his claims. Perhaps he turned to his friends at Alfred House for help. The scholarly wit of its opening gambit is slightly out of keeping with Graham's usual florid style, the casual classical references particularly sophisticated. Figuring himself as the "young and vigorous Neoptolemus", assailed by "the old and talkative Priam" in Virgil's *Aeneid*, Graham deliberately implies that he too is a killer of old kings, by implication those of the medical profession. Graham was so delighted with these paragraphs that he couldn't resist using the best of them again, almost word for word, when he came under attack in the Newcastle press in spring 1779. Of course Turner's letter gave Graham a perfect opportunity for further self-promotion. It would not be the last time Graham used the spotlight of public attack to his advantage. "The ingenious and ingenuous writer... hath said so much in my favour, and so very little to my disadvantage, that I cannot, with the public, suspect him for an enemy. No: I consider him as my friend..." Graham went on to agree wholeheartedly with Turner's (accurate) prophecy that were the effects of ether to be properly attended to, its medical importance would then be recognized. After the "charm" of its novelty had worn off, it had been neglected "till some practitioner of more genius and discernment than the bulk of his brethren", who refused to be lazily led along by "fashion and authority", managed "by dint of PATIENT THINKING" to secure for the world "an invaluable treasure".

He had a point, however immodestly expressed. But challenging the boundaries of medical convention at this time was a hazardous business. Deviations from the norm frequently led to charges of quackery. This was particularly true if medical innovation was accompanied by innovatory marketing techniques. Thanks to both, James Graham had become increasingly conspicuous during these months. His personal as well as his professional life were beginning to come under scrutiny.

Rumours had already started circulating about the nature of the relationship between Graham and Mrs Macaulay. When John Wilkes visited Bath in January 1778, he reported to his daughter Polly: "It is not only my opinion, but that of the generality of Mrs M—'s friends, that her head is affected, and some indiscretions with Dr. G— are the common topic of conversation." To divert Bath society from this kind of scandalous suggestion, Graham turned again to poetry. He was addicted to inserting anonymous panegyrics into provincial papers, their authorship betrayed only by his equally strong recycling habit. In May 1777, the *Bath Chronicle* published a remarkable poem entitled 'The Triumvirate', hailing Graham as the "great and good Benevolus":

> On his fair front, in mingled glory, sit,
> Sentiment, virtue, dignity, and peace.
> No frown severe, nor folly's sick'ning smile,
> Dwell in those eyes, where beauty reigns supreme,
> In beams of wisdom, eloquence, and love.
> Where is the ear, that, at his tuneful voice,
> Whose soft, harmonious chords, mellifluous strike,
> Thrills not with pleasure at the trembling sounds?

The point of this eulogy was not just to attract custom but also to remind the world of the utter respectability of this uxorious doctor. Enter Mrs Mary Graham, in one of very few printed references to her:

> Each female excellence and female charm,
> All that delight, and win the heart to love,
> Are her's; the native inmates of her breast.
> Happy, thrice happy he, who calls thee his!

And to dispel malicious gossip further, a footnote assures the paper's readers that the third figure of the poem is "a most amiable woman, a patient of the Doctor's" who, far from being a jealous rival, is said to be united to Mrs Graham by friendship and "sister-vows".

Dr Graham took himself off to Edinburgh that summer. On his return he sent Mrs Macaulay away from Bath. She was dispatched in late autumn "to the south of France, for the benefit of her health", according to her first biographer Mary Hays. Her travelling companion was James Graham's own sister, Mrs Elizabeth Arnold, who later provided Hays with most of her biographical material. Macaulay was very ill indeed at this point, arguably too ill to endure the discomforts that faced her. Both women wondered whether Macaulay would even survive the journey. Walpole's confidante, the former salon hostess Madame du Deffand, "a blind old lady of wit" to whom he had given Macaulay an introduction in early December, wrote of her alarm at the historian's spectral appearance when she met her in Paris. She was certainly not well enough to continue to Nice as originally planned, and instead remained in Paris for a few weeks (socializing with "persons of the first rank and eminence", such as Benjamin Franklin).

After her return, Wilkes spent the next few months writing maliciously gossipy letters to his daughter about his friends Dr Wilson and Mrs Macaulay. "I saw her yesterday looking very ill indeed… She was painted up to the eyes, and looks quite ghastly and ghostly." A few days later Wilkes reported that "The rage of politics is, I think, more violent at Bath than even at London, and nothing is talked of but America, except Kitty Macaulay, who grows worse daily". Whether he was referring to her health or behaviour is hard to determine.

As for Graham, his social and financial status continued to soar. He had moved to more exclusive premises in Bath's Queen's Square the previous November, and now lived just a few streets away from Alfred House. A few days after Mrs Macaulay's return from Paris in early January, he managed to extract a testimonial from Dr Wilson which all three must have hoped would help ward off gossip. (It declared that there had been no return of Wilson's previous symptoms since Graham's treatments twelve months earlier.) This was quickly included in the fourth, expanded edition of *The General State* published in February 1778. But before the month was out Graham had vanished to Edinburgh, announcing publicly that he had been called there by business.

He stayed until the end of September, during which time he seems to have built up a reasonably well-to-do Scottish practice from his house in the Old Town. Mrs Macaulay did her best to help him. She told the Earl of Buchan, an ardent political reformer and friend of Franklin, that Graham had rescued her from the very brink of the grave:

I do assure your Lordship that I look upon Dr Graham as a happy Genius in the medical line of knowledge and as such very cordially recommend him to your Lordship's notice and patronage in the extent of his practice at Edinburgh where he is now from a prediliction to his native country determined to fix. It is undoubtedly the interest of the public to encourage all men of science and abilities who will venture to step out of the hackneyed road of the medical practice by which thousands languish under the pressure of curable disorders and at length sink to the grave...

Most of the patients Graham treated in Edinburgh in 1778 are recorded anonymously in his own publications. They included friends of his "own worthy father and mother", as well as a young Walter Scott and an old Scottish aristocrat, Lord Hope, the Second Earl of Hopetoun. Scott, then aged seven or eight, had been lame since suffering from polio in very early childhood. It is a measure of the respectability Graham enjoyed at this time, despite Bath accusations of quackery from Philip Thicknesse, that he treated Scott at the recommendation of the boy's grandfather, Dr John Rutherford, the eminent University professor. "The celebrated Dr Graham was an empiric of some genius and great assurance", according to Scott. "In fact, he had a dash of madness in his composition. He had a fine electrical apparatus and used it with skill."

Years later the novelist recalled his uncomfortable experiences with Graham in a letter to Lady Louisa Stuart:

...[T]here was so much suspicion about the operator trying some violent experiment that some cousin or friend that had little better to do at the time generally attended on the very unpleasant hour I spent in Dr Grahams company. This was not without reason for the man was a daring experimentalist. He tried aether and... took an opportunity to pour a very caustick fluid on my limb which gave me excessive pain. Captain Swinton of Kimmerghame was my friendly guard he enterd at my cries and with much wrath for he was a fiery old soldier removd me from the persecution according to medicine.

In the same letter Scott described his encounters with his fellow patient, Lord Hope, a patron of the architect Robert Adam. Graham's treatment of the old man, who arrived in style in a coach-and-six with a running footman, to be decked with magnets by the Doctor till he looked like a Native American, made a strong impression on the sceptical child:

Sure am I, I never saw any thing so extraordinar[y]... he was hung round of strings of common loadstones from head to foot like so many belts and collars and the very weight must have been oppressive to the poor old man, for whom, child as I was, I felt a species of compassion & interest, the rather because he gave his fellow patient [i.e. Scott] sweet meats and I rather think a magnet... He was so bedizened that he was more like a Cherokee Chief than an English or Scottish nobleman. I had, being... a fine sprag boy, a shrewd idea that the magnetism was all humbug, but Dr Grahame, though he used a different method was as much admired in his day as any of the French fops.

James Graham's decision to remove himself from Bath was well judged. It did not remove him from the scandal which erupted later that year, from which Catharine Macaulay's wrecked reputation is only now recovering. The events were still glorious gossip even a full decade after they took place: a scurrilous pseudo-biography of the Whig politician Charles James Fox recorded the relationship between doctor and historian with relish: "As from previous engagements, no hope of a matrimonial union could take place between the *Emperor of Quacks* and the *Queen of Liberty*, she resolved however upon a family connexion at least; and like Queen Christina... she abdicated her throne, left her dignity and state with her excellent friend Dr Wilson, and retired to Leicester, in order to continue in a course of experimental philosophy with Dr. Graham's *younger brother*."

In late November, Catharine Macaulay married twenty-one-year-old William Graham. He had finished his own Edinburgh medical training and was working as a "surgeon's mate", a lowly position but a common career move for young surgeons lacking other opportunities to set up practice. When she wrote to tell her news to Dr Wilson, he was almost prostrated by shock and fury. He assumed it had been a very short courtship:

To the great surprise of the world, Mrs. Macaulay without giving me the slightest notice at the age of 52 [obviously a deliberate exaggeration since she had only turned forty-six the previous year] married a YOUNG SCOTCH LOON of 21 whom she had not seen for above a month before the fatal knot was tied. A mate to an East India Ship, without clothes to his back. She left this place the beginning of October on pretence of the health of her sister at

Leicester whose Husband keeps a mad house, and there she is like to remain for I will never let her come to Alfred House… It is a most beggarly family in Edinburgh. How are the mighty fallen!

Either she had lied to him about the reason for her visit, or Wilson had misunderstood her. It wasn't her own sister who lived in Leicester, but James Graham's. The "House for the reception of Insane Persons" was run by his old friend Thomas Arnold. (Graham often publicly recommended the institution, praising Arnold's gentle approach, but his brother-in-law does not seem to have returned the favour.)

Letters between friends and acquaintances dissecting the surprise marriage criss-crossed the country. Mrs Montagu thought Mrs Macaulay had exchanged Minerva for Venus – in other words, replaced wisdom by lustful love. Walpole referred to the "uncouth match", but commented forgivingly that "Sense may be led astray by the senses". "Poor Mrs. Macaulay!" wrote Edmund Rack to Richard Polwhele, a youthful fellow birthday-party poet who grew up into a vicious enemy of the bluestockings: "She is irrevocably fallen… Her passions, even at 52, were too strong for her reason; and she has taken to bed a stout brawny Scotchman of 21. For shame! Her enemies' triumph is now complete. Her friends can say nothing in her favour. O, poor Catherine! – never canst thou emerge from the abyss into which thou are fallen!" Even the future French revolutionary, Brissot, who met the couple a few years into their marriage and admired Macaulay's "republican energy", commented cruelly that it was like seeing a child attached to a corpse.

At Batheaston Villa in early January 1779, the winner of the Vase competition recited a relatively innocuous poem on the subject of "Winter Amusements", which referred simply to "Folly's vain delusive charms, And Passion's wild career". Instead of repeating it for an encore as requested, its author, Bath's best known satirist Christopher Anstey, whipped out a second manuscript and proceeded to recite verses about Macaulay, James Graham and Wilson, some apparently so lewd they were never printed. So reported Horace Walpole, who had once been much impressed by Anstey's risqué burlesque on the spa town's dissipated visitors, *The New Bath Guide*. Now he considered Anstey to have "tumbled from a greater height" than Macaulay. The sexual innuendo in the lines published in the *Bath Chronicle* on 7th January is clear enough, and Graham's own rhetoric and terminology are easily recognizable. The poet promises a recipe to prevent "Beauty's Decay":

By a sweet pretty Nostrum quite pleasant and new,
Which learn'd *Historians* and Doctors, I find,
Have lately reveal'd for the good of mankind.
A Nostrum like which, no elixir yet known,
E'er brac'd a lax'd fibre, and strengthened its tone.
Nor e'er was so grand a restorative seen,
For bringing back sixty – to lovely sixteen!

The "conjugal blessing" is decreed "the truest specific [i.e. medicine] for *Widows* indeed", and sexual experience with a younger man the ideal cure for ageing. An earlier article in a London scandal sheet made similar reference to the methods of James Graham's medical practice: "she could not resist the *magnetic Influences* of Dr. Graham's Brother…" The sexual prowess of Macaulay's various consorts were suggestively compared in a manner very familiar to any readers of contemporary erotica, accustomed to delight in the sexual resonances easily teased from the ongoing discoveries of natural philosophy.

The event was a source of public titillation for years. Disastrous for Macaulay, it did no end of good in raising Graham's public profile. The Doctor and his ethereal, magnetic and electrical powers were alluded to in a succession of wisecracking defamatory poems, pamphlets and even a Haymarket farce. Knowing very little of William Graham other than that he was young and handsome, satirists simply conflated him with his more famous brother. One print, "The auspicious marriage", shows a diminutive William, looking remarkably like James, leading Mrs Macaulay away from Alfred House. Dressed to the nines, and tottering towards the altar of Hymen, she casually treads underfoot the staff of liberty. Her books, quill and ink have been cast aside and the shamefaced statue of Hymen seems to be carrying an electrical conducting tube. Rumours about Macaulay's previous indiscretions with her "aerial doctor" were further fuel for these scandal-mongers, who lewdly insinuated a panderous role for James. One very vulgar poem, 'A Remarkable Moving Letter, which was Suggested by an Extraordinary Epistle Sent by Her on Her Second Marriage to Her Clerical Admirer' (1779), written in Macaulay's voice, makes no effort to distinguish between the Graham brothers:

When, from a Cloud prolific fancy drew
Astride my *Quarto* Volumes Cupid flew:

Gr–h–m was perch'd behind, and in his hand
A Portly Syringe stood, or seem'd to stand…

The poem ended with a promise to stuff Wilson's corpse into the
marble tomb in Walbrook he had prepared for Macaulay.

It was inspired by an actual letter, which John Wilkes described to
his daughter on 21st December 1778. "I was [at Alfred House] today,
and had a long conversation with the Doctor, who is outrageous, and
is thoroughly convinced *from facts* of the lady's former intimacy with
Dr —, and he thinks her a monster. He read me her *long* letter the day
of her marriage, as supposed just before celebration; it contains every
variety of style: it is indecent, insolent, mean, fawning, threatening,
coaxing, menacing and declamatory. Such words I believe never escaped
a female pen… his love seems turned to rage and hatred… I am treated
as the declared favourite." Wilkes was perfectly shameless in his hopes
of personal financial gain from Dr Wilson's abandonment.

Were it not for the intervention of well-meaning Edmund Rack,
we might now know every detail of what actually went on between
Macaulay, James Graham and his two siblings. Furious at Macaulay's
refusal to relinquish what he had once promised her (the deeds to
Alfred House and a £400 annuity after his death), Wilson threatened
revenge. Rack confided in his journal that Wilson had employed
Clement Cruttwell, a Bath newspaper publisher, "to write a narrative
of her Conduct relative to Dr Graham, in which some Letters would
have appeared that would have blasted her honour for ever. This
work was begun printing, & Advertisd. Her relations and Friends
were alarmd." They were right to be. The book's advertised title was
absolutely tantalizing:

*An authentic narrative of the conduct and behaviour of Mrs.
M—y [Macaulay], now M—y G—m during her residence at
A—d house, B—th; containing a succinct and faithful history of
the extraordinary means made use of by that lady to obtain such
a profusion of expensive gifts from her benevolent patron the Rev.
Dr. W—n. Her acquaintance with Dr James G—m, the famous electrical empiric and her behaviour from the commencement of that
connection, her intimacy and friendship for Mrs A. sister to that
empiric, her journey to Paris with occurrences there, her journey to
Leicester and her marriage with Mr. G, brother to Dr G and Mrs A
with all the original letters, notes, and anecdotes. To which will be
added a dissertation on swindling.*

Cruttwell, the anonymous author of this book, would benefit to the tune of £200 and a ring for this friendship "on a late trying occasion", according to Wilson's newly written will. Cruttwell visited gossipy Wilkes on 10th September 1779, and read out passages of a letter from Mrs Macaulay to Dr Graham, one of a damning set apparently saved from the flames by "a maid, Betty". Wilkes, the author in his Hell Fire Club days of a famously obscene parody of Pope's *Essay on Man*, piously judged its content "too gross for the public eye", which didn't stop him spreading it about. As well as the main protagonists, one of Macaulay's brothers, Mr Wanley Sawbridge, and Mrs Arnold too, were said to be "shown in the most odious colours".

Edmund Rack, a man who generally spent his days pondering whether or not Adam was born with a navel, considering the cultivation of carrots and attending Mr Herschel's "Experiments on Light", was drawn into the controversy by Catharine Macaulay's other brother. The radical politician John Sawbridge went to Bath in early January. Rack agreed to act as "an Arbitrator... & after sitting on it 7 Hours I at length determind, that in Consequence of Dr Wilsons giving Mrs Macaulay Eight hundred pounds, she should deliver up all the securities Dr Wilson had given Her; and the manuscript of the narative, with all the Letters and papers relative thereto, should be burnt in the presence of J Sawbridge Esq on or before the 25th of March next." Rack evidently thought he had done well for Wilson: "I am sure the Dr ought to give me 100 pound in his will for it is a very good bargain for him – the House alone being worth £1400; but I dont expect anything." He got nothing. Wilkes too had suffered the "*frequent* and *powerful* eructations from his holy entrails" at so many dinners in vain. The less than divine Wilson had left in legacies far more than he was worth and a year after his death in 1784, the will was put into Chancery.

Catharine Macaulay and William Graham went on to enjoy a long and happy marriage, and remaining letters testify to a good and enduring relationship between William and his new step-daughter.

Throughout these years, in public at least, James Graham was virtually silent on the matter. It was a great coup to have raised his public profile so triumphantly, yet with so little blemish to his own reputation. He rewarded Rack's domestic diplomacy by subscribing to an edition of his *Essays, Letters and Poems*, which came out in 1781. In Graham's own future publications, he only expressed the greatest of pride in the family connection with the woman he still compared fawningly with the Russian empress. He seems to have continued to wear around his neck a miniature of his former patient, said to have been given him by the historian herself. The Macaulay affair had done its work. Graham was left forever stamped with a reputation for rejuvenating the sexuality of older women. His place in the public eye was secure, his ambitions only expanded. Now it was down to the electric empiric to capitalize on his new-found fame.

Barely a week after the wedding Dr James Graham replied to an advertisement placed in a London newspaper by a company of eminent Scottish architects: "To be Sold, or Lett for any Term of Years, A House, pleasantly situated in the Terrace, Adelphi, late in the occupation of the Mess. Adams. The House is fitted up with a Number of useful and convenient Fixtures, which may be had at a fair Valuation." The future proprietor of the Temple of Health had found its perfect setting. The house's fixtures would soon become considerably more glamorous.

4

The Speculators

D eign to accept the tribute which I owe,
O ne grateful – joyful tear permit to flow;
C an I be silent when good health is given?
T hat first – that best – that richest gift of Heaven!
O Muse descend! in most exalted lays,
R eplete with softest notes, attune his praise.
G en'rous by nature, matchless in thy skill!
R ich in the Godlike Art – to ease, – to heal;
A LL bless thy gifts! – the sick – the lame – the blind
H ail thee with rapture for the cure they find!
A rm'd by the DEITY with pow'r divine,
M ortals revere HIS attributes in *thine*!

The nasal drone of bagpipes drifted across the Thames when the building of James Graham's new house began. At daybreak, the sound insinuated its rhythms into the oozing mudflats on the river bend, and penetrated the sooty constructions of house martins nesting in the eaves of the Strand's shops. The insistent beat of reels, jigs and strathspeys organized the daily ring of pick on stone and shovel in soil as rubble came down and the bases of arching brickwork walls appeared. Perhaps the occasional prostitute, a Covent Garden lady still at work in the small hours of the morning, unexpectedly found a new tempo to her labours.

The pipers had been hired to spur on the efforts of several hundred cut-price Scottish labourers imported by the Adam brothers to realize their ingenious transformation of London's river frontage. John, Robert, James and William were the sons of the architect who had designed Edinburgh's Royal Infirmary. The three eldest followed in their father's professional footsteps, and formed a family firm. The youngest was their business manager. Robert was the creative genius of the family. His architectural vision was daring, his speculative approach no less so. Instead of taking a commission to design or remodel a single property from some suitably wealthy individual,

Adam decided to publicize his architectural skills by building a brilliant new private palace on the waterfront. It was called the Adelphi. (*Adelphoi* is Greek for brothers.) Anyone with enough money could buy an exclusive lifestyle of predetermined taste and luxury. London had never seen speculative building on this scale before.

When the Adam brothers embarked on the Adelphi scheme, they were gambling with their reputations and their money alike. Both barely survived. By the time Graham came to view the house where James and Robert themselves had lived in a kind of show home – it was one of a central pair in the grandest terrace – the difficulties that had dogged its building were a thing of the past. London had more or less forgotten the various debacles over unsecured leases, disputes over landownership, and workforce walkouts that had threatened the Adam family fortunes during the previous decade. William Adam & Co. had just about managed to ride the 1772 credit crisis (auctioning off collections of old masters and antiquities), and had staved off bankruptcy with a national lottery whose prizes ranged from Poussin paintings to property leases. (This was yet another source of controversy, since it was the second time a special Act of Parliament had saved the Adam brothers' skins.) Britain was enjoying fiscal confidence once more – the nation was thriving as a precarious "Paperwealth". Circulation of money was widely viewed as essential for a successful economy, so credit flourished, unhindered by the Government. Everything seemed possible, and anything worth the risk.

For those who needed to borrow, there were more or less scrupulous ways of doing so, and speculation could take many forms. There was often a fine line between so-called "Insurance" and out-and-out gambling. Increasingly complex trading schemes on the popular national lottery were vigorously promoted in the press by the likes of "Messrs Hazard & Co", or "Mess. Richardson and Goodluck". Meanwhile upper-class gamers were having the time of their lives. At Brooks's, White's and other gentlemen's clubs, addicted members set new records for fortunes won and lost overnight. Their wives and mistresses wagered almost as wildly at cards in their drawing rooms. The Bath satirist Christopher Anstey expressed the national mood succinctly:

Whate'er the wretched basedly dare
From pride, ambition, or despair,

Fraud, luxury or dissipation,
Assumes the name of – Speculation.

All in all, there was a climate of acceptability for financial risk-taking on a grand scale which allowed Graham to feel supremely confident about the extravagant plans he was making for his next venture. When Robert Adam had come to London twenty-odd years earlier, fresh from an Italian tour, he had deliberately put on "a face of brass", and set himself the task of seducing polite society. He trudged "doggedly from one nobleman's ante-room to another", as he confessed, trying to impress prospective clients. Adam spared no effort "to blind the world by dazzling their eyesight with vain pomp", finding himself the prettiest horses and most glamorous carriage, to attract true wealth with the appearance of wealth. Now the electric doctor planned to use the same tactics. When he inspected the Royal Terrace property for the first time, its potential as a venue for his Temple of Health must have struck him like a vision.

The Adelphi had already easily earned its place on the rounds of visiting tourists. "The extreme depth of the foundations, the massy piers of brickwork, and the spacious subterranean vaults and arcades, excited the wonder of the ignorant and the applause of the skilful," gushed watercolourist Thomas Malton the younger. Graham later enthused in print about the views from the raised Terrace, "at least a hundred feet from the surface of the river… London, that queen of Cities! lengthening herself, disappears from the incapacious and astonished eye." Looking to the right of the river bend over which the Adelphi looked, Graham and his visitors could admire Westminster Abbey, Westminster Bridge and the Surrey hills. To the left were Blackfriars Bridge and St Paul's Cathedral. By the time the Temple of Health actually opened, Somerset House had been built by the architect William Chambers, to general applause. Instead of urban sprawl, the view across the Thames offered a pastoral panorama dotted with windmills. South London barely existed at this point, though it was edging rapidly away from the river. "[E]very spectator must be struck with the beautiful variety of the prospects in every direction", enthused Malton. "Each of these views is so grand, so rich, and so various, that it is difficult to determine which deserves the preference."

When the Adam brothers had begun work, the site proved even more of a challenge than it first appeared. Steeply sloping and falling erratically from the Strand to the river, the area's tendency to flood at high tide often left it reeking and filthy. Sweeping away semi-abandoned ruins, Adam had constructed the Thames's most elegant embankment. Above this artificial escarpment, four hundred soaring feet of arcades, a magnificent residential development now stood. Its unifying façade, pale yellow new stock brickwork and exquisite white stucco ornament gleaming, could almost persuade onlookers that they were admiring a single stately mansion. The daily business of the working wharves was fed discreetly under the terrace through subterranean streets, and into a surprisingly capacious series of warehouses, stables and underground vaults concealed behind the water-level arcades. The Adam brothers' elegant disguises provoked the barbed comments of the odd dissenter to the general adulation. "What are the Adelphi buildings?" asked Walpole. "Warehouses laced down the seams, like a soldier's trull in a regimental old coat." But for most onlookers, military prostitutes were the last images that came to mind. Both "above & Below Ground", the "noble pile" was widely considered "fit to Entertain princes".

Luxury and modernity arrived at the Adelphi hand in hand. The Adam brothers boasted of the water laid on from top to bottom, and lightning conductors installed to support fire protection "much beyond... any other houses in London". They had built a water tower connected to the river, with pipes designed to keep three fire engines constantly supplied "upon a minutes notice", and added fire escapes to the connecting roofs of the houses. The imposing central block, the Royal Terrace (sometimes called Adelphi Terrace) seems to have been the first known use of that now familiar term for a uniform row of houses. The development was also one of the earliest London districts to have street numbers.

When Graham was being shown around the future Temple of Health, he no doubt kept half an ear open for the well-known tones of his new neighbour, David Garrick (and perhaps heard the yapping of his wife's little dog Biddy). The actor-impresario, next door at number five, had been one of the first to sign an Adelphi lease. An old friend of the Adam brothers, he took this house right in the middle of the Royal Terrace even before it was finished, an encouraging move which buoyed the brothers' hopes for the success of their scheme. A more fashionable or socially successful tenant could hardly have been imagined. Thanks to his efforts, the entire nation had become captivated by the glamour of the London theatre world, and Shakespeare had begun his posthumous transformation from playwright to "industry". When Garrick went abroad for a spell, his absence was said to have been mourned "as a national calamity". When he moved into the Adelphi and cartloads of Chippendale furniture began to arrive, Dr Johnson remarked that he now lived "as a prince rather than as an actor".

Garrick was at the heart of a vibrant coterie of eighteenth-century glitterati, his house one of their regular gathering places. After dinner with the Garricks at the Adelphi one night in 1776, a young Hannah More wrote home to her family that she had "seldom heard so much wit, under the banner of so much decorum". Many of Garrick's circle were in the "Club" originally set up by Joshua Reynolds for the intellectual entertainment of the actor's old Lichfield companion, Samuel Johnson. Membership spanned the overlapping worlds of politics, theatre, history and science, and included Richard Brinsley Sheridan, Charles James Fox, Edmund Burke, Edward Gibbon, Joseph Banks, Adam Smith and Earl Spencer. One fellow member, Topham Beauclerk, a brilliant though lice-infested conversationalist – the illegitimate great-grandson of Nell Gwyn and Charles II – did indeed end up as an Adelphi neighbour. Many others were frequent visitors.

Garrick was certainly responsible for ensuring the close proximity of his favourite bookseller and publisher, Thomas Becket, at the north-east corner of Adam Street and the Strand. "My dear Adelphi", Garrick wrote to Robert and James in 1772, "We shall all break our hearts if [Becket] is not bookseller to the Adelphi and has not the corner house that is to be built... if you can make us happy by suiting all our conveniences we shall make his shop... the rendezvous of the first people in England." By 1780, Mr Becket was printing and selling James Graham's misleadingly named promotion for his grand œuvre, *A Sketch: or, Short Description of Dr Graham's Medical Apparatus... in his house on the Royal Terrace, Adelphi, London*. It ran to 92 pages, and described virtually every candlestick on the premises.

From his description in this long pamphlet, it is easy to imagine Graham's first admiring glances at the double rows of lamps and elegant railings of the Royal Terrace. He must have been delighted to see that the "stately and highly ornamented pilasters" running up the façade already gave number four an appropriately "temple-like appearance". He would then have stepped straight from the narrow pavement into a groin-vaulted passageway, his mind's eye perhaps already decorating its ceilings and doorframes with discarded spectacles, crutches and hearing trumpets collected from successfully cured patients. A grand and pillared entrance hall led towards a generously proportioned stone staircase which wound its way both upwards and downwards. Light poured into the hall from the conical glass dome in the roof. For London, the Adelphi was an enterprising departure in layout. There was obviously no possibility of gardens on the artificial stage on which the densely built streets were constructed. The tall buildings of the Royal Terrace – four stories above street level and two below – relied on light and ventilation shafts from above and from the long narrow internal court between the backs of the Terrace and John Street behind. The arrangements of rooms and discreet passageways would allow entrances and exits to suites of rooms over several stories. The accessibility of water in the development was a further selling point, and there were water closets galore. Graham's neighbour Garrick had generous laundries on the topmost floor, but the Doctor converted these into extensive bathing facilities. "On the sixth or attic story, besides lodging rooms, there is a large reservoir or cistern of very fine water, connected with large boilers, and commodious baths, cold or warm, simple or medicated, of various sizes, for children as well as for grown persons."

Between the main floors of the house and the endless vaults, warehouses and stables below and beyond ("to which the subterranean gloom gives a considerable degree of sublimity") was a double basement. This would become Graham's "elaboratory", where "chemical essences" and "simple or galenical medicine" were said to be prepared under his supervision. In these gloomy depths his apothecary, his "chemical operator" and their various assistants would also live, packed away in a series of small rooms along with his medicines, able to come and go by their own entrance.

As Graham continued his tour of the Adelphi house, each element of Robert Adam's design spoke to his heart and business mind alike. From top to bottom, from detail to ground plan, he had found the perfect framework for his new Temple of Health, just waiting to be transformed into an extravaganza of health and natural philosophy. Looking up, the Doctor was entranced by ceilings that had been inspired by those of ancient Rome and were now the cutting edge of contemporary style. Strong panels of colour, dominated by sorbet pink and pistachio green, were intersected by geometrical patterns of delicate low-relief ornament, and set off by circular or oval panels with mythological figurative scenes. These were painted by well-known artists such as the Italian Antonio Zucchi. "I shall just mention... a pastoral representation of the three graces, in the most charming attitudes, with a cupid reclined under a tree, playing on a flute, with his bow on the ground, and his quiver and arrows hanging on a bough of the tree," boasted Graham, in ecstasies about his "supremely elegant" new ceilings. He was in good company. The bluestocking Elizabeth Montagu was just as thrilled about work done by Robert Adam at her house in Hill Street in 1767: "he has made me a ceiling and chimney piece, and doors, which are pretty enough to make me a thousand enemies; Envy turns livid at the first glimpse of them."

Virtually every interior surface was carved and ornamented in a manner which combined richness and delicacy that, to most people's taste, impressed rather than overpowered. Moulded friezes, architraves, cornices and door frames, even the carpets, continued and unified the neoclassical decorative schemes. On the first storey, in the room which would house the actual Temple of Apollo, ceiling-to-floor windows opened out onto cast-iron balconies overlooking the river, another groundbreaking feature of Adam's work.

Graham would be quick to reinterpret Adam's colour schemes in the light of favourable symbolic meanings, and then adapt to them the draperies and upholstery of the immense series of glass-legged thrones and banquettes that formed part of his medical apparatus: "The hangings, &c. of the room, are composed of a delicate green, rose colour, and pure white: denoting innocence, purity, hope, temperance, and the blooming ardour of good health... The temple is painted light green, because that is most agreeable to weak eyes; and because it is the emblematical colour of hope, and of the reviving spring." Graham also capitalized on the abundance of gold already in the rooms. He would announce sanctimoniously in his publicity material that "pure gold is absolutely incorruptible".

The ubiquitous "elegantly gilt festoons of flowers of almost every kind" that hung about the mirrors and mantelpieces were eventually echoed in tones of gold leaf on every other suitable surface, including the electrical equipment; the circular rings from which these artificial garlands hung were decoded by the Doctor as "symbols of perpetuity" and further embellished with decorative "professional devices", presumably the tools of a doctor's trade. Graham incorporated the floral theme into the very apparatus itself. Electricity-conveying chains which ran down from the huge central column of an electric and magnetic throne in the Great Apollo chamber, (a storey above the terrace level) would soon be covered with "the richest and most beautiful artificial flowers". They decorated a temple within a temple. In the same room, and connected from dome to dome with highly polished brass rods, he installed a treatment centre for one. This glass-legged metal-lined capsule, which Graham called a "curious little edifice... the first of its kind that was ever seen", was entered through a Gothic arched doorway from which sprang a "most magnificent volume of foliage, exquisitely carved and richly gilt". When he came to describe the extraordinary contents of these apartments, Graham reassured the public that "Sufficient support and security [was] afforded to this astonishing apparatus by means of the substantial walls and stately columns in the great hall, and rooms below."

Of course Graham was eyeing up the Adelphi house not just as a doctor, but as a performer and a theatrical manager. Music was a vital element of a good show, and when his first utterance rang clearly through the house, rising up to the double-height gallery-like landing two storeys above, the Doctor must have had one of those "Eureka!" moments. The Doctor had been using music therapeutically, "to alter the tone of [a patient's] mind", for several years. He believed it made them more receptive to other treatments. Here was the perfect spot for the musicians he already regularly employed. Graham would install up here "a large, fine toned organ, with the usual variety of stops", whose tones would bounce off the hard planes and angles of the stairway and resound around the glass and plaster in every room of the house. There was nothing to "deaden or obstruct the sounds; for the sonorous metal balustrades, the polished mahogany rails, and the stuccoed walls painted in oil, undulate[d] and reverberate[d] the sounds in the clearest, sweetest, and most distinct manner". Beside the organ there would still be plenty of room for an accompanying "band of medical music", consisting of "a couple of clarionettes, a couple of mellifluous German flutes, and one of the sweetest female voices in England".

James Graham was prescribing music in the middle of a remarkably inventive period of instrument-making. The fashionable musical aesthetics of the late eighteenth century demanded ever more expressive powers and effects, as drama had become an increasingly important element of performance. The new instruments invented to provide this emotional variety were often short-lived affairs, their practicality undermined by their complexity. There were hurdy-gurdy type keyboards, with strings "bowed" by the action of revolving discs, extended harpsichords for duets, mechanical attachments so that various instruments could be played automatically, early pianos, and cross-breeds of all kinds. The undisputed mechanical genius John Joseph Merlin was developing an one-person orchestra known either as the "Celestial" or "Vocal" harp. It actually sounded "as if all the instruments were invisibly emerging from it", according to Sophie von La Roche, a German tourist who inspected it in 1786. "The work and labour expended on this achievement call for respect, although I should consider my self unfortunate if I had to listen to it daily!"

Another ethereal sounding new instrument, the Glass Harmonica – also known as an angelic organ – drew Dr Graham to its otherworldly tones. Its eerie humming moan will be familiar to anyone who has ever rubbed the rim of a wineglass with a wet finger. In the hands of a practised musician the purity of its tones is haunting, thrilling and inexplicably moving. An update on the "musical glasses", the glass harmonica was yet another of Benjamin Franklin's innovations. Marie-Antoinette's music teacher Gluck used to play on glasses filled with water to different levels standing on a table. Franklin's approach was much more sophisticated. He had glasses blown in different diameters, and fitted sideways, chromatically, one inside the other, each slightly separate, but connected through the centre by a horizontal rod rotated by a foot pedal. A rain-soaked sponge gave enough moisture to sustain a player twice through Handel's *Water Music*, while a handy teacup of powdered chalk helped draw out the smoothest tones from the fingertips – "incomparably sweet beyond those of any other". Thomas Jefferson was so entranced by the sound of the Glass Harmonica he declared it "the greatest gift offered to the musical world of this century". Mozart and both C.P.E. and J.S. Bach were among many who composed for it. Others were horrified by the intensity of the instrument's effects. "Its melancholy tone plunges you into dejection… to a point the strongest man could not hear it for an hour without fainting," wrote one. Another strongly recommended avoiding playing the Harmonica if you were suffering from disturbed nerves, or disappointed in love. It would have made an astonishing impression in the acoustics of the Royal Terrace.

"Were I to have the misfortune to be bit by a mad dog… I would think very lightly of the affair, but would order the musical airs I love and admire most to be sung or played almost night and day for several days, or perhaps weeks." Graham had "thought it proper… to fling together" some ideas for a *Treatise on Medical Music* in the first edition of *The General State* in 1778. The Treatise itself, like all the Doctor's most ambitious projected publications, never actually appeared. But this rambling assortment of contemporary and ancient anecdotes and citations is particularly useful as one of the clearest articulations of Graham's understanding of psychosomatic symptoms. "Can there be anything more incontestably true, than that care and anxiety, disappointment in what we have ardently wished for, and loss of what we have affectionately loved, by preying on the mind, and engrossing all its attention, will disorder the whole frame of the body, and become the source of both chronic and acute complaints?"

Graham enlisted a number of doctors using music in their treatments to promote his cause. Dr John Leake, obstetrician and keen admirer of Shakespeare, Milton and Pope, was convinced that there was a logical explanation at work, that it wasn't just a kind of faith-healing. "THE SALUTARY POWER OF MUSIC AND ITS MANNER OF OPERATING ON THE BODY AND MIND, DEPENDS AS MUCH UPON RATIONAL, AND DEMONSTRATIVE PRINCIPLES, AS THOSE OF ANY MEDICINE in the *Materia Medica*," Graham raucously capitalized as he quoted. He believed, like Leake, that music worked so well because it excited "an agreeable sensation on the nerves of the ear", which in turn communicated with the brain, and thus the "general nervous system". This integrated view of the nervous system as a framework of interacting sensibilities, uniting and controlling the whole body, was an essential characteristic of the theory of vitalism Graham absorbed in Edinburgh in his youth. Unlike most conventional physicians, who were perfectly content to allow a shift from a mechanistic to a vitalistic understanding of the body to take place with little or no change to clinical practice, Graham was constantly alert for alternative therapies that would put to use this theoretical realignment.

Graham described music acting on him "just as a smith's great bellows does upon his fire; it enlarges, melts, and brightens every faculty of my soul, and very emotion of my heart, – with the most delightful and most intense fervour". For him, the moment at which the mind is taken out of the body, the action of being "transported" or "ravished" by sensory experience, is the point at which the corporeal shell can be physically healed. In Graham's vitalistic and visionary universe, this sublime moment seems to be related to electricity, because both are somehow equivalent to his Christian version of the Promethean flame, the source of his healing. Electricity is "the universal living fire which connects and moves the whole solar system... and which you, my courteous reader – this book, and the chair you sit in, the charming object by your side, and everything in the universe is full of… It is the breath of life – the spirit of God! – which he breathed at the creation into man's nostrils, and which gives and maintains life throughout all his other works!"

Like many of his books, *The General State of Medical and Chirurgical Practice* contains some extraordinary digressions, often extending to page after page, which swoop the reader away from the bedsides of suppurating or sore-ridden patients into the heart of Graham's emotional life. To follow his exuberant, spiralling prose is to be rewarded with glimpses of a man constantly swept away by the beauty of the world: striding out at dawn, gazing up at the noonday sun, or moved by an inspirational musical performance. He was led frequently into extended and animated asides. He regularly achieved sublimity with ease.

It is impossible to escape the conclusion that when he conceived the Temple of Health, making music an integral part of the medical process, he was indulging his own imagination just as much as he was consciously manipulating the imaginations of his patients and clients. At least equal to his desire for recognition and financial reward was this urge to share with others the kind of passionate experiences which propelled him through life.

This passion for the sublime even came into play as he assembled the scientific apparatus he needed for the new venture. He was looking for the biggest and the best. But, unusually, he was also seeking beauty.

With a property of the Adelphi's grandeur waiting to be filled, it was just as well that not all of his electrical equipment had to be built from scratch. He had already amassed a certain amount, and brought some apparatuses back from America. As with his publishing ventures, his gift for recycling came swiftly into play. Through the 1770s and '80s, electricians in the vanguard of their field were busying themselves with plates, drums and cylinders, experimenting with more effective designs and materials, and marshalling shellac, mercury, taffeta, cat fur and velvet ribbons in their efforts to increase the effectiveness of their generators. In the main, relations were cooperative rather than competitive. But in 1778 some locked horns in a surprisingly stormy argument about points and knobs. Which shape made the best lightning conductors?

The dispute was largely due to the stubbornness of a respectable if obsessive electrical researcher called Benjamin Wilson, a Yorkshire-born portrait painter whose past patrons included David Garrick and the Marquess of Rockingham. Matters came to a head after

Wilson clashed with Benjamin Franklin and other fellow members of a Royal Society committee appointed to design a suitable system to protect the nation's gunpowder stores at Purfleet, Essex. Here lightning damage had already proved disastrous more than once. Wilson was so determined to demonstrate the superiority of round-ended over pointed lightning rods that he staged a grandiose display to support his argument. The encouraging presence of King George III, well known to be "always disposed to promote every pursuit which tends to the advancement of science and the good of the public", seemed a guarantee of success. Wilson's plan was to "have a scene represented by art, as nearly as might be similar to that which was so lately exhibited at Purfleet by nature".

Representing nature by art was a favourite occupation of artistic scientists. Graham too would soon be drawing crowds to the Adelphi with his claims of Godlike mastery over the elements:

...while I can literally and visibly draw down into the room confining, rendering not only harmless, but even very salutary, the lightning from the clouds of heaven – while I can concentrate the beams of the sun; squeezing the various kinds of air into close prisons, separating, combining, gently dismissing or expelling them with tremendous violence – so likewise, I can exhibit the exact appearance of the forked lightning, and imitate with my machinery the horrible – the awful noise of the thunder storm, so tremendously loud, that if fifty drums were beat at the same time in the room, they could be no more heard than if a bag of wool was struck with a feather, and it is equally well known, that I can here not only equal, but even far exceed, with the electrical fire, &c. the beauty and the brilliance of any – even of the most glorious luminaries of heaven! – and this vivifying elementary LIGHT, with which every thing that we are acquainted with in nature is full, like THAT of WISDOM as described in the sacred writings, never – NEVER GOETH OUT.

Wilson's show for the King and the Royal Society was essentially a hugely magnified version of the old thunder-house demonstrations invented by Kinnersley. To produce enough charge to represent the cloud passing overhead the painter-philosopher built a truly gigantic prime conductor which hung by strong silk ropes about five feet from the floor. Running to about 155 feet, and more than a foot in diameter, it was so long that it had to be arranged in a horseshoe shape. Most of this snaking beast was made from 100 drum rims attached with wooden slats and covered with a huge quantity of tin foil to make it conductive. A simulated thundercloud ("as it is vulgarly called") of these vast proportions clearly could not be made to move over a miniaturized armoury. Wilson disposed of this difficulty in just the way George Lucas did when filming the opening of *Star Wars* exactly two hundred years later, moving the camera rather than the spaceship: the wooden scale model of the Purfleet building was designed to run on wheels along a raised track underneath the cloud to introduce the necessary variables for the extravagant experiment. Nearly seven thousand feet of wire spiralled above to increase the electricity in the atmosphere.

Only one building in London was huge enough to house all this. The Pantheon on Oxford Street had been finished five years previously, to the general delight of "the polite world". A young architect, Robert Wyatt, had designed a classical interpretation of the vast dome of the Byzantine Hagia Sophia in Constantinople. Its specific purpose was to provide winter accommodation for the spirited society crowds which in summer months thronged to assemblies, concerts and ridottos at Ranelagh or Vauxhall. When the Pantheon opened, a foreign nobleman observed "that it brought to his mind the enchanted Palaces described in the French Romances, which are said to have been raised by the potent wand of some Fairy; and, that, indeed, so much were his senses captivated, he could scarcely persuade himself but that he trod on fairy ground". This glorious backdrop to Wilson's display may have helped convince the king of the superiority of knobs – he quickly had all the conductors on the Palace replaced – but it did little to persuade many serious scientists.

It's not clear whether or not Graham actually witnessed the demonstration – he certainly left Bath to go to London at around this time, later describing himself as having been employed "in prosecuting discoveries, in making farther improvements in my art; as well as in new additions to my apparatus, &c". In the Temple of Health, Graham harvested royal and scientific glory by association, installing part of Wilson's electrical machinery in the first-floor room he dubbed "the Great Apollo chamber". Here he set up a large polished mahogany frame with the "two cylinders of brilliant glass... of prodigious size... each... 20 inches in length and 44 in circumference..." from the Pantheon. They were said to be "so amazingly powerful in exciting and producing the electrical fire, that a coated jar which contains ten gallons is charged by them in half a minute, or by a few turns of the wheel". On installing them at the Adelphi, Graham claimed to have improved them "exceedingly". He upgraded their insulation, and devised a way to spin them either individually or simultaneously, thereby, he believed, "producing either positive or negative electricity according to the nature of the case, the constitution of the patient, or the number of persons to be electrified at one time".

Taking the house next door to a national celebrity would have proved rather more of a coup had David Garrick not died just a few months later. London was devastated. The capital's streets were so crowded with lamenting admirers that a fifty-carriage funeral cortège from the Adelphi took over an hour to reach Westminster Abbey on 1st February 1779. The chief mourner was the playwright Sheridan, and the coffin was borne up the aisle by Garrick's aristocratic friends, Earl Spencer, the Duke of Devonshire, the Earl of Ossory and Viscount Palmerston among them. The Garricks had enjoyed an unusually close marriage, and the actor's widow was devastated by her loss. Suddenly the stream of glamorous visitors to the Garricks' house dried up. The couple's close friend Hannah More recorded sadly in 1781: "As to poor Mrs Garrick, she keeps herself as secret as a piece of smuggled goods, and neither stirs out herself or lets any body in."

But Graham was not in London to witness Garrick's funeral orations. He was far away in Newcastle-upon-Tyne, setting in motion the next stage of his scheme. Newcastle barely extended beyond its ancient city walls in 1779. Its fine new infirmary was completely surrounded by fields. Yet it was probably the fourth largest town in England, certainly the fourth most important printing centre. Stretching for almost half a mile along the banks of the Tyne to the east of the city beside the Ouseburn were most of Newcastle's "famous" glasshouses (High, Middle and Low), at least sixteen of them billowing their smoke into the Northumbrian skies throughout the 1770s. Between them they produced every imaginable form of glassware, from the clearest of window panes to the plainest green bottles. The cheap local coal and proximity of raw materials made their prices unbeatable. On the other side of town, just to the west of the city walls in the Closegate, a few specialist "flint" glasshouses stood, their sweaty workers blowing and grinding in fierce, searing heat to produce sparkling crystal glass tableware and other luxuries. These were the "ingenious" glassmakers whose expertise Dr Graham sought to construct the most important elements of his grandest project yet: "the largest and most elegant Medico-Electrical-Aërial and Magnetic Apparatus in the world".

As usual, Graham's particular ambitions made him deviate from the norms of natural philosophy. To do justice to the Adelphi's luxurious interiors, he decided to design the most advanced scientific apparatuses in the latest decorative fashions. Examples of Enlightenment apparatuses survive which still surprise and seduce the modern viewer with their subtle gilt flourishes and the sensuous curves of their mahogany supports. Graham took this instinctive tendency towards educational embellishment several steps further. He wanted to amaze his audiences with form as much as function, to incorporate aesthetics into his ethereal treatments in a way which paralleled his use of music. And while he was obviously out to make a profit from it, he also clearly adored his equipment with the obsessive passion of any ardent collector.

Flint glass had been patented as a technique for making lead crystal a century earlier by George Ravenscroft. It was a lustrous and particularly refractive new glass which acquired its name from the ground, calcined flint used as a source of silica when it was first made. While windows were usually made from soda-lime glass, and bottles from naturally green or brown glass, flint glass was better suited to candlesticks and candelabra. It reflected the smallest flame, transforming a group of candles into a dazzling display. The same naturally applied to the insulated furniture legs and supports required by anybody working with electricity. Flint glass was also valued in making the part of the equipment – globe, cylinder or plate-shaped – that was rubbed to generate the actual electric charge. As long ago as 1738, the Abbé Nollet specified that the glass globe recommended among instruments for a course of experimental physics should be of "*cristal d'Angleterre*", as English flint glass was known in France.

Relatively few items of such fragility have survived the centuries, but descriptions and drawings by Graham and his contemporaries suggest that showmen, scientists and designers were all profiting from the rapid evolutions in glass technology in this period. It did not come cheaply. Excise duty on glass, stable since 1745, had received another hike in 1777, with further legislation the following year. Elaborate chandeliers could cost hundred of pounds, and were often hired for an occasion rather than bought outright. Air pumps and electrical machines were also becoming increasingly expensive, and by the 1780s a full set of electrical apparatus for demonstration purposes required an outlay of at least £400. The best instrument-makers could command £2000. Graham's plans demanded even more serious investment. This was speculation on a majestic scale. It could not have been without danger. The Doctor must have felt very certain that he would be able to recoup and then profit from such a substantial outlay.

Graham appears to have been captivated by the way the glass apparatus he was ordering seemed to materialize the actions of his treatments. It provided a way in which patients could visualize what was happening to their bodies. Describing the superb pavilion for one he wrote that "it breathes health. For by the means of the massive, highly polished and gilt brass rods which connect it with the dome of the temple, so great a stream of the electrical or elementary fire is brought in, that the patient, when the Apollo chamber is darkened, appears enthroned and environed with a visible species of celestial glory! Add to this, that the patient so far from receiving any shock, is exhilerated and delighted with the aromatic aetherial odours, while he cleanses his lungs, purifies and circulates his blood, and fortifies his nerves by breathing the electrical, dephlogisticated and vivifying atmosphere with which he is surrounded; or in other words, while he inhales and assimilates the *materia prima*, or the universal vital principle of all things." This was glass and metalwork whose functional properties extended into an imaginative realm.

Alongside the sparkles from the smooth reflective "cut-glass" facets, Graham incorporated a great sense of movement. He somehow persuaded the glassmakers to enlarge forms familiar to his wealthy audiences from the elegant glassware on their dining tables or at their drinking clubs into the actual structures of the Temple's high-tech equipment. The delicate "air-twist" stems of cordial glasses which pulled and twisted air bubbles into floating helter-skelters imprisoned in glass were magnified into ethereal pillars. The distinctive opaque white or lapis-lazuli-blue "enamel twists" suspended their lacy coloured coils on an undreamt-of scale. The most elaborate were made with multiple twists – some like tape, some like threads, opaque, transparent or coloured. The columns swirled round like geometric figures or organisms seen through a microscope. Doubled, their spiralling forms resembled ethereal memories of barber poles, with their own muted references to winding bloodstained band-ages. They almost seem to anticipate the double helix of DNA, its rungs not yet in place. These magical structures were transformed into the glittering columns supporting Graham's ever-expanding medical apparatus. Quite how the glassmakers managed to achieve these effects is uncertain. The technical difficulties must have been immense.

The Doctor reserved the most astonishing glassware for the columns supporting the Temple of Apollo – that temple within a temple – constructed for the grand first-floor drawing room at the Royal Terrace: "The spacious dome of this stupendous temple is entirely covered with metal, and is supported by six beautiful fluted columns of a kind of open work quite new in this island.—Though they are six feet high, standing on double square plinths, with bases and capitals richly ornamented, yet they are but pedestals as it were for six pillars of brilliant flint cut glass, enriched at top and bottom with flowered borders cut in the glass, and carved mouldings. Each pillar in the centre is strengthened and decorated with a solid stalk of flint glass, with white enamelled lace or net work in the middle, and bound about with a snowy white spiral glass cord, all of which are a complete and effectual insulation to the tremendous conductors or reservoirs which rest on the top of the dome."

The sheer size of Graham's decorated Leyden jars was unprecedented. In the first room at the Adelphi Temple of Health, visitors were impressed by a huge "snowy white enameled glass" cylinder encased in a zebrano wood frame, stripy and exotic, all the way from West Africa. In front of this was a "most elegant and SUPERB PEDESTAL... carved with uncommon richness, and double gilt with superior magnificence. From the top of it rises a large massy tube of pure flint glass, with spiral tubes in the inside of Lapis Lazuli and golden coloured glass; and on each side two triangularly cut brilliant pillars of flint glass of exquisite workmanship". This supported a six-foot fiery dragon, with wings extended, conducting electricity from its forked crimson tongue to the tip of its tail, which rested on one end of the prime conductor downstairs. Its male counterpart upstairs, equally dramatic, rested on "a massy pillar of brilliant glass, with gold, purple, and lapis lazuli coloured spiral tubes in the centre. On each side of this compound and very curious pillar, arise, diverging, two magnificent triangular columns of pure chrystal glass, cut into true prisms, exhibiting all the rich colours of the rainbow."

One of several electric and magnetic thrones in the Apollo room was almost semicircular and boasted a back rail of cut flint glass, "no less than twelve feet long, of immense value and celestial beauty, and...

supported by six great columns of the same – so truly prismatic, – so exactly cut, – and so highly polished, as to blaze and exhibit with the loveliest lustre, the seven primitive colours, diversified with the richest harmony". (Graham's educated audiences would have appreciated these allusions to Newton's *Optics*.) The throne itself was "supported by eight massy pillars of brilliant glass – the bases and capitals richly gilt and ornamented with brilliant ruby coloured foil, &c.". Here Graham seems to have adopted the technique employed by Robert Adam for the extraordinary glass drawing room he designed for Northumberland House. Its elaborate glass panelling was backed with blood-red pigments scattered with chips of metal foil in imitation of Roman porphyry, and was designed to reflect the hundreds of candles used at evening assemblies. It now seems garish – and more reminiscent of a 1970s British-Indian restaurant than anything else. Adam used the same technology when he remodelled the Theatre Royal in Drury Lane for David Garrick in 1774. (Like Adam, Garrick was an investor in the Duke of Northumberland's new British Cast Plate Glass Manufactory in Lancashire.)

The theatrical and the functional would become inseparable – art and artifice impossible to distinguish at the Temple of Health. Even Graham's fakes were the very best quality. He boasted of a pair of "superb brilliant girandoles... with elegant festoons of paste of the first water, and of the highest polish".

Up in Newcastle, it took four months to assemble the new glassware, time Graham spent in amassing a collection of new patients, fees to underwrite his ambitious and expensive commissions, and of course valuable publicity material. In this last task, the Doctor seems to have courted controversy quite deliberately. Though he needed little encouragement, Graham was perhaps spurred on by the radical circles towards which he gravitated during his stay in Northumberland.

As in Bath, he appears to have found friends among others who, like Macaulay and Wilson, based their politics on ancient English rights, looking back to King Alfred and the Saxons, the Peasants' Revolt and what they saw as the "Glorious Revolution" of 1688. On Sundays Graham probably sat among the huge crowds who gathered at the chapel of High Bridge to hear one of his best-known patients, Revd James Murray, preaching an unfaltering fusion of religion and radical politics. "[N]o man could be a real Christian who was not a warm and zealous friend to civil and religious liberty," Murray thundered, much to the concern of Tyneside establishment worthies. In the early months of 1779, condemnation of the war against the

American colonists was Murray's persistent theme. In and out of the pulpit, he was raising petitions to Parliament against Government policy. Meanwhile the situation across the Atlantic went from bad to worse, lists of dead on each side lengthening daily. The previous year, Murray had published two volumes of *An Impartial History of the Present War in America*. Its dry title belied his impassioned tone. Murray wrote Graham a glowing testimonial.

Graham set up practice in Pilgrim Street, merely houses away from several local physicians, and conveniently close to a number of huge coaching inns which vied for trade from the thrice-daily London coaches and innumerable commercial carriers. A few months after announcing his presence with his usual barrage of advertisements in the *Newcastle Journal* and other local papers, the new doctor on the block pushed the medical establishment too far. This was not a body of men to take incursions onto their turf lightly. The previous year they successfully saw off a "French charlatan", who had slunk off into the night when he was ordered to appear before the mayor and "a group of the faculty" in the morning. No doubt the doctors of the city hospital hoped Graham would be equally easily dispatched.

Graham's own account of the public row claimed that "the lucrative emoluments, and flattering applause" which greeted his practice "excited the envy of the faculty so much that not content with propagating little stories to [his] disadvantage, they went so far as to suborne unprincipled people to tell lies in the public papers, with the view of ruining [him] in the opinion of the public". Mark Pringle of Heaton was the unscrupulous patient, a stroke victim whose affliction had left him in agony with monstrously swollen testicles and severe urinary incontinence. Graham claimed to have restored Pringle to health in two weeks. This was after the Newcastle Infirmary and other local doctors had declared him absolutely incurable. Graham also maintained that he had only made the case public at Mr Pringle's own "earnest request". Meanwhile, the Doctor had reprinted his well-worn "Will Graham go?" sonnet, this time under the initials "E.P." and title 'On hearing that Dr. GRAHAM intends leaving Newcastle, on the 8th of April'.

Ye who have seen, have prov'd his skilful Art,
Will feel his absence in a grateful heart;
The echoing sigh, the silent-speaking tear,
Shall grace his memory – to hundreds dear;

Honour'd, esteem'd, he gains a deathless fame,
While Envy sickens at a GRAHAM's name!

Stung by Graham's provocatively repeated boasts of having been
"particularly fortunate in curing the Infirmary incurables" since the
first hour of his arrival in Northumberland, the enraged Governor of
the Infirmary wrote to the Newcastle Journal to defend his institution
in early March. "The indifference with which the faculty have treated
Dr Graham's pompous advertisements since his arrival [has] induced
the Doctor to consider the field as his own," he declared. Then he
rather weakly argued that Pringle's affliction had actually been
relieved by the application of a blister by an Infirmary medic two
days before seeing Graham.

"Paper wars" were a common feature of eighteenth-century medical
life, and hostilities usually only ceased with the departure or death of
one of the protagonists. Combatants entered vigorously into cycles of
disputatious pamphlets, or, like Graham and his opponents, took to
the pages of the local newspapers, indignantly defending themselves
in terms of professional honour and integrity. Only more shameful
than engaging with an upstart inferior was for physicians to remain
silent in the face of a slur. The high-flown principles each party in
these disputes tended to mouth were a poor disguise for what were
invariably, at heart, battles for the economic high ground.

James Graham, MD (now self-proclaimed "Conqueror, under
God, of Diseases"), could not have been more delighted with the
opportunity this attack presented. He openly alleged tactics of bribery,
threats, and "a canful or two of nostrum gin" to get Mr Pringle on
side. He even diagnosed madness on the part of the Governor, and
accused him of meaning "to rob his family of bread, and the public
of his services, by ruining at once Dr. Graham's medical and moral
character". This was woven into an extended and involved "parody
on the *Governor's* Letter", which gleefully developed a rhetoric of
purging and blistering to refer to the accepted medical decorum
of retaliation in print. The themes were enlarged in a curiously
irreverent biblical pastiche that incorporated the system of official
medical certification by the Infirmary into passages from the Acts of
the Apostles to mock the hospital's uneasy protectionism.

Pringle's betrayal, if that it was, he dealt with in Lear-like tones:
"of all ingratitude, it is surely the blackest, not only to deny the fact,
but to attempt to injure and to destroy the reputation and fortune
of the physician who had taken him from the rack upon which he

had been tortured for years, and laid him, DISINTERESTEDLY laid him, on a sweet bed, and his head on a soft pillow." The Doctor mercilessly pointed out that reasons of delicacy and brevity had previously prevented any mention that along with curing Pringle's painful incontinence, he had remedied his "total loss of virility".

The letters and poems that rushed to print in Graham's defence – supposedly by "A Northumberland farmer", a local Newbiggin miner and a lady who praised him as "Gen'rous by nature, matchless in [his] skill!" – share a recognizable style. A typical example is the letter signed "Clerimont", questioning the strangeness of descending "to low methods, in order to crush a brother of superior merit, and one whose conduct, like the rays of heaven's great luminary, are too bright for them to behold... Can they not bear his meridian splendour a few days longer, when his departure will once more suffer *them* to twinkle in their little sphere?"

Graham returned to London certain that he had triumphed in that particular battle, fired by the zeal of the vindicated. His tactics for drawing attention to his methods seem extreme, were undoubtedly inflammatory, and would ultimately rebound on his own reputation. Yet his gall was in many ways understandable. He had reason to be frustrated at the diehard conservatism of orthodox medicine:

> ...very early in life I became exceedingly dissatisfied with what is called the regular practice. I found it too trifling, absurd, and ineffectual. Neither my masters, my fellows, nor myself being able to cure great, vital, or inveterate diseases, vexed and mortified me to the extremest degree; – and some of my most esteemed and most beloved friends dropping prematurely into the grave, drove me mad.

Graham rightly saw that a great many conventional treatments simply did not work. For over a decade he had wondered why, despite "the boasted advances... in every branch of natural science", the cure of disease, particularly the most dangerous, had been so little improved. Since the beginning of the century, he argued, "Fashions, indeed have changed, but the Healing Art hath gained little by the alteration... it hath been rich... very rich, in theory; but poor, very poor, in the practical application of it." This was hard to dispute. Graham was working in an era when controlled trials were such a rarity as to be almost unheard of, and "empiric" was a term of abuse for a physician. The vast majority of doctors still relied on therapeutic techniques which were far more likely to do harm than good. At the same time they guarded their terrain with a jealousy which today seems quite shocking.

If Graham had been less effective at poaching patients, he simply would not have been worth attacking. He did it by emphasizing the "friendly powerfulness" of his methods, and the almost complete absence of pain or shock brought on by his "curious machines". These worked, he now explained, by saturating his patients with "the electric fluid, and with aerial and musical influences, *which no obstruction whatever can resist*; the stagnant morbid matter and humours are rendered fluid, and set in motion, they are repelled with proper applications from the vital or particular parts, while others are defended and strengthened with aetherial medicines, or magnetic plates and bars. In certain cases, magnetic, icy, and other influences, are applied to attract or repel powerfully morbid matter from the upper and vital parts to the lower extremities; while streams of the electric fluid irresistibly pervading, and carrying through the whole system, or home to parts particularly affected, attenuating, aetherial, antispasmodic, and balsamic medicines, subduing and eradicating the disease, and giving new springs to the vital principles." It was all beginning to sound convincingly systematic. Patients were used to this terminology of blockages and irregularities, humours and morbidity; they had seen what electricity and magnets could do at lectures, fairs and assembly rooms.

Graham was clearly convinced by his own explanations. In fact, he probably owed a great many of his medical victories to what has since been established as the placebo effect. Now, of course, it is accepted that patients taking a pill believed to be a painkiller are in fact very likely to feel their pain reduced, as a result of genuine physiological processes rather than any trick of the imagination. Placebos can actually inspire the body to produce pain-relieving endorphins. John Hunter (William Hunter's surgeon brother) had some understanding of these issues. Realizing that gonorrhoea tended to be a self-limiting disease, and that most of the medicines claiming to cure it were utterly ineffectual, he carried out tests on his patients using bread pills. He dosed his own wife with London Thames water masquerading as Bath spa water. The leading "man-midwife" William Smellie was similarly unabashed about prescribing placebos during a lingering labour, suggesting that if clamouring assistants and an anxious or impatient mother cannot be soothed by "arguments and gentle persuasion... it will be convenient to prescribe some innocent medicine that she may take between whiles, to beguile the time and please her imagination."

Graham was fumbling towards a recognition of these ideas, evident from fleeting moments of insight and revelation – such as when he declared that he was "perfectly convinced that prayer is of the greatest benefit to human Beings, *whether God hears them or not*". But he could not travel too far down this road without casting doubt on the scientific basis for his methods of healing. At the same time he was never quite able to explain the science, without getting swept away by the wonder of it all. Electricity, magnetism and air, the principles Graham was busily bringing together in his extraordinary Temple of Health, were, he believed, "the various faculties of the material soul of the universe". He was convinced these must be the earthly manifestations of "the ETERNALLY SUPREME JEHOVAH himself! The GREAT SUN OF THE UNIVERSE". So his mountain of metaphors rose, until finally, overwhelmed by the unrenderable contrast between God's majesty and human littleness, Graham dissolved into silence: "the LIGHT of all light; – The – !!! but here, here at the entrance of intellectual vision – on the very threshold of comprehension we stop..."

5

The Gestation

"Goodness – condescension – and generosity like her Ladyship's should be rewarded even <u>here</u>; Dr G. will strain his best abilities to have the pleasure of presenting to her, in a week or two, perfectly cured, and intirely sound, the offensive object her humanity has snatch'd from pain, rottenness, & death."

Every year, hundreds of well-born young men hired tutors, armed themselves with sketchbooks and watercolours, consulted the latest volumes of travel advice and set off for Paris, the Netherlands and ultimately Italy and the edifying ruins of Rome. The average gentleman traveller acquired more in the way of exasperating foreign affectations and tenacious sexual diseases than the moral and cultural education this rite of passage was designed to achieve. At least so all those satirical portraits of foppish young grand tourists in the works of Sterne, Pope, Smollett and Foote would suggest. Meanwhile, other less privileged individuals were constructing more specialized versions of the Grand Tour. Those who left English shores with less money and more purpose undoubtedly enjoyed greater rewards. The architects Robert and James Adam, William Chambers and James "Athenian" Stuart all travelled to Italy or Greece for their own industrious refashionings of the "Grand Tour", learning from the European literati how best to advance the cause of neoclassicism.

James Graham sailed from England to Holland on 1st May 1779, on a voyage with a different but no less particular purpose. Like the young men with their sketchbooks, "improvement" was his ambition. Before opening his great venture in London, he needed to be certain that the apparatus on which his fortune would depend would not turn out to be passé before it was even unveiled. He wanted to be able to assure his patients that they were enjoying the very best treatments of their kind. So instead of engaging in uplifting conversations with the past, by scrutinizing temples, paintings, mosaics and ancient palaces, Graham made it his mission to foresee the future. He sought out a succession of Europe's instrument-makers, natural philosophers and electrically oriented medics, the leading men of learning who were every day throwing new light on the Doctor's fields of enquiry. At the same time, Graham expressed an interest in "ascertaining the true nature and virtues" of the waters of Europe's smartest spa towns. No doubt he also had every intention of analysing the rich and royal patients from across the continent who flocked to these resorts in the summer months.

In the Kalverstraat, Amsterdam, not far from the City Hall, Graham was delighted to explore the workshop of an Englishman, John Cuthbertson. Cuthbertson and his master-turned-father-in-law had moved from London to the cosmopolitan Dutch capital some ten years previously. His instrument sales, books and public lectures had made him the accepted leader in the field of glass-plate frictional electrical machines. A few years previously, Franklin's friend Jan Ingen-Housz had been impressed by Cuthbertson's explosive experiments with an electric glass pistol. They were inspired by Alessandro Volta's trials using an electric spark to explode methane from nearby swamps. It turned out different mixtures of common air and hydrogen could do the same trick. At the Temple of Health Graham would adapt this idea to salute a portrait of King George III with two "batter[ies] of philosophical cannon… charged with inflammable air [i.e. hydrogen], and discharged with electrical fire", producing explosions, he claimed, as "loud and tremendous" as gunpowder. They were sufficiently striking for at least one artist to include a large cannon in his caricature of the Doctor.

In Amsterdam in 1779, although the Dutch "golden age" had long since drawn to a close, Cuthbertson was reaping the advantages of an unusually well-established market-economy tradition. As a commercial natural philosopher, he suffered none of the unease about the boundaries between "serious" scientific demonstration and popular entertainment which, elsewhere in the world, were more anxiously policed. (Wilson's transformation by his opponents after his Pantheon experiment from a respectable authority on electricity to a charlatan is a case in point.) In Holland the conversion of scientific culture into commodity was neither new nor dubious.

When Graham came to see him, Cuthbertson was at something of a transition point. He was already renowned for his exceptionally efficient English-style twin-plate electrical machines. They used flint-glass plates and increasing numbers of cushions to excite ever greater quantities of electricity. Interest worldwide was shifting towards the possibilities of huge and hugely sophisticated machines, producing ever longer and stronger sparks. In just a few years, Cuthbertson would be commissioned by the polymath Dr Martinus van Marum to build a gigantic electric frictional generator for the Teyler's Foundation, still in the Haarlem museum to this day. A vast battery of 135 Leyden jars was fed by a machine with two parallel glass discs, each 65 inches in diameter, and mounted on a yard-long axle seven and a half inches apart. Two operators cranking simultaneously produced tongues of fire two feet long. Graham seems to have been exceptional among medics in sharing this interest in magnitude. Most physicians using electricity were far more concerned with the convenience and portability of their machines.

Size must have been a topic of conversation in the Kalverstraat workshop. As the glinting glass plates turned, the insulated leather cushions quietly rubbed and the sparks crackled on the sharp steel collecting combs, Graham and Cuthbertson's discussion probably turned to rather a public argument of the previous summer. Preventing the build-up of moisture on the glass of electricity machines and reducing friction without losing electric charge were the two main issues confronting improvers in the field during the '70s and '80s. An amateur instrument-maker in Delft, Gerhard Cuypers, had been following up observations on how different quantities of alkaline salts in the glass affected its electrifying abilities. He found that plates treated by being baked slowly in an ordinary bread oven between thick layers of soft cardboard for several weeks excited more electric matter than a normal equivalent-size plate. Significantly, this was true even in the damp weather which was usually the death knell for electrical experimentation. Cuthbertson had reacted rather heatedly to his claims, though this may have had more to do with competition for patronage from van Marum than anything else. Mindful of the damp riverside situation of his new London home, Graham went to Delft to take advice from Cuypers. Frustratingly, the Doctor recorded the mere fact of this visit, and nothing about what it achieved.

From Delft, Graham travelled to Leiden, where he was quite charmed by Professor J.N.S. Allamand, now an obscure figure, but then a celebrity in the world of electricity. He clearly sat high in Graham's philosophical pantheon. Here was a man who had literally supported Musschenbroek as he staggered back from the shock of discovery of the first Leyden jar. He had been the assistant, disciple and later the biographer of Willem 'sGravesande, another important Dutch Newtonian. (When 'sGravesande's survey of physics began to be published in 1720, the first of its kind, it was instantly translated into English in two competing editions. Sir Isaac Newton's experimental assistant, J.T. Desaguliers, made it into print first by dictating to four copyists simultaneously.) Graham was delighted with "the politeness and science of the learned and indefatigable" Allamand, and admired both his electrical apparatus and what he considered to be "the largest and best natural magnet perhaps in the world", capable of suspending a weight of about two hundred pounds.

Onwards Graham travelled through Flanders and Brabant, "examining every thing that merited [his] attention". In Maastricht he was distracted by the jawbones of the mosasaur, a late-Cretaceous marine predator named after this region, then in the cabinet of curiosities belonging to M. Hoffman. (Hoffman had assumed the strange beast was some sort of crocodile.) But this was a mere diversion for his Scottish visitor. It was Hoffman's ideas about the dangers of masturbation that really caught Graham's imagination. As first surgeon to the city's Military Hospital, Hoffman had become a specialist in the subject with a particularly large caseload on which to theorize.

His views had recently been cited with much approval by the Enlightenment's expert on onanism, a Swiss physician called Samuel Tissot. His enormously successful and much translated book on the subject dealt, as he carefully stressed in his preface, with "the disorders occasioned by... self-pollution", rather than the "crime" of the act. "Hoffman has seen the most fatal accidents flow from a dissipation of the seed," wrote Tissot. "After frequent nocturnal pollutions (says he) not only the powers are lost, the body falls away, and the face turns pale; but moreover the memory fails, a cold sensation seizes all the limbs, the sight is clouded, and the voice becomes hoarse; all the body languishes by degrees: disturbing dreams prevent sleep administering any relief, and such pains ensue as are felt from the blows of a cudgel."

Hoffman was convinced of the close connection between the brain and the testicles. "The seminal liquid," according to him, "is distributed in the same manner as the animal spirits of the brain, into all the nerves of the body: it seems to be of the same nature." As for treatments, for the most part, Hoffman's theories neatly coincided with Graham's own. The important thing was to "animate the languid tone of the fibres". Believing that wasted seminal fluid drained away a man's strength more speedily than loss of blood, Tissot (like Graham, and his influential predecessor George Cheyne) advocated a suitably restorative diet, free of indigestible meats and strong alcohols, and emphasized the importance of "regime". For cases involving "draining and lust", Hoffman prescribed "Asses' milk".

In Brussels Graham had "the honour of inspecting" the electrical apparatus of the Emperor of Germany's uncle in his palace. In Paris, he walked the wards of the vast Hôtel-Dieu on the Île de la Cité, where six or seven thousand patients at a time competed for the attention of harassed doctors, according to Graham. Venereal diseases were here the main attraction for this Grand Tourist.

Graham also managed to get an introduction to Dr Pierre Jean-Claude Mauduyt. Again, he could hardly have sought advice from a more reputable character. Here was an individual who had actually been commissioned by the French Royal Society of Medicine to carry out research on electrical medicine. This was largely in response to demand from provincial doctors, anxious for more information about this still burgeoning field. Mauduyt's work, published by Government order, made it to the library shelves of upstanding members of the British medical establishment, like John Coakley Lettsom, better known for his war against quackery than for any tendencies in that direction himself. In his report on the electrical treatment of eighty-two different cases, being printed at the time Graham met him, Mauduyt made a cautious appeal to his readers: "I am a long way from dictating laws; I merely say frankly and simply what I practise myself and what seems to work best."

Graham described Mauduyt as "a gentleman of ingenuity, learning, and liberality". Not only was he able to converse with him, but he "had likewise the privilege of inspecting the apparatus, and of seeing a number of both sexes go through the operations under the Doctor's immediate direction." Graham made wistful reference to "this great and most important business" being carried out "at the royal expence".

In the report of his test cases Mauduyt's tone could hardly have been more different from Graham's writing voice. This was partly a measure of the two men's different characters, but it also reflected the distinctively different demands of commercial enterprise and state-funded research. Where Graham is typically exuberant, metaphorical, boastful, provocative and often borders on the mystical, Mauduyt is practical, precise and careful. In place of Graham's pages and pages of alarmingly explicit yet deeply sentimental testimonials, Mauduyt supplies a neat fold-out table of electrified patients, with columns headed with the number of days, age, date of illness and so on. He warns fellow practitioners to ensure their patients' feet are dry before treatment on rainy days, to wipe the insulated supports of the banquette each time, and to watch out for pins and brooches sticking out of women's clothes. He suggests alternative regimens and methods (highly reminiscent of bathing routines at spa resorts) and reminds that his aim "is to get patients accustomed to an apparatus of which most of them are afraid". A few years later, when van Marum was experimenting with the effects of electrification on pulse rates and perspiration, he realized that fear could easily become a factor which confused results.

The system Graham was already using in Bath of combining electrical treatment with forms of massage got a subdued thumbs-up: "rubbing" or "frictions", after electrification, or with warm towels during the electric bath. In a later work, Mauduyt became slightly more lyrical, describing the feeling of an electric bath as "a sensation similar to being touched with a spider's web". He suggested a method of drawing sparks in cases of deafness using polished wires, the first the thickness of a crow's wing feather, the second that of a pigeon's and the final one the thickness of a writing quill. The kind of therapy Graham would have witnessed is illustrated and explained: a treatment for menstrual problems shows a woman sitting on a glass-legged stool raised on a platform. Her legs are slightly parted, her hands rest on her knees, her eyes are lowered and she smiles rather bashfully as she averts her gaze from the long pointed poker-like rod aimed at her crotch. From her sacrum emerges a wire which is looped into the ring above the large knob of the prime conductor, about the size of her head.

The Frenchman and the Scot must have had quite precise discussions on their shared interest: the best type of glass to use (Mauduyt favoured that manufactured at Cherbourg as a second best to English glass), the perfect polish required on the yellow copper sticks for applying the "fluid" to patients, the dangers of globes and cylinders breaking and shattering in use and the advantages of the more robust plate machines of the type in which Cuthbertson specialized. Mauduyt possibly inadvertently gave Graham further inspiration for one of the most dramatic parts of his Temple of Health apparatus – the six-foot fiery flying dragon and his mate. Discussing how to increase the force of the machine, he suggested that as well as the prime conductor, made of metal, others could be hung from the ceiling, as Wilson had done in the Pantheon. Mauduyt recommended secondary conductors made of cardboard and covered with tin leaves, suspended by pure silk cords, enclosed in glass tubes to protect them from dust. A showman's leap of imagination and a memory of Wilson's serpentine conductor were all that was needed to transform these into mythical beasts dominating the apparatus at the Temple of Health. If their diamond-shaped scales were slightly separated (rather than smoothly joined as Mauduyt suggested), sparks could leap dramatically from point to point, lighting the creatures up as they apparently breathed electrical fire from their open jaws.

The mere fact that Graham was pursuing electricity as the main tenet of his therapeutic approach did not make him particularly unusual in this period. Electrical machines were by then part of the paraphernalia of many hospitals, including Edinburgh's Royal Infirmary. But in Britain they did tend to be a treatment of last resort. A Gravesend surgeon had been honoured in 1778 with a medal from the Royal Humane Society of London for his essay advocating the use of moderate electric shocks to resuscitate those presumed dead from drowning.

The lack of consensus about how electrical therapy actually worked was a problem for practitioners seeking recognition by the establishment: it largely reflected a lack of consensus in the medical profession about how the human body itself worked. Jostling for acceptance somewhere among the various competing theoretical frameworks was that vague idea promoted by Graham that electricity's power of penetration freed "obstructions" in the nerves and other vessels and so restored the circulation of humours and blood. But medical electricity was never able to escape the strong possibility that its effects derived not from its physical action on the body but from the workings of a patient's enthusiastic imagination. In such a cut-throat professional environment, this made easy targets of its practitioners.

Trumpeting the scientific celebrities he met in the summer of 1779, Graham makes no mention of Franz Anton Mesmer, the animal magnetizer. He had good reason for avoiding any reference to him. It's unlikely though that Graham could have avoided the man himself. During that year Mesmer's presence in Paris was quite impossible to ignore. A jowly Swiss doctor in his mid-forties, expounding his theories in an incomprehensibly thick German accent, he was an unlikely individual to find surrounded by swooning women. Yet one amazed witness had reported of a Mesmer patient as early as 1775 that "when he would point his index finger at her, even though from some distance, she would actually fall senseless to the ground".

He had come to Paris from Vienna the previous year, in the hope of finding serious professional recognition for his intriguing claims about an invisible fluid that ebbed and flowed in the human body, like the tides of the oceans. (Mesmer was also fleeing a scandal involving a young female patient whose sight he had restored.) If heavenly bodies could affect the movements of waters around the globe, so too could they affect the human nervous system, Mesmer argued. Like electricity, gravity and magnetism were by this time recognized natural phenomena, but their precise operation were far from fully understood. In the context of Enlightenment scientific and medical understanding, Mesmer's belief that bodily health could be restored by applying magnets to reharmonize the flow of the patient's fluids sounded perfectly plausible to many minds. Thanks to the imagined "drawing" action of magnets, therapeutic powdered lodestone was already used to soothe injuries. Small artificial magnets covered in cloth or black velvet were worn linked together as bracelets or necklaces, and bare magnets could be tied to different parts of the body or even looped behind the ear. They were a particularly popular cure for toothache and earache.

Mesmer took this notion much further. He transformed the now commonplace idea of healing with actual magnets into a vision of a magnetic "universal fluid", a life-giving force which flowed throughout the world. It had something in common with Graham's rather metaphorical concept of the "electric fire". The startling new therapies Mesmer developed to channel this mysterious force became known as animal magnetism, mesmerism or somnambulism. In effect, he had discovered the power of hypnotism, and he was clearly a master of the art. The inscription below an undated French engraving announced that Mesmer cured numerous ailments, including dropsy, paralysis, gout, scurvy, blindness and deafness. These were, of course, exactly the kinds of chronic conditions in which Graham specialized.

If Graham managed to get into the crowded Hotel Bullion that summer (as he surely must have attempted), he would have seen four oval-shaped, tarred oak tubs standing incongruously on the inlaid floors of an elegantly decorated salon. The tubs, known as *baquets,* were packed with flasks of treated water, magnets, iron filings and scented herbs. Each was surrounded by patients with fingers interlaced, thighs gaping and knees pressed urgently against their neighbour's, all reflected in the vast mirrors which lined the walls. "My initial urge was to go and join the circle," the portrait painter

Elisabeth Vigée-Lebrun wrote of her visit, "but I noticed that my neighbour had scabies, so I quickly withdrew my hand and continued into another room. During my journey, M. Mesmer's followers came towards me from all corners of the room, armed with their little metal wands, and I lost patience with them."

The magnetic fluid that would supposedly unblock these patients was conducted from the *baquet* by metal rods, like those used to apply electricity, or ropes which could be entwined around afflicted limbs. Mesmer himself, in lilac- and gold-embroidered robes, sometimes still brandished a white magnetic baton. But by 1779 he was claiming to be able to direct the flow of the fluid with eyes and hands alone, and his forefinger was notorious. Results were sensational. Patients were literally entranced. Many fainted, or convulsed in spectacular "crises". They had to be led by disciples to specially prepared areas, lined with soft mattresses. Music, sometimes provided by a pianist, sometimes by a singer, evoked a suitably otherworldly atmosphere. Most strikingly the unearthly call of the glass harmonica sounded to summon and direct the celestial forces. Mesmer was a particularly skilled performer on the instrument. His unusual mood-altering improvisations had powerful effects on his patients, and probably influenced Graham's choice of instruments at the Temple of Health.

Although full-blown "Mesmeromania" was still gathering force, most of the French medical establishment was already alarmed at the animal magnetizer's success. By 1779, the *Journal de Médecine* and the *Gazette de Santé* had both run hostile articles, denouncing the practice. Graham's reluctance to mention Mesmer is understandable: he was probably afraid of being tarnished by association. Yet there are numerous parallels between their approaches to medicine and science. Both introduced ideas that were original enough to amaze and impress, but close enough to mainstream understanding not to be dismissed out of hand. Both understood the use of drama, and made persuasive appeal to their patients' senses and imaginations. They also both believed they could control or channel natural phenomena. Both enjoyed huge celebrity and success, only to be denounced as charlatans. And both Mesmer and Graham drew into their theatres of healing a very mixed crowd of cynics and believers.

Their clients included individuals drawn by gossip, fashion or the possibility of experiencing the barely disguised erotic frisson of shared physical encounters. But these doctors also attracted patients who were truly desperate for a cure. They were people who had suffered terribly, and who had been failed by orthodox medicine. These were men, women and children who urgently needed something to believe in. And of course, Graham and Mesmer were both fired with self-conviction of unusual intensity, and propelled by the unshakeable certainty that at some point the world would recognize their true and immeasurable value. They made compelling symbols of hope.

But the differences between Graham and Mesmer were also significant. Mesmer was desperate to be accepted by the Academy, had married sufficiently well to have little need for social or financial advancement, and was delighted to give his name to a movement. Graham was a far more isolated and eccentric figure, a lone maverick who spawned few followers, whose ambitions always exceeded his income.

James Graham's claim at this stage of his grand tour to have "had the honour of an interview" with Benjamin Franklin, "THE GREAT AMERICAN PHILOSOPHER", has been ridiculed. Having returned to America to help draft the Declaration of Independence, Franklin was now negotiating commercial and defence treaties with France in Paris. Why, goes the argument, should one of the most famous people in the entire world have bothered to talk to a little-known upstart like Graham? But of course they had a number of possible connections: Kinnersley, Philadelphia and indeed Catharine Macaulay, who had met Franklin in Paris in 1777. More significantly, they were bonded by one of the single greatest social influences of that century: not an individual or a place, but an organization. Like Graham, Franklin was a Freemason. He had a sworn duty to be ever alert to the claims of brotherhood.

Freemasonry was easily the biggest association in the Hanoverian British world. In Britain at least, although tales of clandestine Masonic rites involving rolled-up breeches, rolled-down stockings and bared chests were already circulating, Freemasonry was far from a secret society. Its members strutted in regalia in lively street parades and met openly in public houses. The Somerset House lodge used to meet behind the Temple of Health at the Adelphi Tavern. Both Graham's younger brother William and his friend Dr William Buchan were initiated into Masonry there in the spring of 1782, so this was most likely to have been the lodge where Graham practised the "craft" during his London years. (Records for the period are too sparse to be certain.)

Initiation into a lodge brought vast social, economic and indeed intellectual dividends for its members. Where else could coopers mix with counts, glaziers mix with gentlemen and vintners drink with viscounts? This was a new way of socializing, and one which bridged deep class divides. As increasing numbers from the aristocracy and royalty joined lodges throughout England and Scotland, Freemasonry became ever more fashionable. Many members were drawn by the merry-making, the food, drink and song that made meetings go with a swing. Others were attracted by the possibility of mental as well as social improvement. Graham must have particularly relished the dramatic ritual and symbolism of lodge ceremonials, elaborately lit by meaningful arrangements of candles. The Doctor eagerly incorporated elements of Masonic imagery into his own performances and pamphlets. When Graham designed the elaborate fake stained-glass windows at the Temple to indicate that he was a member "of that most ancient and honorable body", he made sure that the "ensigns of Masonry" (the level, the square and so on) were emblazoned in a prominent position on the lowest pane of the great centre window on the first floor, grouped together with wings on either side of a putative family arms. This was less surprising than it would be today: eighteenth-century trade cards often included the fact of membership.

Freemasonry made Graham part of a huge cosmopolitan family, linked to an inestimably valuable network of potential friends and equals across Europe and America. Thanks to the vast scale and organization of Freemasonry, this went way beyond any wishy-washy ideal of brotherhood and fraternal love: there were huge opportunities for patronage and mutual aid. This of course had particular advantages for Masons with itinerant careers like Graham. A system of Masonic certificates allowed newcomers to find their social footing and enjoy the recognition and benefits of lodge membership not just throughout Britain, but on the Continent and across the empire.

Enlightenment was a consistent theme running through eighteenth-century Freemasonry. Some lodges offered medical and scientific lectures to their members. One of the guiding lights of early British Freemasonry was the Newtonian experimental philosopher Desaguliers. When eighteenth-century Freemasons spoke, as they often did, of being enlightened, they used the term both intellectually and symbolically.

When Graham reached Paris, Franklin had recently become the "venerable" master of "La Loge des Neuf Sœurs", the Nine Sisters' Lodge, which has been described as the "UNESCO of the eighteenth century". This particular lodge was so dedicated to the diffusion of knowledge that it had formed an educational institution called "Le Musée de Paris". It had a particularly high proportion of foreign members, including Jan Ingen-Housz, Joseph Banks and Joseph Priestley. In the summer of 1779, preparations were beginning for a great celebration of Franklin's election, to take place in August. "No-one was more fashionable, more sought after in Paris than Doctor Franklin," recalled Vigée-Lebrun. "The crowd chased after him in parks and public places; hats, canes and snuffboxes were designed in the Franklin style, and people thought themselves very lucky if they were invited to the same dinner party as this famous man."

Graham was approaching the height of his powers at this point. This tall, handsome and eloquent man in his mid-thirties was himself turning heads quite literally. "I was walking the boulevards with him one day and all eyes were fixed on him," recalled another new acquaintance, Jean-Pierre Brissot de Warville, remembered now as the leader of the Girondists, then just another struggling young writer. He wrote that Parisians were impressed by Graham's noble and majestic expression. He had the kind of looks which commanded respect, all the more so when he spoke. According to Brissot, the splendid way that the Doctor expressed his opinions seemed at one with the ideas he was trying to convey. Brissot first encountered the Doctor at the home of another radical Freemason, Robert Pigott. He was one of Graham's most fervent converts and a member of the Somerset House Lodge. Three years previously, convinced that the outbreak of the war in America was a harbinger of imminent British disaster, Pigott had sold ancient family estates in Shropshire and fled for the continent. There he became infatuated with Voltaire, and moved in circles which certainly included Franklin. He was particularly inspired by Graham's vegetarian philosophy and became a "Pythagorean" – as vegetarians were known at the time – as zealous as the Doctor himself. Soon Pigott would be publicly singing the praises of the Celestial Bed, before getting thoroughly involved in the heady politics of the French revolution, when he became an ardent promoter of the "cap of liberty".

Brissot is the source of the first clue that, even then, Graham's disorganized approach to financial matters was beginning to get him into trouble. Waiting in prison to be guillotined at the height of the Terror in 1793, Brissot remembered his former friend: "Graham was poor and nearly always submerged in debt. These debts pointed to the enormous chaos of his business affairs, and this was something from which he needed to divert attention." Back in London, rent alone on Graham's Adelphi property was costing him £154 a year, the highest in the terrace, and he was pursuing quite extraordinarily grand plans for its interior. The Doctor's expenditure was spiralling all the time, and he urgently needed to begin to recoup his costs.

It was time to work his extravagant charm on extravagant new patients, now flocking to the spa resorts of the Low Countries. What had worked so well in Bath might prove even more successful at the watering places of all Europe's nobility. While Graham was sharing his philosophy of life and health in Paris with a young revolutionary in the making, the Spencer family was journeying slowly towards Aix-la-Chapelle.

Lord Spencer was one of the richest young men in England when Lady Spencer married him for love nearly a quarter of a century previously. Intelligent and remarkably well-educated, she soon used her enormous new wealth to distinguish herself as a committed and systematic philanthropist. Benevolence gave her life meaning, and mitigated her guilt about succumbing too often to the thrills of high-stakes gambling. "[W]hile I from many fortunate circumstances enjoy credit and reputation," she confessed a few years later in one of her almost daily letters to her son George, sobered by the sight of a cartload of prisoners on their way to the Tyburn gallows, "... my Conscience tells me how often I have swerved from my Duty and broke through my firmest resolutions." In another letter she exhorted him to make it a rule to set aside a suitable sum for charitable purposes four times a year, every quarter day: "If no objects present themselves you will soon amass a little fund of Charity which is the pleasantest thing in the world as it enables you freely and liberally to contribute when necessary... it will be less likely to make itself wings & fly away."

Her daughters inherited her gambling addiction with little of her self-control. The elder, now Georgiana Cavendish, the Duchess of Devonshire, had wed similar quantities of wealth but rather less love at the age of sixteen. Marrying into a powerful Whig dynasty in 1775, she entered the heart of the select and tyrannically fashionable group of aristocrats known as the "ton". Overnight, the Duchess became an adored national arbiter of taste, exerting her influence on hats, hairstyles and the ballot box alike. As her most recent biographer wrote: "the mere association of her name with a performer, a play, a book, or piece of china could ensure success." As one of her mother's friends once wrote, complaining of a lack of correspondence from the Duchess, "as I never hear of her I look in the newspapers to see if she has broke a leg or an arm…"

By the summer of 1779, the Duchess was exhausted by "racketing", politicking and a series of miscarriages. She arrived at Aix to recuperate with her parents and sister on 16th June, and after a tedious final leg through the woods along hilly unpaved roads they took lodgings at "La Court de Londre", a little way out, but "quiet and roomy". This small fortified town, now called Aachen, boasted an abundance of hot water springs, good company and picturesque scenery. It was also a favourite haunt of courtesans, full of appeal to those not too sick to socialize, and particularly successful in attracting the syphilitic. Georgiana Cavendish settled down into a routine of purging, enemas, early-morning bathing and drinking the recommended quantities of mineral water. Meanwhile her father gambled at cards (breaking the faro bank on occasion) and her mother took painting lessons and went walking on the ramparts and in the countryside with the Duchess's sister, Lady Harriet: "It is curious to see Mills turn'd by hot water and rivulets running smoking through the grass." Lady Spencer recorded every "bloody stool" her elder daughter passed, and anxiously evaluated the progress of her "evacuations".

Nowhere could the Spencers escape requests for their well-known compassion. The newly arrived Dr Graham was intriguing and plausible enough for Lord Spencer to recommend into his (fellow Freemason's) care a man who had approached him in desperate circumstances, financial and medical. Thirty-year-old David Nugent had suffered several sleepless years on account of a leg so swollen and ulcerous that surgeons at the Whitechapel Hospital had recommended amputation as the only cure. All the doctors in London had failed to help him; a very long course of Mr Norton's Maredaunt's antiscorbutic drops proved equally useless, his ankle became "thick as his thigh" in Brussels, and his pains only increased at Claude Fontaine. Arriving at Spa "in so putrid a state" it was feared he would infect the whole town, he pressed on to Aix-la-Chapelle, by this time so weak he fainted each time he bathed and "could scarce creep about on his crutches".

By the sixth day of Graham's ethereal and electric "medicines, applications and influences" the crutches were abandoned. The patient was reborn. It seemed miraculous. "Dr G.", as he referred to himself, ordered Nugent back to the clear warm waters of Spa, where the Spencers were now destined.

This is one of the rare moments when any information about Graham's family emerges. There is evidence he had a son and two daughters, but their dates and places of birth have proved impossible to trace. It is fair to assume that they were accompanying him on these European travels, since at this point some unspecified emergency involving one daughter took Graham back to Paris, at a cost of 35 guineas. Three weeks later though, he was rendezvousing with his new patrons in the celebrated Ardennes valley.

Spa was revelling in its most brilliant era. The diamonds adorning noble visitors in the ballroom and at the card tables of the recently built "Redoute" glittered as freely as its crystal-clear mineral springs. A nineteenth-century guidebook claimed that at least "thirty sovereigns and princes of the blood" assembled here in the resort's glory days, and "in ordinary years there were seldom less in Spa than 14 resident physicians". It was ridiculously easy to meet everyone: "the custom at Spa is to have [locally printed] cards delivered round by a man to announce your arrival, the compliment is immediately acknowledged by the visiting Tickets of those who have received them, by the same man. Thus you are introduced to persons of all nations... Ladies here are not at a loss for partners as they change every dance."

"Spa is doubtless the great rendezvous of Europe," effused Graham on his return to London, "yet such is the genius of the place, such the politeness of those who resort thither, that they seem all of the same country, and even of the same family. In that charming place, all is cordial unanimity, delicate attentions, gaiety of heart and brilliancy of spirit: for there the animal spirits mount up and sparkle like the waters of the Prouhon fountain! To soften, brighten, and embellish every scene, and to strew flowers in the general path, seems the general delight; and, in one word, to live happy in society, is *there* the only science, (gaming excepted) that is studied and practised in every company."

The Spencers were, of course, on easy terms with many of the other visitors, and it was a simple matter for a woman of Lady Spencer's social and fund-raising calibre to set up a "Subscription... for putting several poor under Doct. Graham's care." Here was a splendid and laudable diversion for wealthy holidaymakers. National differences were obliterated. This was despite what Lady Spencer described as the "horrid news from England, of the Spaniards having join'd the French so that we now have a War to support against the united forces of Spain in France and America, and much disturbance to quiet in

Ireland where their distresses and discontent are arisen to the highest Pitch." Marie-Antoinette's favourite and Georgiana's great admirer, Countess Jules de Polignac, her family and their friends began to balance their expenditure at cards with worthy contributions to the collection for Graham's unfortunates. Every guinea was carefully noted by their meticulous benefactor, Lady Spencer, and filed under "G". ("Method, you know, is my hobby-horse.") The Countess of Dammartin and the Marquis de Serent proved particularly generous.

Political leanings also had to be put aside in this idyllic retreat. Self-promotion was always necessarily coupled with pragmatism. Graham gratefully accepted a guinea from the "tall, lusty" and haphazardly progressive despot, "His serene Highness Frederick Prince of Hesse-Cassel". He also secured the Prince's valuable signature on a witness statement. But Graham, like all Europe, knew full well that the Landgrave's spare shillings were largely raised by the hiring-out of 12,000 "Hessian" mercenaries fighting at that very moment alongside his nephew George III's troops in the war in America, a war of which Graham never approved. The ambitious Doctor's bids for the attention of Europe's royalty required the kind of compromise familiar to his old friend Brissot, who has been romanticized by many since his execution as the epitome of Enlightenment idealism. Brissot persuaded his publisher to send specially bound copies of his first book to Frederick II of Prussia, as well as to Graham's other favourite continental monarch, Catherine the Great. "I am making my debut in literature, and my name is not at all known," justified Brissot in 1781. "As I want this work to cause a sensation, it must have the most publicity possible, it must be sent out everywhere, to all the crowned heads, and I will spare nothing to that end."

These were busy days for Graham. His supporters' contributions bought each of them a peculiar form of rational entertainment as well as a good conscience. Whiling away the empty hours in their prescribed "regimes", between carriage rides through the gardens surrounding the Geronstère spring and strolls in the shady Promenade de Sept Heures, Spa's temporary residents diverted themselves with inspections of Graham's "curious apparatus". It was considered no intrusion to settle down at the Château de Limbourg where he was staying, (now become "a crowded hospital") and watch the Doctor perform his daily operations – on monstrous prolapses, paralysed or gangrenous limbs, children with leprous scurfs or ghastly occupational injuries. This was taking the popular diversion of "medical recreation" to unusual heights. Dressing changes were apparently attended with fortitude, though the stench of "acrid, putrid matter, and bloody gore... flowing constantly" from the mouth and nostrils of one thirteen-year-old orphan was so bad that Graham insisted Lady Spencer surveyed the "shocking spectacle" from the doorway, a lavender-water-soaked handkerchief to her face. A paralysed painter's wife was one day cured of her palsy, but then a week later also relieved of "a considerable quantity of blood", and twenty-seven "long thick round LIVING WORMS".

(Two summers later, Lady Spencer's portly gambling friend Rachel Lloyd, a great fan of Dr Graham, took it upon herself to check up on this patient. "I have enquir'd after the poor woman that Graham cur'd of the Palsy, she is quite well, and has been so ever since, only in the very cold weather she had a little numbness in one of her hands, but it was very triffling, and did not hinder her from doing any sort of work. She prays for you every day of her Life. I can't hear of the other Patients yet, as they live at a distance, and I don't know their names, you will send them when you write next...")

Wherever Lady Spencer and her family went, "all the diseased of the place, and for many leagues round, flock[ed]... and crowd[ed] about... in a constant succession", frantic for their share of her "goodness" and "charity". Not surprisingly, throngs were soon forming around Graham's own house. It became a matter of daily routine for Lady Spencer, Lady Clermont, the Duke de Coigny, the Marquis de Serent and other grandees to pick out from the mob "such diseased objects as they judged most worthy of being relieved, such as the father or mother of a large family, or young worthy like person", and present their chosen cases to Graham for treatment. As far as Lady Spencer was concerned, "the best charity that can be done to a diseased or crippled poor person, is to restore them, if possible, to health, and to the proper use of their limbs so as to enable them to be useful members of society." Any deemed definitively incurable by Graham were dispatched with money and generous condolences. He described the sums handed out at his house in this cause as so huge that his own servants regularly burst into "tears of admiration and delight". Meanwhile the Devonshire and Spencer family staff "stood seemingly quite insensible and unconcerned; for to them, such scenes were no novelty".

In Spa, Graham achieved his best ever success in ensuring credit-worthy authentication for his cures. Surviving correspondence with Lady Spencer shows him summoning her urgently to look at particular patients prior to treatment, so that she could bear crucial witness to their before-and-after states: "Her Ladyship will find that the old woman has the looks – (sweetness and serenity) – of an Antediluvian Saint, or Dowager Angel," he wrote of one patient. The Marquis de Serent, who took a keen interest in curiosities, was, like Lady Spencer, assiduous in monitoring the progress of Graham's patients and his "Godlike acts" upon them. Lady Spencer's records match Graham's own accounts of his cures. Allowing for his usual hyperbole, Graham was undeniably responsible for transforming the lives of a significant number of individuals in a very short time.

Before Spa's illustrious visitors went their separate ways, and the patients at the Château de Limbourg went back to being useful to society, Graham staged one last triumphant public-relations exercise. He assembled at his house the now healthy men, women and children, newly clothed and with pockets lined, and invited their benefactors for a final inspection. "This was, indeed, a heavenly sight... which angels must applaud... the poor, but now happy people uttered the most expressive thanks." Lady Spencer was said to have turned from the company and exclaimed with tears of joy in her eyes: "'Is it possible that they can be the same creatures! How much true pleasure may thus be purchased at a small expence!" Thirteen of the group of observers volunteered their valuable names to bear witness to Graham's achievements: "seen, and certified, by us, as completely true and having happened before our very eyes during a very short time, which does great credit to the knowledge, zeal and humanity of Doctor Graham". Writing afterwards in thanks, Graham underlined his gratitude three times and begged leave to assure Lord and Lady Spencer, the Duchess of Devonshire, and Lady Clermont "that, he will earnestly pursue and improve every means to become, daily, a better Physician, and a better man". He almost certainly meant it.

Graham's publicity coup in attracting the attention of the Spencers and their well-connected European friends was immense, its immediate profitability less so. The subscription had raised nearly seventy guineas. This was a figure which one of the Spencers or their friends might win with ease on a good night at the card table. It would only have made a small dent in the bills mounting up in London. Having managed to keep up appearances with a wonderfully altruistic façade through late July and early August, he eventually came clean in a begging letter to Lady Spencer. "I left England... with 140 guineas expecting both money and honour as a Physician at Spa," wrote Graham in a letter obsequious with honesty. "In the same proportion that I have been disappointed of the former, I have been supremely fortunate in obtaining the latter, in being known to SUCH a family as my Lord Spencer's..." Yet even after the strictest economies, he now found himself seventy-five pounds short of the sum needed to clear "everything" at Spa and transport himself, his family and his apparatus back to London. He had tried selling his equipment, and various gold trinkets and jewels, with no success. "What chance have I of his Lordship attending to the impertinence of my little private concerns?!" Every chance, happily for Graham. The money was lent, but it was never repaid.

Back in London, Graham had too many other demands on his purse. He tried, as he had before, to underwrite his costs by offering an apprenticeship to any pupil-assistant willing to pay 1,000 guineas up front, and a hundred pounds a year "for board, &c., while he remains in my house". The Temple of Health was taking shape, but there was still much to be done. To "embellish" the wonders of his new apparatus, he was gathering together "the most precious treasures of nature and of art".

No aspect was neglected. Ingen-Housz, van Marum and other experimenters had recently been exploring the possibilities of electrobotany: what effect might electricity have on the germination and growth of plants? Pierre Bertholon, an inventive French priest and physics professor, would soon publish his ingenious designs for increasing crop production through special electrifying watering machines, and other intriguing devices, none commercially successful. Others tried to hatch chickens' eggs faster with the help of electricity. Alluding to developments like these, Graham began to assemble pots of "curious rare, and valuable plants, such as the balm of Gilead, roses, pineapples, &c." on the huge dome of his magnificent new Temple, installed upstairs in the Adelphi in the Great Apollo chamber. Being covered in metal, the dome functioned as yet another vast prime conductor. The point was to show electricity's amazing power in encouraging plant as well as human growth. In glass containers placed amongst these exotic fronds, gold and silver fish swam in impressive shoals. Whether these were alive or artificial, a silent shifty homage to Kinnersley's Philadelphian fish, is not clear.

He was also devising his uniquely eye-catching concoctions. Three types would be exhibited, continually brewing up in great, metal-lined, thirty-six-gallon globes, their names inscribed on each: Electrical Aether, Nervous Aetherial Balsam and Imperial Pills. None were patented. They were so inimitably complicated to make, he thought it unnecessary. (This also meant he escaped the tax on patent medicines imposed in 1783.) Medicinal powders had been mixed with water in Leyden jars ever since they were invented, in the belief that when the electric shock was administered, the medicine would somehow penetrate the patient's body along with the electric "fire". There had been some controversy in the late 1740s over a Venetian lawyer's invention of *intonacature*, as these medicated tubes were called. Benjamin Wilson was so intrigued he sent for special glass from Venice so that he could replicate the experiment down to the last detail. Nollet denounced the technique, but Priestley described Gianfrancesco Pivati's experiments as "a manifest example of the virtue of electricity". Pivati had concealed the strongly scented "balsam of Peru" in a glass cylinder, so that not a whiff of it could escape. Then a patient was electrified by the cylinder. When he later fell asleep at home, and began to sweat, he woke to find the whole room perfumed by the balsam, which had penetrated his clothing and bedclothes. Running a comb through his hair, he discovered it became strongly scented too. Clearly, making medicines by electrifying substances in tubes was nothing new. But until Graham, no one had dared make such a spectacle of it, incorporating the actual manufacture of medicine into the performance of healing.

Graham could only describe the extraordinary properties of his medicines by ascending to "the regions of metaphor", as he put it. "[I]f thro' extreme bodily fatigue and anxiety, I feel myself as it were crampt in a cold dark room, in a moment, by the means of the electrical aether, and nervous aetherial balsam, I find myself saluted as it were by love, joy and harmony! who in a moment fling open celestial scenes – and smiling, transport me on soft waving wings – with balmy and melodious gales, into the sweet, brilliant, and flowery palace where they, the handmaids of HAPPINESS, reside! illuminated with ten thousand lights of virgin wax! or warmed and gilded with a vernal, a meridian sun!"

One possible cause of these powerful effects could be seen bubbling away in apparatus in the first room of the Temple. Since Bath, Graham had been dabbling in pneumatic chemistry. Now it had become the height of fashion, a regular topic of newspaper discussion, and Graham put together a suitable array of equipment to display his expertise in the new gases that were causing such excitement. Meanwhile, his writing began increasingly to show the signs of a mind altered by the effects of inhaling them.

All through the 1770s, different "airs" were being produced, from saltpetre, brimstone, iron filings, mercuric oxide, liver of sulphur and other substances, each discovered to have different effects on candle flames, kittens, mice and mint plants. Joseph Priestley's crucial realization that atmospheric air is made up of different components, and his identification of oxygen and nitrous oxide, helped lead the way towards a host of other breakthroughs in the field. Listing his scientific heroes, Graham pronounced his indebtedness to "the great, judicious, and indefatigable Dr. PRIESTLEY", as well as John Pringle, expert on jail fevers and Priestley's champion at the Royal Society. Others key players in chemistry not named by Graham included the Duke of Devonshire's paralytically shy cousin Henry Cavendish and Antoine Lavoisier, who lost his head in the French Revolution, but gave oxygen its name and was proved right in his argument that Priestley's beloved "phlogiston" did not actually exist.

These were "surprizing" times, as Priestley kept noting, as he and his contemporaries continued their investigations into aerial chemistry. Rodents were gassed or suffocated in their hundreds. The first inklings of the process of photosynthesis emerged, and the fizzy-drinks industry took the first steps towards its rapid climb to world domination. The names that were bandied about – factitious airs, fixed air, aether and phlogiston – were unfamiliar, unstable, bewildering and impressive. Graham eagerly incorporated them into his vocabulary. Others wrote to the newspapers for elucidation: "What is the simple, clear, and unequivocal meaning of the term *fixed air*?" begged "A novice" in Lincoln's Inn, noting that such was "the present fashionable rage" for Philosophy that "even the Ladies consider this branch of science as a sure road to conquest".

Under Priestley's influence, the "goodness" of the air became a matter of medical and even moral concern. His invention of the nitrous air test to determine it had allowed the development of a popular new tool, the "eudiometer". At last the "salubricity" over which Thomas Short had agonized could be scientifically tested – or so it was briefly believed. Throughout Europe, the enlightened marched off with their eudiometers on environmental tours, monitoring the air quality in graveyards, factories, sewers, coastal areas and marshes.

Graham proudly displayed several at the Temple of Health, along with other intriguing new pieces of equipment – troughs of water, with air bubbling through into inverted bottles and tubes, oiled silk bags for administering these strange gases, bell jars and burning glasses. These were arranged in the first room visitors entered at the Temple of Health, on the terrace level. In another part of the same room, he placed metal shelves along a giant eleven-foot-long prime conductor, and lined up on these rows of vials and strangely shaped vessels, each with its own mysterious contents. All were supposedly being "acted upon" by the combination of electrical fire, magnetic influences and "various kinds of factitious air... and in such prodigious torrents, that [the Doctor and his colleagues claimed to be] capable of performing almost every process in chemistry, in a manner far superior to what is done by common culinary fire".

Standing on a table below canopied prints of Catherine the Great and the Grand Duke and Duchess of Russia was a glass-globed apparatus for carbonating water, a recent invention that had proved a great commercial success. (Graham's equipment was naturally far bigger than the standard.) Various hookahs were available for imbibing "aether condensed with nitrous or magnetic influences". An Indian one was inlaid with fine silver flowers, and its thirteen-foot brown-and-gold tube had a mouthpiece made of agate. Another was bright purple, decorated with gold, with a twining tube of crimson and gold, and a mouthpiece that could be changed according to the nature of patient's disease. Graham's displays publicly signalled his place at the cutting edge of technology and style alike.

Graham experimented with some caution, but possibly not enough. While he was in Newcastle, "two beautiful young ladies", probably suffering from a streptococcal throat infection, had been "hurried out of this world" by a physician trying to treat them with carbon dioxide. This was the "common fixed air" (discovered by Joseph Black) which Graham claimed had "killed so many people since it became fashionable to use it". The story was that the Newcastle doctor had filled the room with gases produced by pouring "some spirits or oil of vitriol" into a tub of chalk and water, so that the patients choked to death as the contents of the pail fizzed into the fetid atmosphere. Their family only just escaped. Happy to condemn, Graham is characteristically less precise about his own methods of making what he called his *vivifying and tempered fixed air*", or indeed what exactly he meant by this description. Since he so often lumped all his therapies together – ethereal effluvia, spirituous aromatic baths and musical influences, together with more straightforward magnetic and electric "fluids" – it is impossible to identify the independent or exact effects of any of them. But even allowing for his adventurous advertising strategies, the sensations he described after taking "electrical aether, and nervous aetherial balsam" are extraordinarily intense. They bear a striking resemblance to the effects of nitrous oxide:

> A thrilling extending from the chest to the extremities was almost immediately produced. I felt a sense of tangible extension highly pleasurable in every limb; my visible impressions were dazzling and apparently magnified, I heard distinctly every sound in the room and was perfectly aware of my situation... as the pleasurable sensations increased, I lost all connection with external things; trains of vivid images rapidly passed through my mind and were connected with words in such a manner, as to produce perceptions perfectly novel. I existed in a world of newly connected and newly modified ideas. I theorified; I imagined that I made discoveries. When I was awakened from this semi-delirious trance... [m]y emotions were enthusiastic and sublime... I exclaimed... *Nothing exists, but thoughts! the universe is composed of impressions, ideas, pleasures and pains!*

Humphrey Davy, the dark-haired poetry-writing young Cornishman who experienced these novel sensations, was employed by Thomas Beddoes to investigate "the physiological effects of the aëriform fluids" at the newly founded Medical Pneumatic Institution in Bristol in 1798. Davy described the impact of breathing twenty quarts of unmingled nitrous oxide in a closed box a few years after James Graham's death. It's now popularly known as laughing gas, but in 1794 was sometimes called "vital air". Thanks largely to Davy's meticulous records of experiments with the gas on himself and others, his enticing pamphlets and his spellbinding skills in public speaking, laughing gas became a widespread craze in the early nineteenth century. Medical students giggled legitimately in lectures, members of the public queued up to inhale the stuff at glitzy theatres, and Davy himself was addicted. But when Graham was designing the Temple of Health, its effects were barely known.

"[W]e must either invent new terms to express these new and particular sensations, or attach new ideas to old ones, before we can communicate intelligibly with each other on the operation of this extraordinary gas," declared James Thomson, after experiencing "that peculiar thrill" of becoming one of Davy's experimental subjects in Bristol. Another compared the feeling with that of ascending some high mountains in Glamorganshire. A Mr Wansey experienced "sensations so delightful, that I can compare them to no others, except those which I felt (being a lover of music) about five years since in Westminster Abbey, in some of the grand choruses in the Messiah, from the united powers of 700 instruments of music". A paralysed patient said after breathing nitrous oxide, "I felt like the sound of a harp." The effect on a Norfolk rector whose ulcerated leg improved after inhaling "the VITAL AIR diluted with a portion of atmospheric" was to produce "a constant gaiety, as if I had been drinking champagne". Others agreed, and H. Cardwell confessed to "feelings so pleasurable as almost to destroy consciousness"; he was "almost convulsed with laughter".

Beddoes and Davy made the first systematic study of pneumatic chemistry in relation to medicine, but described it as "an art in infancy" over two decades after Graham first began to practise it. It wasn't until 1848 that ether was first publicly demonstrated as an anaesthetic. To judge from their records, if the electric doctor was regularly submitting himself and his patients to nitrous oxide, it was hardly surprising they were all feeling better. "I am certain that my muscular strength was for a time much increased," noted Thomson after Davy's dose. The poet Robert Southey experienced "a sensation perfectly new and delightful", but more significantly, "during the remainder of the day, imagined that [his] taste and hearing were more than commonly quick". He was sure that he felt himself "more than usually strong and cheerful". Southey told Davy that he supposed "the atmosphere of the highest of all possible heavens to be composed of this gas". It was a remark that could have come from Graham's own pen.

Graham's visual demonstrations of elemental forces had a persuasive part to play in building up the scientific mystique of the Temple. He also displayed electrometers, lodestones, ornamented rods and tubes for various purposes, magnetic bandages, medicine cups made of horn, silver, glass, wood and magnetized materials, and other intriguing pieces of equipment. The "treasures of... art" had less obvious relevance to its philosophical themes, but were selected with a similar eye for taste and function. Even the family Bible, used for daily dawn worship led by Graham in the Great Apollo Apartment, was a fine Baskerville folio, "printed on royal polished paper, elegantly bound in red turkey leather, and very richly gilt". But the most dramatic elements came from "Mr. Cox's stupendous Museum itself".

Anyone who had gasped at James Cox's towering, bejewelled automata when they were showcased in his fashionable museum in Spring Gardens in 1772 and 1775 would have been delighted by this selective re-staging. One contemporary observer of the London scene, D'Archenholz, saw the Cox collection several times,

> ...always with fresh admiration. Never was taste and grandeur, all the skill of mechanics, and the magic of optics, united in such a high degree of perfection. The eye met with nothing but gold, diamonds, and precious stones which were shaped into the forms of a variety of animals; assumed their gestures, and seemed to be alive; birds of different kinds and of exquisite plumage sung the most ravishing notes; the swan of Europe swam in artificial rivers; the hare and partridges ran about in groves, planted by the hands of the most cunning workmen; while camels, elephants, and other productions of Asia, stalked around, and imitated nature with a scrupulous exactitude.

Cox was another of the eighteenth century's great entrepreneurs, a spectacular speculator who was also briefly the owner of Oliver Cromwell's embalmed head. He had successfully exported nearly three quarters of a million pound's worth of luxuries in the late 1760s and early 1770s, mainly to the Far East. China and India briefly went wild for his breathtaking musical automata and richly ornamented objets d'art, known as "sing-songs". But it was a risky market, particularly since these expensive items were rarely commissioned, but made "on spec". When demand in the East fell, Cox opened his museum in London. As a skilled retailer, who shared Graham's genius for publicity, he was quick to add his voice to those who defended luxury for its contribution to the national economy. His productions, he claimed, afforded employment to an army of "ingenious artists", and gave "pleasure to every friend to commerce and the elegant arts".

The doors of a disused Huguenot Chapel in Spring Gardens, off the Mall, had opened in February 1772 to reveal a magnificently decorated and carpeted room, warm air wafting through it. It was packed with huge mechanical music boxes, in the shape of exotica like temples and elephants: one took the form of a twelve-foot-high bird cage, moving and singing and executed in gold, silver and jewels. Vast sparkling velvet sofas, crimson and gold, mirrors and "convex glasses", thrones, altars, vases, fountains and cascades completed the effect. For years, the building would be known as "formerly Cox's Museum". His catalogue's motto reflected the uneasy convictions of his generation: *Quid est quod arte effici haud queat?* ("What is there which cannot be achieved by art?") This was as ambiguous as the lifelike movements of his animated figures.

An exorbitant entrance fee and lines of visitors were not enough to save Cox, heading rapidly for ruin for the second time in his life. Neither was a national lottery. Eventually, Cox was declared bankrupt in November 1778, and so freed from the pressures of his creditors. Graham returned from his grand tour of Europe in time for a sale in Fleet Street "of fittings and fine embellishments" from the Spring Garden's Museum advertised for 6th–7th October 1779. Cox's 1772 catalogue referred to Johann Zoffany's paintings "on ovals of copper" of George III and his wife, Queen Charlotte, which sound remarkably similar to those Graham saluted with his philosophical cannon in the Temple: "These Royal portraits are magnificent beyond description, they are plac'd in frames of metal finely wrought and richly gilt, from whence issue numberless rays forming a glory or irradiation like beams of the sun, in various reflected colours of light, some of which, when in motion, appear like liquid fire extending on every side."

Would such a splendid backdrop enable Graham to make the crucial transition from worthy medical entertainer of the nobility to personal physician of the truly rich and mighty? Lady Spencer had her doubts. Georgiana, on the other hand, was now quite desperate to conceive. It was unthinkable that she should not provide a son and successor for the formidable Devonshire estates. Five and a half barren years were doing little for a marriage that had never been very convincing. Her own husband was rumoured to be the only man in England not in love with the Duchess of Devonshire. In October, Georgiana Cavendish consulted Dr Graham on her own account. A more desirable celebrity client could hardly be envisaged.

Four years later, Graham alluded to her treatment in his *Lecture on Generation*. He does not mention Georgiana by name, but refers to "a beautiful and truly virtuous lady, of rank and of immense fortune, who... had unfortunately been married when too young, even at the age of sixteen... A great estate, many virtues I believe on both sides, and noble titles, demanded heirs". The regimen was more sophisticated than that prescribed to the Dutch wife in Philadelphia. It consisted of daily electrifications for an hour or two, bathing on alternate days in deep cold water strongly scented with aromatic herbs, and drinking sage and liquorice root juice washed down with Spanish wine or sparkling German spa water. Wine and spa water also had a crucial topical application. The Duchess had "the good sense and the resolution" (and she must have needed an awful lot of the latter) "every night and morning, I believe for several months, to pour a whole large flask of the same water, or of the Champaign wine, cooled in ice, into and upon the fountain of life!" Another patient told to douche and wash her vagina in the same way, to pour "the icy cold vivifying clement into and upon the bower of bliss", was alarmed at the oddity of the advice. "She startled at the seeming danger of complying with the eccentric, or rather concentric prescription! – and I believe, more innocently than archly exclaimed, 'dear doctor! will that not give *it* cold! – will it not make IT sneeze? – surely it can never be safe!'" This patient persevered with the prescription, and apparently experienced "the most excellent effects".

In the autumn of 1779, though happy to continue to give financial support to some of Graham's most needy patients, the discreet and ever watchful Lady Spencer cautioned her daughter not to listen to Dr Graham "with regard to internal medicines", but rather to take advice from the family physician, dependable Dr Warren. The rest of this letter has since been tantalizingly torn off, so it is impossible to know whether Lady Spencer was trying to warn the Duchess away from Graham per se, or if she was happy for her to make use of his electrical, magnetic and "aetherial" treatments. Nor, of course, is it clear what her definition of "internal" might have been. But after a few months, Georgiana's appointments with Graham came to a speedy end anyway. Her husband had at last given her a child to love. It was just not her own. But with surprisingly rapturous pleasure, Georgiana adopted little Charlotte, the nervous, affectionate and illegitimate daughter of the Duke's late mistress.

That winter saw a near-endless stream of workmen trooping in and out of the Royal Terrace. In were brought hookahs and air pumps, electrometers and Leyden jars, fumigators and decorative tripods. Antique busts arrived, followed by china cockerels, statues, prints and allegorical oil paintings featuring cornucopias and willow branches, rabbits and mules. Fake stained-glass windows painted on fine white silk appeared behind the first-floor balconies. Their inscriptions and vivid images – altars, moons, suns, planets, gods, temples, owls and doves, serpents and phoenixes – were so extravagant with symbolic import they had to be decoded at length by Graham in his publicity material. A sign was put up over the front door, with "TEMPLUM

ÆSCULAPIO SACRUM" in gold letters, to show that the building was consecrated "to the great purposes of preserving and restoring health".

Inside, just by his favourite chair, a trapdoor and a huge, hollow, flint-glass tube with gilt brass mountings were inserted in the middle of the floor. They connected the terrace-level front parlour where Graham received his wealthy patients with the laboratory below. The Doctor needed only to call down to his apothecary, or to drop down a written prescription into the box waiting on the table in the room underneath, and, on the tinkling of a bell, an underling could pop up with whatever was required through the trapdoor. "[T]he servant springs up and descends thro' the floor in a moment..." Even further down, a forty-foot-long green baize bench was built for the subterranean street that ran nearly a hundred feet below. This linked the river bank to the Strand, and gave inconspicuous access to the servants' hall in the basement. Here "the poorer sort of people" could be kept safely out of the way of grander patients when they queued for free advice and electrical treatments (and expensive bottles of medicine) from six till nine, morning and night.

But it was not just furnishings, apparatus and what even those most generously disposed towards Graham and his methods might call "props", that were required. Graham was on the hunt for employees, robust models of health and happiness who could illustrate his medical theories in their very persons.

Graham advertised for a female assistant. He needed a "genteel, decent, modest, young woman" who was "personally agreeable, blooming, healthy and sweet-tempered... She is to live in the Physician's family, to be daily dressed in white silk robes with a rich rose coloured girdle. If she can sing, play on the harpsichord or speak French, greater wages will be given. Enquire Dr Graham, Adelphi Temple." More would be required of this paragon than merely sitting demurely before an audience, like the young Quaker girl he had employed in Philadelphia.

The Doctor certainly had good taste. From among the streetwalkers and actresses who jostled for trade and patronage in the bars and theatres near the Strand, Graham picked out a young girl whose face would soon be familiar to every man in England. Emy Lyon, who eventually became Emma, Lady Hamilton, wife of the British Ambassador in Naples and finally Nelson's mistress, had spent a childhood tediously confined to a poor mining village in North Wales. At the age of twelve Emy Lyon bravely made the long coach journey

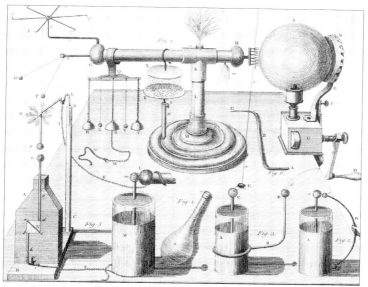

Eighteenth-century electrical apparatus of the kind
used by Ebenezer Kinnersley in his lectures.

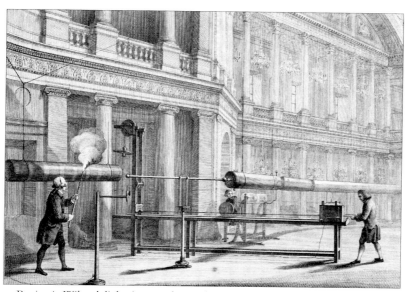

Benjamin Wilson's lightning-conductor demonstration at the Pantheon, 1778, as
shown by Michelangelo Rooker, the scenery painter who later reproduced the
Temple of Health on stage for the show *The Genius of Nonsense*.

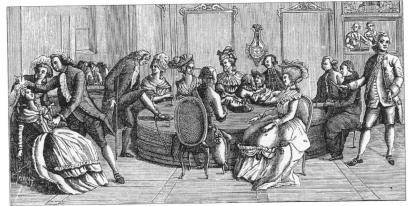

"Mesmer's Tub": animal magnetism in operation in Paris.

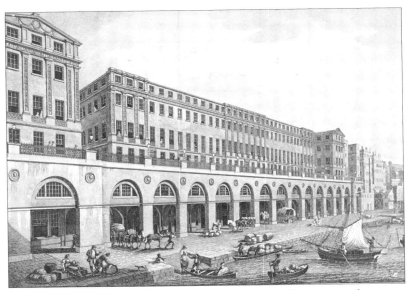

The Adelphi, the speculative development built on the Thames waterfront
by the Adam brothers, where Graham opened his first Temple of Health.

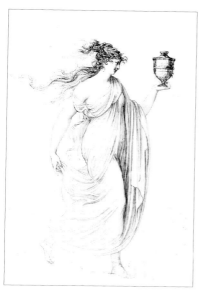

Emy Lyon, who later became Emma, Lady Hamilton, posing as Vestina, the Goddess of Health.

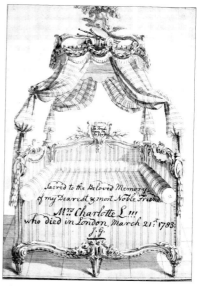

A print signed by Graham and labelled "the Celestial Couch or Sofa".

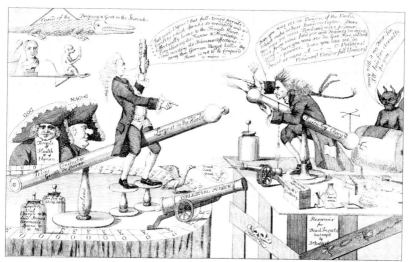

A caricature showing Graham electrically duelling with his chief rival in the field of entrepreneurial medicine, Dr Katterfelto.

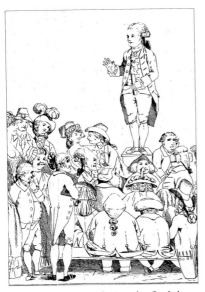

Graham lecturing during the final days
of the Temple of Hymen, with Fox,
Wilkes and Perdita among the audience.

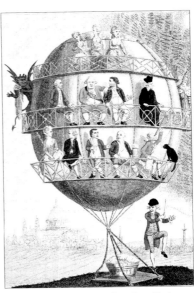

A cartoon from 1783 showing Graham
and his Vestina about to ascend to the
heavens along with Dr Katterfelto and
other assorted has-beens.

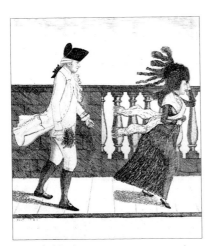

Probably the most accurate portrait
of Graham in existence, by Edinburgh
artist John Kay.

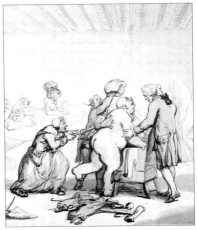

Satirical view of Graham's
earth-bathing establishment.

to London, where she found domestic work first in the home of a doctor in Blackfriars, then with a musical and theatrical impresario called Thomas Linley. Before long though, her pretty face, sociability and lively ambitions had pitched her into the myriad temptations of London's seamy nightlife.

She thought she could become an actress, trading on her voguish beauty. After all, she did look as though she had just stepped out of a classical-revival painting. Her straight nose, wide-set eyes and heart-shaped face, not to mention a rounded and well-proportioned figure, were exceptionally striking. But she only made it to wardrobe mistress's assistant in Drury Lane before getting the sack. Prostitution was the only livelihood left to a country girl at loose in London with no connections. At the mercy of pimps, pickpockets and sex tourists, Emma would have leapt at this job at the Temple of Health. Here was an unrivalled opportunity to leave the streets. A handsome and charming doctor who was confidently predicting that she would soon be entrancing the leading lights of London's nobility and aristocracy had offered her work, board and lodging, some family life and a daily dose of the Bible. For Emma this was a chance to claw her way back towards respectability. Ironically, in the hands of satirists, journalists and later biographers, her work with Graham would become a mocking symbol of her sleazy past.

At the Temple, Graham dressed her in Grecian sandals and fine flowing drapery which both revealed and concealed her flawless body. While William Hunter displayed the insides of dead, diseased and decaying bodies at his anatomy classes in Great Windmill Street, Dr Graham planned to do exactly the opposite. He wanted to educate his audiences with a living specimen of physical perfection. He taught Emma how to pose gracefully as Vestina, the Goddess of Health, and produced her like a showman. She was the epitome of health and wholesome fertility. Her movements were reflected in every gilded mirror, glanced off numberless shiny surfaces, and curved round the vast silver ball at the top of the fourteen-foot-high grand electrical-magnetic throne in the Apollo chamber. In a pen-and-wash sketch by Richard Cosway, Emma appears as a perfect fusion of classical, medical and erotic archetypes. Her luxuriant wavy hair flies out behind her, and she gazes, smilingly and modestly, not at the audience, but at a votive urn. In true celestial style, Vestina even seems to be walking on air.

Her future husband, the diplomat and collector Sir William Hamilton, eventually bought his second wife from his own nephew like just another objet d'art, paying off his debts in exchange for his mistress. "After many years of devotion to the arts and the study of nature, Hamilton found the acme of these delights in the person of an English girl… she lets down her hair and, with a few shawls, gives so much variety to her poses that the spectator can hardly believe his eyes," wrote Goethe when he encountered her in Naples. Sir William developed the "attitudes" Graham had taught her until Emma's *tableaux vivants* were celebrated throughout Europe. He tutored her in antique gesture, drawing on expertise derived from a superb collection of vases and Graeco-Roman sculpture, so that her emotion-laden poses were instantly recognizable to fellow connoisseurs. He even had a life-sized box made with a black border so that she could be framed as a living work of art. Emma revelled in these performances, adored the publicity, and loved nothing better than to be painted, as indeed she was, over and over again.

It seems appropriate that while Emma was earning a living as a goddess, promoting fecundity among the sparkling pillars and shining domes at the Adelphi, Sir William had stumbled on a more obscure erotic sideshow. On the streets around Naples he noticed poor women and children ornamented with unmistakably phallic amulets. (It was his "taste for antiquities" and their similarity to ancient Roman ones which attracted his attention, he claimed.) These were meant to ward off the evil eye and work as fertility aids. Then, to the ambassador's astonishment, he learnt of a three-day festival of the modern Priapus, St Cosmo, celebrated each year in Isernia, near Abruzzo. A new road had made the town more accessible, and priests soon began to stamp out the tradition, but in 1780 an acquaintance reported the sales of huge numbers of wax votive offerings "representing the male parts of generation, of various dimensions, some even of the length of a palm". They were mostly bought by women, who took their "Vows" to church, kissed them devoutly, and presented them with a financial offering to "Blessed St Cosmo", with the words *così lo voglio*, "let it be like this". At the great altar, sick members of the congregation would uncover any unhealthy part of their body, penises included, to be anointed by the reverend canon.

Had he but known of it, this phallus worship would have made an excellent footnote to James Graham's forthcoming *Lecture on Generation* – although the Catholic backdrop might have alarmed some of the audience. In his palatial new premises, Dr Graham, cheerfully writing lectures, lyrics and publicity for his new venture, was brimming over with excitement. On either side of the fireplace, his expanding medical notes were now alphabetically filed away behind green silk curtains and latticework doors, separated by sex, with a male and female antique bust guarding each. His glass chute was to hand. His apparatus gleamed invitingly. In the absence of an audience, the female dragon was taking a rest from breathing out fire, but continued to fly across the room, wings outstretched. And two storeys above, in the airy front room just to the right of the orchestra, Graham had installed his "completely insulated magnetico-electrical bed, the first and only one that now is or ever was in the world". The Doctor felt thoroughly equipped to deal with his affairs with all the "prudence, attention and dispatch which form the soul of business".

The extended promotional "Sketch", which described the Temple in every splendid detail, resounded with the glorious self-assurance of a man about to take the world by storm. In just a few years, he confidently declared, he would probably give up practical medicine, and start teaching medicine and philosophy in public "academical lectures" (intended "for the good of the human species of every nation and clime, even for the children of those who shall be born a thousand years hence"). Graham's ambitions were extensive. He would publish "a complete System of Prophylactic and Practical Medicine", to contain "the whole art (without even a shadow of reserve)" of preventing *and* curing disease. He was also considering giving the benefit of his attention to religion, and publishing "a complete and rational Body of Divinity". This would articulate a "true vital religion", prey to none of the inconsistencies or prejudices of existing forms of Christianity. But this was not all. Having reformed medicine and religion, there was still Law to be rewritten: "I may send into the world... a manual of Human Prudence, and a SIMPLE, yet full and naturally digested code of laws for civil, political and ecclesiastical government." These works would all naturally be submitted with great deference to the relevant powers-that-be. In his zeal for reform, he even tried to inaugurate new forms of punctuation, suggesting that an inverted exclamation mark might express "abhorrence or contempt".

His aspirations were born of a sensation of power and control. In this uncertain world, where disease swirled invisibly in every crowded assembly room, where war tore families apart and divided nations, where weakness bred weakness, and death picked its victims from slave ships and battlefields, Dr Graham believed he had discovered a way to organize the very elements. "I have it in absolute command

and subjection," he wrote of his scientific apparatus. It was a fantasy of intellectual and physical control over the natural world almost certainly partly fuelled by nitrous oxide. There were also less tangible forces at play

Graham was a man who hovered hungrily on the edge of acceptability. But his social ambitions were not entirely straightforward. Despite his fondness for show and pomp, his desire for personal wealth was far outstripped by his longing for recognition – Brissot backed up Graham's assertion that he could live perfectly happily on a few potatoes. The Doctor's desire to improve the lot of his species was genuine and he was writing about it at this point with all the nervous excitement of someone on the verge of a huge achievement. Yet his claims to have complete dominion over mankind seem to have been generated by something more pathological than either ambition or social anxiety. His characteristic exuberance was beginning to shade into a kind of mania, even delusion.

Graham boasted that he had ransacked "the four quarters of the globe" to assemble his unequalled collection of "healing influences", and make it the best perhaps "ever thought of" (always a favourite phrase). "[A]nd the four elements themselves, air, earth, fire and water have been courted so as seemingly to blend or even alter the immutability of their respective natures – living imprisoned, jaring and reluctant, or dying in tortures on a human rack – acquiring new powers, or assuming new natures in the mighty – the tremendous conflicts! Thus subjecting as it were, NATURE herself – to Man!"

6

The Bed

"I cannot fail of acquiring a fortune equal to my highest ambition and I look forward, delighted, at the prospect of immortal fame!!!"

"Here is charming weather come again for my Lord Spencer," wrote plump Miss Lloyd in early June 1780. Thunderstorms had followed a month of overpowering heat, and the Spencers were in Bath, tending the head of the family's dreadful gout: "…a full south wind and not a cloud in the sky. I hope it's the same with you. I am going to Dine at Lord Waldegrave's, but I am not without my fears, on account of Lord George Gordon being to Present a Petition to the House of Commons to repeal some Acts in favour of Roman Catholicks, to day, at the head of twenty thousand people, who he has summoned to meet him in St George's fields, that I wish I was not to be so near them as Whitehall."

She had every reason to be concerned. That twenty thousand quickly swelled to well over twice that number. From the terrace of the Adelphi, bagpipes and the tramp of multiple marching feet could be heard as a sea of blue cockades steadily swarmed over the bridges at Blackfriars and Westminster. The processions converged ominously around the Houses of Parliament, having been joined en route by yet more crowds, now thickened with opportunistic troublemakers. As the legislators began to arrive, their carriages were efficiently surrounded. Peers of the realm were attacked, pelted with mud, and forced to cry "No Popery!" Lord Gordon, the deeply eccentric and fanatical MP who had whipped up this frenzy, could do nothing to control the situation. His anti-papist demonstration exploded into an incoherent, violent and drunken riot, long remembered afterwards with real horror as "a time of terror". Over the next five days, London came close to anarchy. By day the crowds seemed to simmer down, only to bubble over with fresh vigour each night. Catholics rich and poor, suspected sympathizers and unpopular figures of authority were all targeted. Chapels and private houses were besieged, looted and burnt with little discrimination, and even "popish canaries" were condemned to the flames, still singing wildly. Prisons were destroyed and over sixteen hundred convicts set free, some reluctantly. Irish immigrants were particularly victimized. The Bank of England itself was attacked.

On the Tuesday evening, Lord Mansfield, astonished to find himself a target, escaped with his wife through a back door minutes before his house was stormed. Pictures, fine furniture and every book he owned, along with legal reports and priceless manuscripts – "the choicest... ever known in the possession of an individual" – came hurtling through broken windows onto the bonfires below in Bloomsbury Square. Lady Anne Erskine lived with a leading Methodist, Lady Huntingdon, whose chapel was said to be marked out for destruction on the same night:

> We were surrounded by flames! Six different fires – with that of Newgate among the rest towering to the clouds – being full in our view at once, and every hour in expectation of this house and beautiful chapel making the seventh... The flames all around had got to such a height that the sky was like blood with the reflection of them. The mob so near we heard them knocking the irons off the prisoners; which, together with the shouts of those they had released, the huzzas of the rioters, and the universal confusion of the whole neighbourhood make it beyond description! Every moment fresh reports coming in of fresh fires being broke out some true, some false; some that Parliament House was on fire, others the Archbishop's Palace at Lambeth; but all agreeing in our danger.

As the rumours and smoke reached James Graham, who had always been outspoken about his tolerance for all religions, he must have been praying that the rioters were unaware of either his political views or the valuable contents of his house. The sound of smashing glass was everywhere a precursor to the burning and looting. Graham had a lot to break. The glorious future he had anticipated for himself suddenly looked as fragile as the apparatus on which it was founded. Did Graham bite his tongue, adopt a blue cockade, light up his windows, and chalk "No popery" on his own front door? Or was the Adelphi enough of an island to escape the worst, its exceptional fire precautions too well publicized for rioters to bother testing? One wealthy neighbour, Wilke's lawyer John Reynolds, certainly made plans to flee to France, moving family and possessions to Kent in readiness. "Many noble and other families were employed all yesterday and last night, in removing most of their valuable effects, expecting their houses to fall a sacrifice to the ungovernable fury of the mob," reported *The London Chronicle*. Graham at least had the advantage of basements and nearby underground vaults where his most precious furniture and apparatus could be moved for relative safekeeping. But he also had alarmingly clear views across London from the roof of the Royal Terrace. By Wednesday night the area between Holborn and Fleet Street was burning "like a volcano". The resented tollgates on Blackfriars Bridge had been destroyed. The dead, drunk and wounded were tumbling into the Thames, down steps that had launched a thousand transportations. Several fire engines were pumping gin from the cellars of a Catholic distillery in Holborn, to the profit of a few, until the stills themselves exploded and raw gin and rum poured out freely over the cobbles. Unable to believe their luck, men and women fell to their knees to gulp it up, but the fiery unrectified spirits burned like acid. Soon they were seen motionless, in contorted postures, with swollen tongues and blue faces, oblivious to the songs of intoxicated carousers all around them, senseless to the screams of abandoned babies and terrified children.

Walpole, who later referred to that day as "black Wednesday", reported that lines were drawn across the Strand and Holborn that night to prevent the mob from coming west again. This action probably saved Graham and the Adelphi. London and Westminster were put under martial law. 285 rioters were killed, and hundreds more wounded and arrested over this short period. Over the next few months or so, the trials, convictions and hangings of rioters were reported in the newspapers on a daily basis and makeshift gallows appeared all over town. A wax effigy of Lord Gordon became a popular attraction in Paris, but his life was eventually spared, after a spell in the Tower of London charged as a traitor. The work of rebuilding the ruins began. By 17th June, the first of many versions of events had been rushed to press: "This day is published 'RIOTS IN LONDON' price 1s... A plain and succinct narrative of the late riots and disturbances in the cities of London and Westminster, and Borough of Southwark." Other letters and advertisements for newly published pamphlets quickly followed, addressing every conceivable aspect of the topic – one from "a staunch Whig", another on the subject of "The Romish Horseleech".

"You may insert your opinions on any public matter in the newspapers, with a certainty of being read a thousand times," wrote a Prussian visitor to England that year. "Every thing in London is made known by means of hand-bills or advertisements in the newspapers. One person informs you that his MAD-HOUSE is at your service; a second keeps a boarding-house for ideots; and a good-natured man-midwife pays the utmost attention to ladies in *certain situations*, and promises to use the most scrupulous secrecy… Physicians offer to cure you of all manner of disorders, for a *mere trifle*, and as for the money to pay them, you need never be at a loss; thousands daily making tenders of their services to procure you, *at a moment's notice*, any sum that you may stand in need of."

Graham of course went one step further. As soon as London seemed sufficiently settled, he employed two of the largest men he could find, dressed them in the finest livery and huge three-cornered hats trimmed with gold lace, and sent them round town with his new handbills. Samuel Curwen, a Salem loyalist self-exiled to England at the outbreak of the American revolution, spent nine long, lonely years on the other side of the Atlantic from his unhappy wife. One cloudy day that summer, he rambled up the Strand to call on his shirt-maker before passing by the Adelphi:

[T]he object that met my eye was 2 remarkably large and fullfaced men whose fierce countenances in length and breadth resembled Satan's shield by Milton compared to full moon. They were habited like an Oxford Music Doctor in his gown, and standing on either corner of Adam street, with each a paper bundle standing erect in a grave thoughtful posture with a face soliciting look; on taking one a penny was demanded, it was a sheet and ½ pamphlet containing, "a sketch of the Temple of health!, in Center of Royal Terrace Adelphi." N.B. the priest is a Doctor Graham of as consummate appearance as ever dealt in mockery.

Delighted Londoners quickly dubbed Dr Graham's vast porters Gog and Magog, after the enormous wooden statues at the Guildhall of two legendary pagan giants associated with Albion's ancient origins. They are considered the traditional guardians of the City of London and appear in the Lord Mayor's annual show to this day. Here was a new take on the clowning "Merry Andrews" traditionally used by workaday quacks to drum up custom. Graham's Gog and Magog attracted such crowds that they ended up at the Guildhall several times themselves, arrested for causing just the kind of "Nuisance" that alarmed the authorities in the wake of the recent riots.

It was all good publicity for the Doctor though, who through the spring and early summer had been so busy gathering patients and supervising electrical treatments that he claimed not to have had "leisure for even the necessary refreshments which nature requires", let alone "the honour and pleasure of waiting on the nobility, men of learning and science, and gentry" who came to see his apparatus. On 1st July he officially opened the Temple of Health "for the inspection of the Public". For 2s 6d, anyone could come to marvel, from six in the morning till nine at night. For twice that price, Dr Graham himself would exhibit "a most brilliant display of the Apparatus". This took place every evening, from half-past eight till half-past ten, and advance tickets could be delivered by the porters.

The "solemn dedication" began at noon, making the most of the Temple's south-facing aspect. As the eerie tones of the glass harmonica sounded offstage, combining with organ, flute and the plucked notes of a little harpsichord, the room was filled with light: Graham's stage direction commanded "*The Sun [to blaze] in its Meridian Splendour*". Two Grecian-robed young women and their priest-like male companion burst into an extraordinary recitative:

Hail! Vital Air –Aethereal! – Magnetic Magic – Hail!
Thine Iron Arm – thy bracing sinewy Arm! is everlasting Strength!
Hail! Harmony! – Music Divine!!! – thrice Hail! – Thy Soul is Love – Joy – Peace – and Health!
And thou, celestial Fire! – Thou, FIRE ELECTRIC! – GREAT RENOVATOR! – THE LIFE OF ALL THINGS! Hail!

The music then changed and suddenly the room was bathed in a soft pinkish light, as "rose-coloured silken Curtains" were quickly swept across the window. A sprightly song piled more praises on sacred Health – "The Monarch's Bliss! The Beggar's Wealth" – before the organ began to swell once more, a "GRAND CHORUS" rang out, and the audience was suddenly enveloped in darkness. As Graham described it, the apartment was instantly lit up, Kinnersley-style, with thousands of electrical stars and heavenly bodies shining brightly. The singers burst out with yet more paeans to the "Fire Electric", whose hand "flings the Rose of Health o'er the pale Cheek of Sickness", and then the Doctor rose to deliver a "poetical address" to the assembly.

He spoke of "the whole art of enjoying health and vigour, of body and of mind, and of preserving and exalting personal beauty and loveliness; or, in other words, for living with health, honour, and happiness in this world, for at least a hundred years".

A newspaper report that appeared eventually in Berlin and finally Moscow described the regular evenings that succeeded this launch in some detail, inflating the entry fee considerably for dramatic effect:

> Garlands, mirrors, crystals, gilt and silver ornaments are scattered about with profusion, so that from all parts they reflect a dazzling light. Music precedes each lecture, from 5 o'clock till 7, when Dr Graham presents himself vested in Doctor's robes. On the instant there follows a silence which is interrupted only at the end of the lecture by an electric shock given to the whole audience by means of conductors hidden under the cushions with which the seats are covered. Whilst some jest at the astonishment of others, a 'spirit' is seen to emerge from under the door of the room; it presents the appearance of a man of gigantic stature, thin and haggard, who, without uttering a word, hands the Doctor a bottle of liquor which, after having been shown to the company, is carried off by the spirit. To this strange apparition succeeds a pretty woman under the form of the Goddess of Music, who after singing six pieces, vanishes in her turn. Dr Graham having finished the lecture, the audience breaks up without daring to express regret for the six guineas expended on so extraordinary a spectacle. Before the sittings the Doctor makes a public offer to dissipate melancholy and mitigate extravagant gaiety.

Graham's lecture had yet to develop into the "libidinous" one that got him into so much trouble the following year. Before long Graham would be delivering a breathtakingly direct explanation of how to have babies, which radically equated sexual health with sexual pleasure. At this stage Graham tried to confine himself to "explaining the true nature and effects of Electricity, Air, Music, and Magnetism, when applied to the human body". His insulated magnetic and electric bed was only fleetingly mentioned in promotional material. It even took a few months for "Vestina, the Rosy Goddess of Health" to make her appearance in newspaper advertisements. But soon sealed copies of "private medical advice to those married ladies and gentlemen, who are not blessed with children" would become available for a guinea to be read discreetly at home, where spouses could discover in privacy "such Precepts as will, if duly attended to, make Man and Wife *Sweeter, Lovelier* and more *Desirable* in each other's Eyes". And of course how best to populate the nation with healthy, beautiful offspring who could legitimately inherit their parents' wealth and titles.

Rachel Lloyd was an early and enthusiastic visitor to the Temple. After a morning out with Lady Carlisle and Lady Waldegrave – they went to inspect the King while he inspected the military camp that filled Hyde Park at the time – she and Lady Carlisle went to see "Dr Graham's Electrical Machinery". They judged it "a most curious sight". Spurred also by the astonishing tales of Spa medical heroics she had heard from the Spencers, Miss Lloyd recommended Graham to another aristocratic friend, Lady Gower: "He is a most wonderful man... and... might be of great use to you, in recovering your hands to their own shape, and when you come to Town we hope you will go and see, and hear him, at least."

Letters about the new quasi-medical sanctuary and its unusual proprietor were crossing the channel within weeks of its opening. Benjamin Franklin heard the news from Rudolph Erich Raspe, the beaky-nosed, carrot-haired curator employed by the Landgrave of Hesse-Cassel, one of Graham's best Spa benefactors. By then Raspe's pilfering of coins and medals from the museum he had remodelled had been discovered, and he was on the run; even the Royal Society had expelled him for "deficient character". Hence, perhaps, his ambivalent take on the Doctor: "Dr. Graham, the Prince of Quacks, has set up in the Adelphi a Temple of Health and pretends to do and does wonders with his electrical, magnetical, aerial, aetherial and musical influences – in open defiance to the Faculty. His house is crowded, he gets money and the Faculty begin to follow his example in setting up electrical mills for the sake of health and money." (Raspe was a man inexorably drawn to others who lived on the borderlines of illusion and authenticity. He had championed James MacPherson's fraudulent Ossianic epics in Germany, and later anonymously published the travelogue of that model semi-fictional travel liar, Baron Munchausen.) He concluded: "Though there is a great deal of madness in that, it will be productive however of some good experiments, and at the end turn out an improvement of Science; for good comes of evil, which I hope and wish may be the case of this and of Your Excellency's country."

Within a few weeks, Graham contrived a wonderful puff in the *Morning Chronicle*, far more valuable than a straightforward advertisement. Long before the article's end, its fanciful prose style revealed Graham as its unmistakable author. (Less instinctive self-promoters could easily hire specialized puff-writers.) "The Temple of Health is now so much a place of the *ton*, that no lady or gentleman can possibly confess they have not seen that elegant place, especially the celestial brilliancy of the evening exhibition of the apparatus, without being looked upon as shockingly deficient in taste." London's latest fashionable venue was lauded as a "museum" – *utile* and *dulce*, as Hanoverians were fond of saying – a site of "the highest mental gratification to ladies of taste, as well as to men of science". And this was a mere bonus. The main draw was meant to be physical rather than mental improvement – every tour brought with it the supposedly restorative effects of breathing in the Temple's ethereal air for a few hours.

Graham set out to be all things to all people. Individual or group medical treatments were still available by appointment. The Temple of Health, "that stupendous, that magnificent mansion", boasted the next paragraph, "is to all intents and purposes an attick school, where wit and repartee and tender pleasantry sparkle and seem concentrated as rays of light in the focus of a burning glass… The polite and excentric proprietor of the Temple, or rather that son of science and of the healing art, has at last convinced the world that it is the real interest of every sick or debilitated person to repair to the Adelphi, in order to be cured with ease and elegance in that terrestrial paradise. There we see the infirm smiling away their infirmities, hypocondriacs holding their sides laughing, and even the most excruciating and most confirmed diseases flying away, like cold and darkness before the genial beams of the vernal, of the morning sun."

Henry Angelo, the Royal Fencing Master, and obviously no stranger to opulence, remembered the house at the Adelphi "splendidly" lit up, its apartments "magnificently furnished". The equally worldly traveller D'Archenholz, described Graham as joining "all the wonders of art to the precious secrets of his profession. Nothing, indeed, could be more superb than this temple; the electric fluid, managed with uncommon skill, was darted around in beautiful irradiation; transparent glass of various colours chosen and placed with taste; valuable vases filled with the most exquisite aromatics, which awakened the soul with a soft languor, were the first objects that presented themselves to the observation of the curious."

Graham's decorative use of glass had never been seen before in England, and would not be witnessed again for some decades. The world over, only a few isolated instances of anything remotely comparable had ever been built. The notoriously eccentric Prince of Palagonia had recently covered walls, ceilings and other surfaces in his bizarre Sicilian villa with elaborately coloured glass plating and mirrored panelling. He also raised Goethe's eyebrows with his fractured multicoloured stained-glass windows (not to mention disguised torture chairs that welcomed visitors with nails hidden under their upholstery). Catherine the Great of Russia would soon be picking out Adamesque motifs on the blue-and-gold glass ceiling of her dressing room, and commissioning glass columns, tabletops and even doors from her Imperial Glass Works near St Petersburg. In 1795 John Blades, one of Graham's own cut-glass suppliers in London, was said to have created an emerald-green glass mausoleum for the Nabob of Oude, a full fourteen feet high. In another half a century or so Maharajahs in India began ordering from English manufacturers something like the kind of furnishings Graham had on display at the Temple of Health. Eventually their distant palaces would sparkle with colossal chairs, sofas, beds and thrones, made of solid cut-glass and upholstered in coloured velvet. Glass bookcases, banisters, torchères, dressing tables and even swings, not to mention the obvious chandeliers, became the rage among the super-rich of Patiala, Gwalior, Udaipur and Hyderabad in the late nineteenth century. But in 1780s London, Graham's tall twisting transparent columns were utterly without precedent. Set amidst Adam's sugary filigree and lit with coloured sunlight beaming through fake stained glass by day, and endlessly reflected flickering candle flames by night, they were awe-inspiring.

In his memoirs, Angelo also backed up Graham's claims that his lectures "were attended by ladies as well as gentlemen of the highest rank". While lines of carriages drew up to the front door, eager hoards of foppish young men crowded around, craning to identify the latest visitors. Gog and Magog's tall ornamental silver-headed staffs were put to practical use holding back these "gaping sparks", as colourful and noisy as parrots in their silks, satins and affectations. Graham introduced a one-way system for vehicles, and had to limit the number of companions tagging along with genuine patients coming to daytime consultations. After a shock on the scale of the Gordon riots, well-heeled Londoners were more ready than ever to embrace a diversion as attractive as the Temple of Health. They longed for fun and novelty to draw a veil over fear and destruction. Although the ruins on their doorsteps – in some cases the doorsteps themselves – were already being rebuilt, coffeehouse and ballroom society still had to confront the lists of British deaths and casualties across the Atlantic and nearer at hand in every newspaper. Each lurch between victory and defeat was reported in detail. Danger seemed to lurk everywhere. Even fashionable French hairdressers, imported from Paris by the Duchess of Devonshire and her set, were denounced as spies, accused of corrupting the English servants with whom they mingled with their papist principles and politics.

A young neighbour of Graham's remembered the fun of living so close to the Temple and its "overflowing audiences". Frederick Reynolds, who grew up to be a prolific and successful playwright, was a lively sixteen-year-old at the time. One of his best friends became quite besotted with the Goddess of Health. The role of the Goddess seems to have been played by a succession of young women, and this one was probably not Emma Lyon, who by 1781 was established at the Sussex country home of Sir Harry Fetherstonhaugh, and was reputedly dancing naked on the dining table at Uppark. Reynolds records his friend's passion ending with the illness and death of the Goddess he had loved.

Since the Reynolds family house in John Street backed onto Graham's, Frederick and his three brothers could simply lean out of their first-floor rear windows to enjoy a free view of the Temple of Health's performances. The Doctor was infuriated, and issued regular rebukes. When the boys began to entertain themselves by flicking "with all the force of fingers, thumbs and arms, and with an unerring aim, paper pellets, full against the eager visages of the Doctor's patients", his fury intensified. In the belief that these missiles contained pins, Graham wrote to complain that he and his spectators were compelled "to the positive detriment of their systems" to keep the windows shut on the hottest day. He received a rude little verse in reply.

DEAR DOCTOR,
'Tis not true that our pellets are charged with a pin,
But supposing they are, pray where is the sin?
Grant we put *out* your eye, well, you'll *put* it in.

While the beau monde opened their purses, the satirists sharpened their quills. "[T]he present object of the muse is one of the finest subjects shot flying these many seasons. Satire may fall to like an Epicure, and feast upon the pure, aetherial, electrical green fat of nonsense." Grub Street got instantly to work. Editors were hungry for material to leaven the bitter news that so often dominated their newspapers, and there seemed an endless appetite for press pastiches of the Doctor. Graham offered a wealth of different angles, together with a style of writing and oratory that was instantly recognizable and easy to reproduce. Such a rage for public speaking had recently developed – commercial debating clubs and courses and books on eloquence and rhetoric all swiftly multiplying – that everyone suddenly felt qualified to deliver opinions on this subject. Graham's hilariously high-flown language was an obvious way to signal that he was getting above himself ("…he's inspired! He is a man divine! / Because he madly mounts above his line"). The electric doctor's social-climbing crimes were considered all the worse for having been committed by a "Caledonian".

The *Gazetteer*, particularly funny and ferocious in these early days at the Adelphi, immediately promoted Graham to Prince of Quacks. Within weeks of the Temple's opening, parodies of his "Christian's Universal Prayer", his musical interludes, his poetical orations, his medical claims, his patients' testimonials, even his convoluted footnotes all appeared in the papers. He must have been a genuinely ubiquitous presence, since it was clearly taken for granted in the press that the tiniest nuance would be recognized and laughed at by the reading public. Graham-related "characters" even began to appear in costume at masquerades. One satirical print complete with verse and music called "The Quintessence of Quackism" featured the broad figures of Gog and Magog, on either side of their master, "a Doctor rare, who travels much at home", and claimed to cure everyone and everything. The well-known speaking tube linking Graham's reception room and his laboratory had been transformed into the tail of a monkey. It perched on the Doctor's head and waved a telltale quacking duck in the air. Graham held out a large "Ethereal Pill" in his free hand, and wore a clearly identifiable medallion with Catharine Macaulay's head around his neck. The song was dedicated to the "Emperor of Quacks".

Quackery had been a target for self-righteous satirists for centuries. Inevitably, every era believed itself to be exceptionally overrun with the species: "The present Gang of Quacks, who infest this Metropolis, are almost as dangerous to Society as the late Gang of Rioters." Simply to advertise medical services was virtually to admit to "irregularity" in the professional field: it was self-promotion, and often geographical mobility, rather than the survival rate of patients that defined quackery.

When Dr Graham burst onto the London scene, he offered more in every respect than any of those run-of-the-mill pedlars of patent medicines, routinely denounced en masse. His elevation to quack royalty had little to do with the details of his therapeutic techniques and everything to do with his personality and marketing methods. Few entrepreneurs in any profession had mastered the language and techniques of advertising quite like Graham. In quantity and quality, he excelled. He even promised ten guineas to anyone who had taken his Imperial electrical pills and not felt the benefits. These were said to include fragrant excrement and urine that smelt of "sweetest and freshest roses, lilies, violets, pinks and wall-flowers". The strength of his convictions alone – so passionate, so vocal and so public – put him in a category of his own.

Graham's instant success in attracting the rich and fashionable was another easy target. Leaping on the multiple associations of brass – nerve or gall, money and natural philosophy – the satirists returned again and again to images of the "electrical doctor" drawing coins from his patients with magnetism, bleeding their bodies of "that filthy ore", or shocking their purses with his "electrical magnetic plan". His literary aspirations were mocked with equal vigour. One letter reads as startlingly knowing in its recommendation of the "electrical aether" as a cure for writer's block: "If I find myself *faint* and *exhausted*, or *void* of *poetical images*, I immediately draw the *vapour* of the Doctor's *electrical aether* with great force into my nostrils… and I find my vigour *restored*, my mind *enlarged* and *illuminated* in one moment. I am transported with balmy and melodious gales into the sweet, brilliant, and flowery fields of *poetry*! All the *learning* in the world can neither give a man the *genius, taste*, or *knowledge*, that this *electrical aether* affords…" The youth of England would no longer need to waste time at the universities, nor poets in penury even bother to eat. With the help of electrical aether, British Homers and Virgils would soon be as plentiful as "potatoes".

Sex was less of an issue at this stage. It still hovered decently in the background of portrayals of Graham in late 1780, and the assisted reproduction he offered was firmly associated with his own verbal productions: "Come all ye steril old! Ye tepid young! / I'll make ye as prolific as my tongue!" His mannered speech encapsulated not just his pretensions as a doctor, but his pretensions full stop. It was attacked with such spirit because social and literary obfuscation were seen as equally contemptible, and required exposure.

The kind of anxieties that had vexed a fictional Matthew Bramble a few decades earlier in Bath had lately intensified. That year marked the moment when courtesans suddenly began sharing the social columns of newspapers with aristocrats and royalty. The hairstyles, dress and carriage design of the leading "impures" and actresses were as trendsetting as Georgiana's, and their appearances at public amusements as frequently noted. To the establishment, this shuffling for social dominance was as alarming as it was fascinating. "And what of the society of which you boast?... A mere chaos, in which all distinction of rank is lost in a ridiculous affectation of ease... In the same *select party*, you will often find the wife of a Bishop and a sharper – of an earl and a fidler... one universal masquerade, all distinguished in the same habits and manners." According to Angelo, the electric doctor had managed to buy and charm his way into the best houses. "Dr. Graham kept his equipage, maintained a splendid retinue, and, for a short time at least, was invited to many of the first tables; and in return, contrived to give his claret and champagne."

On Saturday 2nd September, Dr Graham cancelled his engagements and went out for the evening. He settled himself a little nervously in one of the highly visible stage boxes at the Theatre Royal, Haymarket for the opening night of "an original, whimsical, operatical, pantomimical, farcical, electrical, naval, military, temporary, local extravaganza". It was called *The Genius of Nonsense* and Graham was under no illusions about its target. Barely had the Temple's evening exhibitions been launched than rumours of a stage show began to emerge from the "spies of the Green Room", along with much talk of the "shock" that would soon be felt at the Adelphi. Now the audience, who sat as fully bathed in light as any of the actors, hardly knew where to look. Should they keep their eyes on the stage or watch instead the reactions of "the real Doctor" to the night's performance?

George Colman (the elder), the play's writer-producer and an old friend of David Garrick, had saved the best till last. Graham had to sit through numerous scenes of topical ribaldry involving Harlequin and Columbine before Gog and Magog appeared in their laced hats for the final act. According to Colman's son, Graham was keen to get hold of a copy of the porters' fake leaflets so that he could pursue a threatened libel prosecution. The Doctor "protruded his arm, repeatedly, from the stage-box, to procure a hand-bill from the representatives of his own Porters, which they as repeatedly refused to give him". Eventually Graham stood up in his box and leant forwards to offer some coins to the theatrical versions of his gigantic servants. But the audience in the pit were so outraged at this new display of "brass" that they booed him back to his seat with one voice, and Graham was forced to sit back and watch his own portrayal on stage without further intervention.

After the Gog and Magog impersonators had left the scene, counting their takings, the "most numerous and brilliant Audience" at the Haymarket watched their gullible Adelphi equivalents gathering on stage for the imitation lecture. Racy Mrs Cargill, acting again to great applause after a runaway marriage that summer, made her second appearance of the night. Transformed from the Genius of Nonsense into the Goddess of Health, she sang the actual air printed in Dr Graham's handbill.

Come then, ah come, oh sacred health,
The monarch's bliss, the beggar's wealth...

The blossoming comic actor John Bannister, nervous about the news of Graham's musings on legal action, had hoped to get away with "a broad outline sketch'd after his own fancy, of any ideal *Charlatan*" for his own performance. Colman was having none of this. The very evening before *The Genius of Nonsense* opened, he sent Bannister to the Adelphi with his son to see Graham first hand. The next night, when Bannister entered as the "Emperor of the Quacks", his "mere entrance upon the Scene, as the Doctor was wont to present himself in his *Temple*, – his grotesque mode of sliding around the room, – the bobbing bows he shot off at the Company, while making his circuit, – and various other minutiae, were so ridiculously accurate, that he surpass'd his prototype in *electrifying* the publick, – and the whole house was in a roar of laughter".

Less partial reports support Colman junior's recollections. "The Emperor of the Quacks [delivered] an empyric oration, so poignantly severe, and interspersed with such real wit, that the roar of laughter, and the thunder of applause alternately echoed through the house." Isaac Reed, a friend of William Blake, loved the show so much that he returned repeatedly. He likened the amusing Grahamesque dialogue to "an ancient gossip's conversation, viz., a string of questions with an insipid remark at the end of them".

The plot was hardly sophisticated. After some business with glass tubes and medicine appearing through the trapdoor, the Emperor asked for the Goddess of Health, only to be informed by a servant that she been taken ill, and gone to a "doctor" for advice. Mortified, the Emperor sneaked off, and an Irishman from the lecture audience jokingly tried to open a huge book, supposedly full of Graham's medical recipes. This too turned out to be a fake, merely a wooden box from which tumbled oyster shells, apples and lemons. At this, the enraged Irishman set to demolishing the electrical apparatus and the curtain dropped.

The Genius of Nonsense was the first full-scale representation of the Temple of Health to reach the London stage. The reviewers adored it. "The Prince of Pantomimes", the *London Chronicle* pronounced it. Other wits renamed it "The Nonsense of Genius". The staging of the "*quack hospital*", the work of Michael Angelo Rooker, was so perfect that one "Theatrical Intelligence" column declared "all spectators who have visited the Doctor's rooms must suppose, that for the moment they were actually in the Adelphi. Nay, the appearance is so exactly copied, and so excellently burlesqued, that apparent fire is brought out of wooden conductors; whilst canvas balls of painted quicksilver sparkle with *electricity*. At least to the eye there is no difference between the mock and the real representation." The "elegant apartment", exactly copied from the Temple itself, displayed "all the pomp and parade of electricity", concurred *The Lady's Magazine*'s, and other papers. Colman had even incorporated a speaking tube and trapdoor into the action, while "the female voice that is heard in the attic storey of the Doctor's house" warbled offstage. Naturally the real Graham was also reviewed, gleefully described with all the usual puns: he was reported as appearing "shocked", having "never before felt so strong a power of *electricity* – the *charge* was a great one". Yet although the satire was levelled at the impositions of quackery, as one correspondent commented, "the witticisms were at the expence of public credulity".

Graham's medical establishment was a particular gift to impresarios, who were operating in an excitingly transformed theatrical era. Scenery had been moving towards centre stage at British theatres ever since Garrick had appointed Philippe de Loutherbourg as the designer at Drury Lane in 1772. De Loutherbourg had begun his career as a much admired landscape artist in Paris, only coming to London when sexual and financial scandal had put paid to his prospects in France. Thanks largely to his interventions, creaky old theatre sets – identical, flat, dull interiors previously reappearing in show after show – had been abandoned in favour of picturesque and naturalistic constructions. Elaborate backdrops and slips were now being designed for different acts of specific plays, and arranged to produce previously unimaginable perspective effects. Suddenly scenery painters were getting newspaper billings in advertisements for new productions.

De Loutherbourg also revolutionized costume and lighting. He used coloured silks in front of oil lamps, switching light sources and screens to imply time passing. Images miraculously appeared, vanished and dissolved into one other. Ever alert to new possibilities for heightening drama, Graham found these early experiments with transparencies inspirational. Spectacle thrillingly fed spectacle. The reincarnations of the Temple of Health at London's theatres were an irresistible challenge to designers itching to try new effects. They also allowed audiences to enjoy impressive versions of the Temple's decorative splendours – Graham's own imitations of some imaginary Royal Palace – without appearing to have fallen for a charlatan.

The next time James Graham appeared on stage, he had shrunk to a singing wooden marionette, a foot high, and had been renamed "Dr Adelphi". He was the star of an elaborate puppet show. Ironically, Walpole had already privately described his former gout apothecary as "a wooden thing on wires", after grumpily attending his medical lecture soon after it was launched. Charles Dibdin, the ingenious dramatist, composer, musical director and actor for the Patagonian Theatre, recreated Graham's Temple in miniature in a Lilliputian playhouse. (The joke, of course, was that Patagonians, as far as Hanoverian Britain was concerned, were a race of giants "discovered" by the sixteenth-century explorer Magellan, supposedly sighted more recently by a 1760s sea captain.) This puppet theatre, originally from Dublin, had been established a few years earlier in a hall above the arcade of trinket shops in Exeter 'Change, a building on the Strand opposite where the Savoy Hotel now stands. The theatre's stage was only six feet across, but its "scenes" were regarded as always *"remarkable for their excellence"*. The auditorium boasted boxes, pit and gallery, and could fit two hundred full-sized spectators. (Between seasons, the same room was often occupied by the exotic animals of Gilbert Pidcock's travelling menagerie.)

On 11th November, *Doctor Adelphi, or a Hit at the Late Riots* opened the Patagonian Theatre's winter season with "a great variety of new scenery; particularly a view of Newgate in Ruins; and also the Terrace of the Adelphi, and the Apartments in the Temple of Health". The third act featured "A Crutch dance in the Temple of Health, by some of the Doctor's patients". The critics loved the new production, which wove the tale of Dr Graham and his puppet porters into a satire "admirably pointed" at the Gordon Riots. The newly launched *Morning Herald* observed that anyone who had read Graham's publications would "clearly see, that the whole of his character has been (as we may say) written by himself", and considered that it was "excellently blended in the counter-plot of the piece". The composer of Colman's Haymarket entertainment, the staggeringly prolific Dr Arnold, was also vigorously lampooned, and the puppets performed a much admired "glee" that had also been in *The Genius of Nonsense.*

A few weeks later Graham gave his female assistant an even grander title: "Vestina, the Rosy Goddess of Health". She presided over the evening lecture at the real Temple, "assisting at the display of the Celestial meteors, and of that sacred vital fire over which she watches..." Although he had not yet advertised the *Lecture on Generation* as such, Graham was clearly discussing its subject. *The Gazetteer*'s send-up of his poetical address included the lines:

> Does any rich old feeble want an heir?
> Let him to my gay Temple quick repair:
> Etherial balsam shall his strength restore,
> And make him vig'rous as he was of yore.

Ever topical, Dibdin and his equally multi-talented partner in speculation, Hubert Stoppelaer, quickly got going on a new three-act comic operetta: a pastiche of the Doctor's marital advice called *The Nuptials of Venus.* The Patagonian Theatre's new skit was performed in the same witty doggerel as *Hudibras,* a mock-heroic poem about a conceited and bumbling knight errant written by Samuel Butler over a century before. *Hudibras* was immensely long, vastly popular and frequently imitated. The original was a polemic satirizing the parliamentarians in the English civil war. Dibdin and Stoppelaer spotted Dr Graham as a dead ringer for the arrogant knight. The Doctor's bizarre pompositities cried out to be adapted to the multi-syllabic rhymes and absurdly lavish praise associated with Sir Hudibras. The theatre company announced "a great variety of new Celestial Scenery, emblematically representing the paraphernalia of the Heathen Deities". The "view of the Temple of Destiny, and the High Hall and Throne of Jupiter" were obvious spoofs of the Temple of Apollo and Graham's obsession with classical symbolism at the Adelphi.

Competition for London's audiences was increasing all the time. Graham's newspaper advertisements jostled for front-page space not just with announcements of theatrical satires that featured or mentioned him and his Temple, but a cornucopia of other entertainments. Astley's Amphitheatre at Westminster Bridge offered an ever-changing roster, including the "Little Conjuring Horse", dancers performing horseback "attitudes", feats of "manly agility" and airs on a double set of musical glasses. There was also a live zebra at which to wonder, and Astley junior could ride two horses at once. Elsewhere, Mr Breslaw was bringing new life to his "magical" card deceptions and a mind-reading act with the help of "Mr Rossignol", an Italian birdsong imitator. The thickly accented Prussian, Dr Katterfelto, had taken up evening residence with his black cats in Spring Gardens to display his "most surprising and wonderful experiments". Another aggressive advertiser, Katterfelto claimed expertise in a perplexing array of different arts and sciences: "philosophical, mathematical, optical, magnetical, electrical, physical, chemical, pneumatic, hydraulic, hydrostatic, poetic, stynagraphic, palenchic, and caprimantic". One of his more dramatic tricks involved attaching a steel helmet to his daughter's head and lifting her to the ceiling with a giant magnet. His usual puffs in plodding verse were supposedly composed by his admirers, and he was well known for his cries of "Wonders! Wonders! Wonders!"

Nearby at Leicester House, an eccentric archery enthusiast, Sir Ashton Lever, had become something of a sideshow to his impressive private museum, the Holophusikon. Lever was a serious natural philosopher who had opened his doors to a paying public when he could no longer fund expansion from his own pocket. His sprawling collection was crammed with stuffed peacocks, "sea-monsters", a young elephant, a whole roomful of dressed-up monkeys frozen at work at different human trades, as well as shells, antique medals and curiosities from Cook's expedition to the South Seas. Visitors who came to marvel at the Holophusikon were often distracted by glimpses of its owner in the gardens, dressed in green from head to toe and firing arrows from his bow with accuracy and abandon.

These were just the longest-running successes of a metropolis spoilt for choice for amusements. Others came and went: on street corners, entrepreneurs enticed passers-by with promises about the varied performances of their life-sized automata. Ephemeral infant prodigies played their harpsichords or sang at the Pantheon. The patriotic occasionally dressed up for anti-Gallic masquerades, where French wine was shunned. And of course there were always the pleasure gardens of Vauxhall and Ranelagh.

At the end of February 1781, a select London audience began "going to the pictures", Georgian-style. They were so thrilled at what they saw they could barely keep to their seats; bobbing powdered wigs blocked the sight lines of the back rows. After years in the planning, according to its swaggering mastermind, Philippe de Loutherbourg, the Eidophusikon opened at his house in Lisle Street, Leicester Square, to unanimous amazement and admiration. Like Graham, de Loutherbourg had to negotiate a precarious path through high and commercial culture. He took care to package himself as a fine artist rather than some vulgar showman. Like Graham, he strove to impress visitors with the elegance and good taste of his luxurious little theatre.

For the past six or seven years the artist and stage designer had been setting new standards for spectacle at regular theatres, trumping himself with every effort. Mechanical re-enactments of military events and masquerades used clockwork automata designed by James Cox's former employee, John Joseph Merlin, and other immensely skilled specialists. A tour of the Peak District in the late 1770s had led to a sensational show appropriately titled *The Wonders of Derbyshire,* for which de Loutherbourg had come up with yet more innovative special effects. It featured exquisite mountain landscapes, vivid meteorological illusions and above all striking changes in mood and atmosphere. In the "moving pictures" of "natural phenomena" at the Eidophusikon, Philippe de Loutherbourg's technical and artistic skills reached their apotheosis. Dawn, noon, sunset and moonrise appeared in dreamy succession, with moody musical interludes, the scenes moving from Greenwich Park (with London in the distance), to the Port of Tangier and the Rock of Gibraltar. Views of Naples and the moonlit Mediterranean followed, and the show culminated triumphantly in that Romantic favourite, "a Storm at Sea, and Shipwreck", this one based on a well-known actual event.

Sir Joshua Reynolds himself applauded on the opening night. Thomas Gainsborough, one of London's most fashionable portrait painters and a friend of de Loutherbourg, was "so wrapt in delight with the Eidophusikon" that he spent evening after evening in its darkened auditorium, sometimes helping operate the machinery.

"Gainsborough, himself a great experimentalist, could not fail to admire scenes wrought to such perfection by the aid of so many collateral inventions. Loutherbourg's genius was as prolific in imitations of nature to astonish the ear, as to charm the sight. He introduced a new art – *the picturesque of sound*," wrote William Pyne, artist and art critic. Pyne described in detail the magical effects de Loutherbourg conjured up with the help of slips of stained-glass, lamps, rain and hail sticks filled with beads and seeds, parchment tambourines and copper thunder sheets. Moving clouds painted on linen stretched diagonally across the stage were illuminated from front and back simultaneously for greater naturalism. One night, when a real thunderstorm broke out mid-performance, Pyne and his friends opened the door of the gallery so that they could compare the genuine with the artificial. "Man was an extraordinary creature, who could create a copy of Nature, to be taken for Nature's self," declared one of his party at supper in Pall Mall later that evening.

These were impressive rivals for public attention. Yet though some of the initial amazement at Graham himself had begun to wear off, he was far from being neglected. Instead, London's fantastic new celebrity was swept up with great delight to be used as a vehicle for sending up a host of other aspects of 1780s British society. The week *Doctor Adelphi* opened, Graham was incorporated into a second edition of a shilling publication called *A Satire on the Present Times*. In the months that followed, the figure of the Doctor would be used to make arguments about polygamy, fashion, hypocrisy, the American Revolution and public gullibility. But the best was yet to come.

Elevated by the success of the Adelphi venture, Graham decided to expand. He took on smart new premises in Pall Mall, not far from where he had practised before settling in Bath. The property, Schomberg House, was not quite as stylish as the Adelphi, but it was richly decorated with intricate plaster cornicing and mouldings, boasted some unusual architectural features, and was well placed for a West End clientele. It had been divided into three: the east wing was a fashionable textile shop, the west wing was the home and studio of Thomas Gainsborough and the central section would be occupied by Graham. Its owner and previous occupant, the artist John Astley, had added to the top floor a light-filled, dome-roofed studio overlooking St James's Park. Dry and airy, it must have been ideal for Graham's electrical apparatus. "Take me, O take me to thy roof, / And give my soul the raptur'd proof!" exhorted one skit.

Dr Graham's plans for Schomberg House could hardly have been more ambitious. The new venue would be daringly dedicated to marriage and fertility. He called it the Temple of Hymen, and then quickly renamed it the Temple of *Prolific* Hymen. Centre stage would be the electric bed, in an extraordinary new incarnation, more impressive than anything that had preceded it. Couples would be able to pay Dr Graham to spend a night in the bed, and conception was supposedly guaranteed. The whole scheme was a logical development of the ideas and techniques on which the Doctor had been working for years and Graham passionately believed in their moral and national value.

Graham threw everything he could muster, philosophically, medically, emotionally and above all financially into the Great Celestial State Bed – or "medico, magnetico, musico, electrical bed". His aspirations were exalted. Graham made the bed, he said, not just "to insure the removal of barrenness... but likewise to improve, exalt, and invigorate the bodily, and through them, the mental faculties of the human species". This was no cynical attempt to capitalize on the public's credulity. Graham was convinced it would work. At the same time though, he was undeniably eager for the fame and fortune he was certain the bed would bring him.

To construct the world's most erotic and elaborate fertility aid, Graham is thought to have commissioned a mechanical mastermind called Thomas Denton. They may have first encountered each other when they were both living in Denton's native Yorkshire, where he had been apprenticed in boyhood to a tinman. In York, Denton opened a bookshop specializing in works on mechanics. His ambitions soon took him, "an adventurer, to the great mart of genius, London". Walking the streets, Denton's attention was apparently soon captured by a speaking figure, exhibited by some unnamed foreigners. Already intrigued by Enlightenment theories of robotics, Denton immediately "paid his admission, and took a very correct examination of the automaton. Returning to his lodgings he fancied he could construct a similar machine, equal to that of the ingenious foreigner's; and he determined, without farther search, to set about his work." Once Denton had managed to acquire access to a workshop, tools and materials, he produced "a far superior figure to that of the vaunting German", a realistic speaking robot which he toured around Britain, collecting "vast sums of money at each city". This was followed by a "writing automaton", equally impressive.

While small-scale automata frolicked on late-eighteenth-century clocks, watches and music boxes, a number of full-height living dolls such as these were beginning to stir their limbs in the workshops of a little group of men obsessed with artificial life. One "modern Prometheus" after another struggled to animate uncanny moving statues. These eighteenth-century androids could play the harpsichord or the flute, their heaving chests actually appearing to breathe. Alarmingly, a few were even fashioned using human skin. Jacques de Vaucanson, a star in this field, spent years trying to make an artificial man who could bleed. Wolfgang von Kempelen's famous chess-playing Turk was only unmasked as a fraud after decades of success.

Tiring of his "artificial penman", Denton next took up chemistry, yet another field in which he excelled, and one which would have made him an ideal collaborator for Graham in the design of the Celestial Bed. In the years that followed his work for the Temple of Hymen, Denton set up as a bookseller in Holborn, translated and edited a book of parlour magic, and invented improvements to coach-harness plating. Like Graham, Denton clearly possessed that "tint of charlatanism so necessary in this century if one is to obtain the vote of the masses"; this was the opinion of the author of another contemporary handbook on magic.

Descriptions of Graham's electrical bed vary somewhat, and there was certainly more than one elaboration of the Philadelphian prototype. Incredibly, even this, the most splendid, the Grand State Celestial Bed, fell short of the Doctor's original ambitions. Still, he described the final creation as twelve feet long by nine wide, and supported by "forty pillars of brilliant glass, of great strength, and of the most exquisite workmanship, in regard to shape, cutting, and engravings; sweetly delicate, and richly variegated colours, and the most brilliant polish! They are moreover invisibly encrusted with a certain transparent varnish, in order to render the insulation still more complete, and that otherwise, properly assisted, we may have, in even the most unfavourable weather, abundance of the electrical fire."

Above the bed was a vast dome containing the highly fragrant and "aetherial" odours and essences which somehow wafted out "with the breath of music", filling the bed with oriental perfumes and, no doubt, a quantity of near-pure oxygen, ether or nitrous oxide. This "grand magazine, or the reservoir of those vivifying and invigorating influences" had multiple sensory functions. While lovers breathed in its unfamiliar and stimulating scents, their erotic impact was heightened by the inlaid mirrored plates which covered the underside to reflect "the various charms and attitudes of the happy couple who repose in bed, in the most flattering, most luxurious, and most enchanting stile!"

The top of the dome was a work of art in itself. At its summit, the figures of Cupid and Psyche, symbols of everlasting love, adoringly entwined. A statue of Hymen, the god of marriage, watched over them, a torch "flaming with electrical fire" raised in one hand, while the other supported a sparkling crown, electrically "beatified" by Bose's technique. Offering another image of marital fidelity, and also fertility, a pair of live turtle doves billed and cooed beneath this diadem, settled somehow on a small bed of roses. Festoons of fresh flowers also covered the dome, while music was provided by groups of moving mythological figures ("– the Cupids! – the Loves! – the Graces!") playing flutes, guitars, violins, clarinets, trumpets, horns, oboes and kettledrums.

Mechanical music was hugely in vogue, and serious composers and clockmakers were joining forces to produce wondrous and intricate devices to allow music to be enjoyed without the necessity for live musicians – even Mozart wrote 'A Piece for an Organ in a Clock'. Timepieces were becoming ever more incidental to the display around them. Barrel-organ technology was now so sophisticated that weights or clockwork could control the speed of the mechanism turning with great precision, and shift the barrel automatically. This meant that a greater variety of tunes could be played for longer. The tiny automata that so often featured as part of these elaborate music boxes, usually made of painted and gilded copper alloy, were partly there to divert spectators from the noise of the operating machinery, but mostly to amaze them with their lifelike movements.

In the Celestial Bed, pillars constructed out of functioning organ pipes and other instruments supported the dome, and played "in sweet concert" with the mechanical musicians above. The organ itself, integrated into the head of the bed, incorporated all the latest and most sophisticated clockmaking and musical-instrument technology. Meanwhile a shifting painted panel on its front entranced each private audience of two with yet more exquisite automata. Their backdrop was a picturesque rural landscape, complete with the requisite fountains, waterfalls and peasants. Birds flew in the sky and swans glided on the waters. Into this idyll a moving procession of "village nymphs" emerged, strewing flowers in the path of priests, brides, bridegrooms and their attendants. One by one, the enchanting figures disappeared from view into a miniature Temple of Hymen. A tiny clock face on a little church in the background discreetly gave the time. (This small working timepiece may also have served as a subtle nudge to set the couple in the bed to thinking about what might be going on out of view. So-called "libertine watches" which concealed thrusting erotic scenes behind respectable faces and backs were at the height of their popularity.) Above this private pageant, "in the full centre front, appear sparkling, with electrical fire, through a glory of burnished and effulgent gold, the great, first, ever operating commandment, – BE FRUITFUL, MULTIPLY AND REPLENISH THE EARTH!"

Even the mattresses evoked the promise of fertility and fecundity. Feather beds would have set altogether the wrong tone, associated as they were with idleness and luxurious dissipation. So these were rejected in favour of the hearty natural touch – fresh sweet oats or wheat, symbolically including the grain, mixed with scented rose leaves, lavender flowers and oriental spices. An even more suggestive alternative offered by Graham was horse hair, procured at vast expense "from the tails of English stallions", which he straight-facedly claimed made the springiest base. The pulse-quickening association between stallion tails and any other impressive equine apparatus was left to the imagination.

But the biggest bounce was somehow supplied by magnetism. "About fifteen hundred pounds weight of artificial and compound magnets, are so disposed and arranged, as to be continually pouring forth in an ever-flowing circle, inconceivable and irrestistably powerful tides of the magnetic effluvium." It is hard to imagine exactly how this could have worked, but Graham claimed that the magnets, "being pressed give that charming springyness – that sweet undulating, tittulating, vibratory, soul-dissolving, marrow-melting motion; which on certain critical and important occasions, is at once so necessary and so pleasing". As with his stallion tails, the symbolism of these huge magnets was at least as important to Graham as their practical use. Magnetism had long been linked with love and sexual attraction, in the fairground as much as in philosophical treatises. "Aimant", the French word for magnet, also means loving. In the seventeenth century magnetic poles had been labelled as male and female, and the word "coition" used to describe this attraction of opposites. William Harvey, best known for his discovery of blood's circulation, believed semen possessed a kind of magnetic force. A century later, midwifery texts attributed a similarly powerful quality to the womb, to which the male seed was shown attracted like so many iron filings to a magnet. And in literature, high and low, magnetism was an indispensable romantic and sexual metaphor.

Yet one more new-fangled device awaited lovers seeking sure-fire conception in the Celestial Bed. These were the years in which the "ingenious Mechanick" John Joseph Merlin was cavorting at masquerades on his newly invented roller skates, smashing into wall mirrors with his violin in hand, or dressing as a quack doctor, and deliberately shocking guests with his secretly electrified handshakes. He was also making a name for himself with multifunctional and highly adjustable drawing-room furniture – a mechanical tea table "by which any Lady can fill twelve Cups of Tea, and shift them round by the Pressure of the Foot, without the Assistance of her Hands", "gouty", "morpheus", and "Valetudinarian Chairs" (these last could weigh their occupants accurately while they ate, drank and perspired) and an Oscillatory Machine which turned sofas and chairs into indoor swings. Competing with these novelties, Graham promoted his new bed's double frame, the inner section mounted on a pivot which allowed the pitch of the mattress to be altered in an instant. The "gentleman" could operate this at will, so that "he can follow his lady down-hill; as it is called, which is certainly the most favourable posture for the great business of conception, or propagation, in difficult cases, especially in cases of corpulency". (This is a theory which still has its adherents today. Plenty of women trying to get pregnant perform shoulder stands after sex.)

When the Celestial Bed was set in motion by the copulating couple, they had yet more treats in store. Their very exertions controlled its musical accompaniments. As the "tender dalliances of the happy pair" got under way, the instruments on the pillars and dome of the bed began to "breathe forth celestial sounds... lulling them in visions of elysian joys! opening new sources, new sluices... of pleasures, and untwisting all the chains which tie the hidden soul of harmony!" A glance upwards, at their own arousing reflections, tangled in silky coloured sheets, and a stimulating lungful of scented narcotic gases must have increased any lovers' passions. But "as the ardour, – the intenseness of the mighty conflict increases! – the soft notes, – the plaintive tones – the tender aspirations, – the sweet undulating, – tremulous cooings, – the convulsive, agonizing blessedness of the melting and transported pair! – are moderated, increased, or prolonged by the corresponding music which flows or bursts forth from the pillars, from the dome, and from every part of this Elysium! – ... at length, in the fierce but sweet conflict, the gentle milky emotions, which at first fluctuated in their breasts, are sweet constrained by the magical force of music and other influences, to give way to more sublime and more intense enjoyments, excited by the swelling sounds – the noble tones, and the home-strokes of the full organ, which on violent motions being given to the bed, peals forth, bracing and invigorating every spring and principle of life! – coiling up the latent courage of the soul! and as it were, producing a new creation! – yes, life and identity are generally produced by those blissful collisions."

When Graham referred to the sensations of orgasm as "sublime", he was completely in earnest. Defined by Kant a few decades earlier as "a magnitude which is like itself alone", an unimaginable and incomparable power, the "sublime" was already a buzzword. For Graham, it was also an instantly understandable shorthand for the kind of out-of-body sexual ecstasy he was promoting. Graham's sexual take on the sublime may have owed something to Emanuel Swedenborg, the Swedish Christian mystic whose writings on conjugal love were central to an esoteric psycho-erotic counter-culture bubbling quietly away in theosophical London. Swedenborg used complex "Kabbalistic-Yogic techniques to transmute physical orgasm into visionary *nirvana*". (William Blake and the miniature painter Richard Cosway and his wife Maria were among his acolytes.) Swedenborgians as far away as Scandinavia who heard about Graham were struck by the parallels between the two men's cosmologies.

A later, less partisan description of the blissful bed explained more prosaically that "for nearly an hour that the concert lasts one sees in the bed streams of light which play especially over the pillows. When the time for getting up has come, the magician comes to feel the pulse of the faithful, gives them breakfast, and sends them away full of hope, not forgetting to recommend them to send him other clients." It was hard to know what to make of Graham, even then. "It is difficult to say without doubt whether this invention reveals more reason or the Doctor's stupidity. Be that as it may, still the rarity of this discovery and the innate curiosity of everyone have gained for it great success." With the maturity of adulthood, Frederick Reynolds concluded that Graham had in fact possessed a certain kind of self-serving wisdom. "'Every man at forty,' it is said, 'is either a fool or a physician'; some are both, but this doctor was neither. He knew the town, and knew, that, only by glaring deviations from the common path, and by alarming or surprising the multitude, he could pass the regular practitioner. Without doing any public harm, I believe, he certainly did himself much good; and in truth, if there be blame in these transactions, it should rest with the audience, not with the performer."

One of the many frustrations in piecing together a life from such fragments is the fact that, despite a wealth of detail, some of the big questions can never be answered. What, for example, did the Doctor's wife think about these new developments? Charles Kirkpatrick Sharpe claimed that "during his splendour in London" Mary Graham "lived neglected at Islington, supporting herself by her own industry", but there is no other evidence to support this. On the contrary, Graham invoked a household routine of daily family prayers in his publicity material. And given how minutely the press seemed to scrutinize his every move, it seems unlikely any sexual irregularities in the Doctor's personal life – hidden wives, mistresses or any other shady business – would not have been written up triumphantly. So it is fair to assume that he kept to the conjugal straight and narrow. In matters of diet, Graham practised what he preached. His descriptions of sexual pleasure, strikingly different from the rollicking bawdiness in which most Georgian sexual imagery revels, suggest that his marital advice was drawn from experience.

As intriguing and unknowable as his family life are the details of his business plans, such as they were. How exactly did Dr Graham raise the money to pay first for the contents of the Temple of Health, and then for this bed? However successful the Adelphi Temple may have been, it seems unlikely that its revenues could have covered these vast costs. But Graham left no accounts. Though he would soon be forced into making some embarrassing revelations on the subject, he was hardly likely to be completely straightforward about the exact details of his financial affairs in newspaper advertisements or promotional literature. His approach seems to have been to try to buy his way out of trouble with yet another extravagant scheme. This kind of compulsive spending was part of the zeitgeist, and widely available credit made it particularly easy. But it is also now recognized as a common feature of certain types of personality disorder.

Throughout the spring of 1781, Graham juggled with organizing his new Temple, while still trying to keep the money flowing into the old one. He tantalized patients and voyeurs with a well-orchestrated teaser campaign. From early February 1781, the Doctor's newspaper advertisements announced that he would "delicately touch" upon the soon-to-be-opened Celestial Beds before each evening's electrical displays at the Adelphi. The fact that he was publicizing them in the plural suggests that, as well as promoting the new and exceptionally grand "State" bed, he was now referring to the earlier prototypes of his magnetic and electric beds as "Celestial" too. By March, Graham found himself so overwhelmed with patients, he claimed, that he stopped exhibiting his apparatus during daylight hours, confining displays to eight-o'clock shows on four nights a week. Graham was also busy writing up case notes and statistics in his latest self-promoting manifesto, *Medical Transactions at the Temple of Health*. When it was eventually published, he expressed his disappointment that Parliament had so far disregarded "the salutary propositions" he had laid before them, and began to hint that he might be obliged to take his cause to another, more liberal nation. "Alas! alas! we dream that we are free, mighty, and respectable people; while in reality, our national stem and branches are feeble and corrupt, and decay and final declension are feeding and gnawing away our vitals!"

As his friend Brissot pointed out, financial management was never his strong point. The Doctor was beginning to run into serious difficulties. Work on the new premises needed to be paid for and he had yet to cough up the rent for the Adelphi. He quickly advertised for three more "gentlemen" to be taken on as assistant-apprentices, requesting the premium of a thousand guineas apiece. Graham continued to trumpet the imminent opening of the Temple of Hymen and the Celestial Bed still under construction, but the doors of Schomberg House remained firmly shut.

Public curiosity was uncontainable. While Graham was wrangling with workmen, landlords, ailing Goddesses and the nation's conscience, the squinting Yorkshire poet and part-time satirist William Mason semi-anonymously fed speculation by publishing a long and very successful poem he called 'The Celestial Beds'. He dedicated his "bagatelle" to the Doctor in tones unmistakably redolent of the musical performances at the Temple, mock-praising his literary flair and persuasive charms to the hilt:

> Haste, haste, th'immortal Doctor crown;
> Publish his fame throughout the town!
> Enthrone him EMPERICK THE GREAT!
> The conqueror of villain Fate!

Mason, a well-connected Whig clergyman in York, a garden designer, and later one of the earliest abolitionists, betrays in this satire a more than sneaking admiration for Graham. He is impressed, despite himself, by Graham's success in apparently winning over all of London. The "wond'rous art" of "England's demi-god" is said to fascinate the "chastest heart", while his "gilded metaphoric pills / Can cure Disease of all its ills". Graham is the "Etherial Lord" whose death-defying medicines sweeten the very sewers, and whose hygiene advice has transformed Covent Garden's prostitutes into fragrant, blooming milkmaids. The poet pillaged the Doctor's promotional materials at such length in so many elaborate explanatory footnotes that it even seems conceivable he might have written the poem as a misguided favour to the Doctor, whom Mason perhaps encountered during Graham's years as a Yorkshire apothecary.

If so, any promotional mission seems to have backfired. Mason's real target was not the Doctor, but the fashionable, witless crowd who had fallen for him, the "votaries" of his Temple, the "slaves of the *bon ton*". These were the "barren does" who went en masse to the "Quack's imperial court" to try to get pregnant, and the ancient wives, married only for their money, who glimpsed their young husbands "with a frown / 'Bout twice a year when he's in town" but still mournfully hoped and wished "for an heir, / To cheer the bosom of despair". They were the aristocrats who simply loathed their "husband's fetid kiss", and "the mincing Miss, and gouty fool", who thronged to "Graham's magic school". Mason freely sketched brothel-keepers and peers, sycophants and libertines, all rushing mindlessly to be sexually renewed by Graham's electrical and celestial forces:

> Limberhams and debauchees,
> Thither haste with knocking knees;
> Genial and prolific fires,
> Shall wake your pulse to new desires;
> Tho' your embers should be dead,
> Stretch on his celestial bed;
> Soon you'll feel the vital flame,
> Rushing thro' your icey frame!
> Fann'd by agents all divine!
> Who condescend with him to dine.

This "splendid crowd" could not help but wince at the vision they presented. As a reviewer in the *Morning Herald* observed with some pleasure, "the personages the most distinguished... are finely contrasted and satirized with such severity, that it is generally imagined the Doctor will not have an overflow for some time at his nocturnal sports."

The cast of notables Mason described at Graham's court included many of the most prominent figures of the day. The Duchess of Devonshire was naturally singled out, her ludicrously overdressed hair and fawning followers dissected without mercy: "Behold the Graces in her train, / And Folly plum'd above her brain!"

Perdita was another name rarely out of the press in the early 1780s. When the seventeen-year-old Prince of Wales had fallen for young Mary Robinson on stage in *The Winter's Tale* in December 1779, he signed his love letters "Florizel". A convenient shorthand for the season's most famous couple was instantly born. This Royal attention both made and broke Robinson. The young actress and poet quickly became, as Mason put it, the "sweet martyr of her sex's spleen!", as reviled as she was admired. She was the acknowledged leader of the "brimstone corps", as London's most famous courtesans were known that year, thanks to their butterfly-yellow carriages. There was even now a hat named "the Perdita". But she was also the target for much press venom.

By this time, the Prince had dropped Perdita for an older rival, Elizabeth Armistead. In 'The Celestial Beds' Mary Robinson is shown seeking the Prince in the crowd, hoping against hope that a royal baby might at least bring her the £20,000 he had promised her on becoming his mistress. A few months after the poem was published, Perdita was indeed (inaccurately) reported as pregnant in the *Morning Herald*, and Armistead was said to be seeking the help of Graham's bed for the same purpose. Though one of Perdita's recent biographers believes that Graham did no good to Robinson's reputation, the reverse was equally true.

Another actress in 'The Celestial Beds', Ann Barry, Britain's acknowledged Queen of Tragedy, is portrayed as so bad-tempered offstage that she required Graham's purging powers merely to render her human. Respectable but "wither'd" Lady Harrington, mother of seven but now about to turn sixty, appears in the poem as a new version of the stale jokes about Catharine Macaulay, unseemingly panting after sexual pleasures in old age. Her male equivalent is the impotent "old Lecher" John Montagu, the Fourth Earl of Sandwich, now best remembered for throwing a piece of meat between two slices of bread. Montagu was a somewhat rakish cricket fan who had been hated by most Whigs since his prosecution of John Wilkes. As First Lord of the Admiralty, he had been much blamed for naval blunders at the outset of the war with America. His opera-singer mistress of eighteen years' standing had recently been murdered by a deranged admirer.

> Dost thou too want celestial fire
> To light a flame of new desire?
> Does nature in thy pulse stand still?
> Won't she delight thy wicked will?

The Duchess of Cumberland escaped lightly from Mason's pen, imperiously commanding "due homage from the scene", in the style of Helen of Troy. The Temple of Health had decisively established itself as a place where the *bon ton* could cause diversion as well as divert itself. The Duchess, a commoner whose marriage to the Prince of Wales's favourite uncle had caused one of many deep and public rifts within the Royal family, was an enormously ambitious woman. She was described by Walpole (not necessarily a dependable witness of female character) as a "Coquette beyond measure, artful as Cleopatra, and completely mistress of all her passions and projects". Cumberland House was only a few doors away from Graham's new premises in Pall Mall.

> But who can this plump Goddess be?
> What – sweet Louisa C[onnolly]!
> Lur'd by the great magician's fame,
> And sick with twenty years of shame,
> She mingles with the sighing crowd,
> And almost vents her grief aloud…

This was a cruel dig at a woman who had never put herself forward. Louisa Connolly was far and away the most reserved and retiring of Charles James Fox's Lennox aunts, always the family diplomat. Now in her late thirties, she was still sadly childless, having miscarried in her youth not far into a marriage with a husband whom she adored. She must have been mortified at this kind of publicity. Almost as humiliating for their subject were the lines about Eva Maria Garrick, who seems to have been witnessed slipping through the door of her Adelphi next-door neighbour, tempted out of her secluded mourning after months of furore on her doorstep. Mason suggested that she came ready for another shot at connubial bliss. (In fact, the proposals she received the following year from the eccentric Scottish judge, Lord Monboddo, were firmly turned down, and she never remarried.)

Stung at this poem's portrayal of his Temple as a licentious harem, and the implication that he supported Revd Martin Madan's recent and controversial proposals about male polygamy as a solution to the evils of prostitution, Dr Graham quickly announced that marriage certificates were required for use of his bed. Later advertisements repeatedly assured "the Nobility and Gentry, especially the Ladies, that everything [was] conducted with that decency and decorum, which cannot fail effectually to silence envious, ignorant, or malevolent tongues". A new handbill included a testimonial poem addressed to Dr Graham, all too obviously written by the Doctor himself:

> Proceed, great Sir, in spite of pedant fools,
> Who judge from what they call establish'd rules;
> Hold up the mirror of thy matchless skill,
> And prove, that NATURE is your object still;
> Fame join'd with fortune shall the truth advance,
> And prove your doctrines not the work of Chance.

Far from staving off public mockery, the new measures simply increased it. Ever inventive, the Patagonian Theatre quickly tagged a "magnificent representation of the TEMPLE OF HYMEN" to a comic opera already running. The following month the puppet company raised its little curtain on a new three-act comedy seductively entitled *A PEEP into the Temple of Hymen; or, the Celestial Blanket*. An unnamed "lady" – perhaps the Duchess of Cumberland, whose income by then largely depended on funds raised by extravagant social events and in-house gaming organized by her sister – had meanwhile invited Graham to preview his "celestial beds" at a ticketed masquerade, "entertaining her visitors in a manner no less agreeable than novel". At the Haymarket, *The Genius of Nonsense* was revived, a royal-command performance took place, and a new song was added, including a witty reference to King Lear's "let copulation thrive!" speech:

> To't Luxury, Pall-mall! The Dead,
> Entranc'd in a Celestial Bed,

Revive, and rear again the head,
So pow'rful is the Doctor!
Old Age again its sports begins,
Old Dames renew their ancient sins,
And at a Hundred bring forth Twins,
So pow'rful is the Doctor!

But Graham was not powerful enough to prevent a bill of indictment from the magistrates for exhibiting naked figures on the façade of Schomberg House. And unlike de Loutherbourg, who was rescued from prosecution for unlicensed musical entertainments by Sir Joshua Reynolds, he didn't have friends in high places willing to save him. "If one may judge of the interior curiosities of Dr. Graham's *Temple of Hymen* from *exterior* appearances, they must be very extraordinary indeed," the *Morning Post* had surmised when these adornments first appeared. Master of the long campaign, Graham had mounted nude statues of Roman deities like giant billboards, along with plenty of gold paint and a giant golden sun, ready to tempt the right kind of visitors inside the Temple as soon as it opened. *Procul! O Procul este Profani!* was translated into golden Greek capitals and emblazoned over the grand entrance: "Hence, ye vulgar herd!" (This, he later explained, was to "deter the wantonly lascivious – the mere votaries of pleasure, from polluting the Temple".)

Graham's extravagant decorations provoked endless smutty jokes about the precise interpretation of their symbolism: Venus was on top of Mercury, "her *chaste hand* a full yard from any part of her *lovely body*". Was Graham already urging couples to conceive by "riding St. George", as the woman-on-top position was commonly known? Were the gods' relative positions and sizes related to the planets, to show how "scientific" the Doctor was in all his "proceedings"? A mock letter from Mercury to Venus appeared, complaining of his misery at "being a mark for the insolence, ridicule and contempt" of every passer-by, as he stood "like a pimp at the door of a bagnio". Analyses "*of the outside of a certain* AMOROUS TEMPLE" appeared in newspaper after newspaper. "Whatever the Doctor's intention… may be," wrote one correspondent, after speculating that Graham was simply signalling his skill at the cure of venereal disease, certainly one of his advertised specialities, "we think Mercury does him not great honour; for he is universally known to be the God of Thieves and Imposters…" Graham dutifully replaced Venus with a bust of Galen, moved the offending sculpture to the Temple of

Hymen's entrance hall, and wrote on her newly acquired fig leaf: "By the order of the Middlesex justices". Aesculapius, Alexander, Alfred and Britannia were left on the Temple's rooftop and façade to proclaim to an impatient public Graham's true allegiances.

The mood was shifting. The "Aesculapius of the Adelphi" found himself the sitting target of an increasingly foul-minded public. Instead of lovers meeting at Ranelagh, they were said already to be arranging rendezvous at the Temple of Hymen. Doctor Graham was named as the umpire of one mixed-sex "duel" due to take place in Pall Mall on the opening night. The Temple's proximity to the elite brothels in King's Place provoked inevitable jokes about its function as a training ground for prostitutes: "that pure seminary is to serve as barracks for young recruits. Colonels Windsor, Matthews, and Adams, are to be made *Staff-Officers*, and Carrotty Kitty is to be *Drill-Serjeant*; they will learn their celestial exercise under the Doctor's own inspection, and be cleansed from all impurities." Graham was presented as the general in charge of the gang of high-class madams who operated in the area. "Great numbers of nuns are kept for People of Fashion, living under the direction of several rich Abbesses," wrote D'Archenholz. "You may see them superbly clothed at public places, even those of the most expensive kind. Each of these Convents has a Carriage and liveried servants, since these ladies never deign to walk anywhere except in St James's Park."

The well-dressed Doctor certainly seems to have shared many of the customers of these "convents", including the Bishop of London (said to have "exercised" rather than "exorcised" the celestial beds), and numerous peers. To Graham's horror, Lord Abingdon brought up the subject in the House of Lords, arguing that "the attack made upon the molten image of venereal lewdness on the outside of the door of the *medico electrical* doctor, was but to cover the adultery and fornication within." As the Doctor later indignantly swore, "The Temple... had not at that time been used, to his knowledge, even once, for any purpose whatever, either good or bad: How then, could a Peer of Great Britain have recommended the suppression of it, and declared it to be an infamous house of cuckoldom and adultery?" Surely the report must have been a printer's mistake? Luckily Abingdon was too well known for his "*practical* knowledge of the brothels *celestial* and *terrestial*" for the press to take his calls for reform very seriously.

7

The Lecture

> "I must myself take the liberty to say, that I deserve a civic crown, a comfortable annuity from government, or even a golden statue in every kingdom, for the real, the high, and most essential services I have done to mankind..."

Graham could wait no longer. The finishing touches to his new Temple would have to be postponed. Every defamatory report risked losing him customers of exactly the class he sought. Enormous bills were stacking up, and he was being accosted for payment on a daily basis by "a set of rascally fellows", apparently bent on overcharging him. It was time to face up to the fact that the Temple of Health and the Temple of Hymen could not both survive. He began to move his possessions to Pall Mall. Before long, the Adam brothers, keen to collect their unpaid rent, and financially precarious themselves, started threatening to dismantle and sell off the remaining contents of the Adelphi premises, including the Medico-Electrical Apparatus. A lawyer even advised Graham to take up residence in the King's Bench Prison to shake off his creditors.

The press gleefully suggested that the Medico-Electrical Doctor was finding the air of Pall Mall too unwholesome, and reported him on the point of reopening the Temple of Health at the well-known debtors' prison near St George's Fields. "There Venus may go uncovered without a blush, and Mercury riot in every species of plunder." Dr Graham would have been in perfectly good company. Debtors outnumbered felons in England's prisons by two to one, and credit was so ubiquitous that for most people, insolvency was an ever-present risk. Voluntary imprisonment under a "friendly action" actually offered debtors the best protection for their belongings – once the person had been "seized," their property was safe. Jails like the King's Bench were even regarded by thwarted creditors as sanctuaries for the spendthrift. With surety from friends, they could continue to live a more or less normal life, confined merely to a few square miles around the Southwark prison buildings.

("Imprisonment" was certainly no bar to the work of Revd Henry Bates, recently confined to the King's Bench on a libel charge. He continued to edit the *Morning Herald*, and kept up his attacks on Graham in its pages, for the rest of that year.) Prison benefactor William Smith thought five out of six of imprisoned debtors were shams: "When they can carry on their trade no longer, and some of their frauds are likely to come to light, they run to gaol... where they live in luxury and riot..."

Graham had more pride than that, or as he put it, "a soul above it". He also knew that the only way he could claw himself out of permanent debt would be to make a success of the new enterprise. He promised to "continue to labour day and night, as usual, in his profession... and... with the blessing of God!... pay every one in a very few months; and in a few years become himself, perhaps, one of the richest and most useful of his Majesty's subjects". By now, he was so open about his dire situation that before the following month was out his personal debt crisis had been versified at length in the *Morning Herald*.

In the event, all publicity did prove good publicity. When Graham threw open the doors of Schomberg House to the public for the first time on the evening of Wednesday 26th June 1781, curiosity triumphed over circumspection. "The grand *Hymenean Forge* for the formation of future *heroes! demigods!* and *goddesses!* was opened by the magnetic Tallisman of the puissant *Medico-Electrico Doctor* himself, when a select assemblage of *unbraced Bucks*, and pining *barren Does* attended the all-promising solemnity." An illustrious crowd rolled up in their carriages and descended from their chairs at Pall Mall, many faces still familiar today from their elegant portraits by Reynolds and others. The visitors were greeted with a fanfare from a couple of French horn-players standing on the roof, "pretty loudly proclaiming the *Cornu-copian* system that was to compose the amusements within."

All those seductive devices employed at the Adelphi Temple were given full rein at the Temple of Hymen too: "Scarcely has one set foot on the first step of the staircase than one hears harmonious strains of wind instruments which reach the ear through the hidden openings in the staircase, while the sweetest perfumes flatter the sense of smell till the entrance of a magnificent apartment is reached." But the fact that Graham saved his descriptive powers for the Grand State Celestial Bed, rather than offering a room-by-room survey of Schomberg House as he had done at the Adelphi, suggests that the furnishings were for the most part recycled from the Temple of Health.

The opening of the Temple of Hymen was unmistakably a social rather than a scientific event, the audience dominated by prominent Whig politicos. Charles James Fox, MP for Westminster and at this point the acknowledged leader of the opposition to the Tory North administration, was the most famous of these. He had recently been designated the "Man of the People" and was conducting a fervent campaign against the iniquities of the Marriage Act. Fox was, for good reason, the most caricatured man of the late eighteenth century. Hairy as a monkey at birth, a dandy in his youth, he had somehow reached a dishevelled and corpulent middle age without losing any of his charismatic charm. Politically, he stood for reform, and had been associated with the American cause since before the revolution. But Fox was equally famed for his scandalously unrestrained personal life, and loathed by the King as much for the Falstaff role he played in the life of dissolute Prince George as for his blue-and-buff politics. Fox's uncle, the Duke of Richmond (brother of conciliatory Louisa Connolly), was also there with his wife. Their handsome cousin, Admiral Keppel, whom Reynolds had painted in the 1750s in the pose of the Apollo Belvedere, joined them in Pall Mall.

Also among this fashionable throng was the Twelfth Earl of Derby, a moderate Whig who was the talk of the town that summer for his pursuit of the actress Miss Farren. He eventually married her after his wife's death. Renowned as a sportsman rather than a politician, he had a particular passion for cockfighting. The previous year, in a game of chance, Derby had won the honour of naming the Epsom race which still bears his name. Had the coin tossed that day fallen the other way, racegoers today might be betting each year on the Bunbury. There is no record of Derby having been joined at the Temple by his racing friend, Sir Charles Bunbury, but his money-loving mistress Poll Kennedy turned up. She may have come in the hope that Graham's ethereal assistance would save her life. Poll Kennedy was dead a few months later. Stage performers also came to watch Graham's bobbing bows – among them hefty Lydia Webb, the sixteen-stone comic star of the Haymarket, and short fat Signora Giulia Frasi, a retired Milanese singer who had been Handel's favourite oratorio soprano.

They came to spy out the territory and plot future routes to pleasure, rather than to throw themselves instantly into action; they arrived "less with a view of an *immediate sacrifice* at the altar of the presiding deity, than to reconnoitre the harbours on this *amorous coast*". The Duchess of Richmond was as happily married but as childless as her sister-in-law, Louisa. (Possibly both were as ignorant of their husband's infidelities.) She got into the spirit of the Temple by throwing herself onto one of Graham's celestial sofas and playfully pulling her husband to her with the words: "Let thy stern virtues yield to gentle Love!" At this moment, two of the silken ropes holding the glass conductor were seen to snap, and the tube was shattered into a thousand pieces, causing mayhem.

Other leading ladies of society soon became associated with the Temple. The most respectable of these was Mary Isabella Manners, the exquisitely beautiful Duchess of Rutland, a highly influential Whig political wife on the Shelburne side of the party. Also murmured to be among the Graham cognoscenti was Lady Spencer's younger daughter Harriet, now Lady Duncannon, who had grown up into a gambler as hedonistic as her sister. In a few years' time she would act as Georgiana's glamorous lieutenant in the Fox campaign for the 1784 Westminster election, which mired the whole family in an infamous "kisses for votes" scandal. The witty widow Bridget, Lady Tollemache, whose husband had been killed in a duel near New York, was something of a court jester in the household of George III and Queen Charlotte. She made an obvious candidate for gossip about Graham's Temple, delighting as she did in double entendres and coarse jokes. The indiscreet affairs of Lady Craven, the Margravine of Brandenburg-Ansbach-Bayreuth, had already featured in press "crim. con." reports and other salacious articles: her association with Graham must have done little to save her marriage, which collapsed definitively in 1783, leaving her free to pursue her literary, theatrical, geographical and sexual pleasures. As a mother of six she certainly had few excuses for resorting to the Celestial Bed for its prescribed purpose.

These decadent aristocrats and their hangers-on were the perfect audience for Graham in terms of wealth and social standing. The Doctor might have hoped for a little more interest in philosophy rather than pure pleasure. But this was a gathering ripe for moral reform and appreciative of his political slant. Perhaps taking his cue from Revd Murray's Newcastle sermons, Graham's lectures were as well punctuated as his former patient's with references to global politics. "The State's disorder too he mocks," sang Harlequin, in *The Genius of Nonsense,* in an echo of earlier sneers about Catharine Macaulay's "constitution". "The Doctor's plan is a political scheme, endeavouring to introduce an Herculean race in Old England, to enable us to fight the French, the Dutch, the Americans, the Spaniards, and all the world together," one newspaper correspondent baldly and inaccurately asserted. This simplistic interpretation of Graham's somewhat contradictory but essentially pacifist doctrines was a popular one:

> Britain, through thee, shall boldly stand,
> And bid the world defiance;
> What nation, but must dread the hand,
> Of such a race of giants.

Sex, according to Graham, was indeed a patriotic act, procreation a national duty. The ideas on which he had been musing during his apothecary days in Yorkshire seemed to be vindicated further with every passing year. Now at last Graham felt he had developed a social and scientific system to tackle the country's population predicament. With further ballast from the prominent dissenter Richard Price's latest book, which brought the horrifying (if utterly inaccurate) news that the British population was waning fast, Graham pointed the finger at war. By 1780, not only were the American Revolutionary forces looking invincible, but Britain was also at war with Holland, Spain and France, and sporadic fighting was erupting in India, Africa and the Caribbean too. The Doctor made it quite clear that his vivid detours to the world's battlefields weren't mere digressions, but essential elements of his argument. There was little point in educating his visitors about the nuts and bolts of procreation until they understood why it was so important. "My soul shrinks with horror," he declared, " nay, 'tis fired with indignation, even at the thoughts of the havock which has been made among the more innocent part of the human species, and at the millions of gallons of innocent and useful human blood, which have thus wantonly been poured forth, and which have dyed oceans, in every quarter of our terraqueous globe... there is not a man in the world, – there cannot be a woman on earth, who dares to assert, that any of the Belligerent Powers have gained the value of one straw, by these long and unnatural conflicts. No."

The cannibalistic Doctor gobbled up contemporary arguments popular with his predominantly Whig audiences and spewed them out with overwhelming passion, in a style that was all his own. His pacifist principles were hurled at bishops and press gangs alike.

In approving the war against America, the Anglican bishops had, according to Graham, in effect given the go-ahead for unprecedented slaughter: "Let us deluge... the world with human blood," they might just as well have said, "... for nothing at all... for the pretended, the ideal honour of this little island..." As for each victim of the press gangs, every innocent father snatched from his wife and children, each was "made to swear on the sacred word... that he will madly, impiously, fruitlessly pursue, all over the globe, by land and by water, with fire, famine and sword; yes, he is made to swear, that under the penalties of dishonour and of death, armed with every implement of murder, ruin and devastation, that he will chase, harrass, rob, sink, burn, capture or destroy, his neighbours and fellow creatures, who never hurt or offended him, his family or his friends...!" It was a source of terrible national shame, a horrific contrast to the era's advances in intellectual progress: "if the demons of war must still be let loose, in these comparatively humane and enlightened times!... let it not, O God! be recorded, that they were Britons... who perpetrated such enormities..."

Alongside the decline in numbers, Graham detected a deterioration in the physical quality of Britons. In rousingly millenarian terms he evoked a land of puny, enfeebled, inbred creatures, on the point of extinction. They had no one to blame but themselves. Graham lavished his most violent attacks on extravagance and dissipation. Once again, he was not expressing a new idea, but tapping into debates which had been raging through most of the century. Graham particularly picked up on ideas that luxury could injure mental as well as corporeal powers. The ever-increasing circulation of luxury goods was an issue of huge national importance for its detractors and defenders. For decades, entrepreneurs, economists, novelists and other writers had been arguing about the moral and political implications of the consumer revolution. Britons' declining powers – physical, intellectual and numeric – were regarded by Graham as a threat to their country's very existence. The state's "measure of follies and misfortunes seems now to be full", he pronounced, and the sun "either totally obscured by the foul vapours of luxury, and by the thick mists of universal corruption, or for ever set upon Britain, and now rising on transatlantic worlds!!!" The Doctor was apparently oblivious to the irony of making his case from the very site of luxury's headquarters.

The tide could be turned, he argued, with legislation. Prostitution – for which men, not women, were squarely blamed – had to be suppressed. A bachelor tax should be imposed, parents of three or more children rewarded and the ludicrous practice of sacking servants of either sex when they married had to be abandoned. Graham proposed mass public divorces for couples whose marriages were effectively bankrupt. He called these "JUBILEES, or *matrimonial insolvent acts*, for the relief of wretched, discordant, and BARREN couples". Graham made explicit those parallels between economic and sexual commerce that were often merely implied in eighteenth-century writings on the subject. Polite society was in the throes of embracing a new model of marriage, in which love and companionship were supposed to triumph over dynastic or financial concerns: "Matrimony is in fact a kind of co-partnery business, which requires a joint stock of fidelity, affection, prolific powers, and so forth, to carry it successfully and happily on: in all, or in any, of which requisites to be *deficient*, is certainly to be insolvent; and this is a species of insolvency which in my opinion has a much greater claim on the commiseration of parliament, than those bankruptcies which arise from pecuniary misfortunes."

Graham went on to address reforms in the clergy and the national diet, and to advocate a rather hideous form of eugenics drawn from observations of agriculture. Consciously "crossing the breed" was recommended in matrimony as in animal husbandry, and he suggested that sickly, diseased or malformed males should either be castrated in childhood or married off to post-menopausal women. Finally, a good twenty minutes into his three-act lecture, Graham began to discuss how babies were actually formed.

Even the orthodox medical jury was still out on this question. There had been leaps and bounds towards the truth arising from developments in microscopes and advances in anatomical knowledge over the past century or so. But enough contradictory theories were still circulating for Graham to consider carefully each of the essential arguments in turn. (To examine every minute shade of opinion that existed within each would have taken all night.) There were two main schools of thought. Supporters of epigenesis, as it is now known, believed that life arose from formless matter. Preformationists held that all life, but particularly human life, was "preformed" at the moment of Creation. This second group of thinkers was divided into "spermist" and "ovist" camps.

Graham took a broadly historical line in his explanation to his audience. Notions that went back as far Aristotle, Hippocrates and Galen had been perpetuated in popular sex manuals well into the middle of the eighteenth century. Compared with the modern, scientific theories now emerging, these old ideas seemed increasingly lewd and vulgar, and Graham was keen to distance himself from them. He dismissed as impossible the ancient notion that the mother's womb was a mere seed bed, and that all the responsibility for forming the embryo lay with the father's sperm. How could this be, when children resembled both parents? Graham also argued that progress in anatomy had now rendered implausible the Hippocratic theory that a foetus was formed by a mixture of the semen of both sexes. This assumed both men and women had to orgasm – and possibly even ejaculate – to conceive. A seventeenth-century French royal physician had vividly envisaged the woman's womb "Skipping as it were for joy" as it went to "meet her Husband's Sperm, [to] graciously and freely receive the same, and draw it into its innermost Cavity or Closet, and withal bedew and sprinkle it with her own Sperm, and powered forth in that pang of Pleasure, that so by the commixture of both, Conception may arise". But Graham didn't buy this. Though clearly in favour of female sexual pleasure, he argued that in fact "it is well known that there are many women who do not sensibly emit in the act of generation, but who nevertheless bring forth at the full time, stout, healthy, compact children."

The idea of preformation got round the eternal question of where and at what point life technically begins by implying that it is always already there. Although it would be nearly half a century before any-one actually laid eyes on a human ovum, images of an opened-up human egg had been reproduced since the 1670s. In its centre stood a tiny figure whose umbilical cord led into a network of lines, apparently in the heart of an unfolded flower bud. Graham's description of this "ovist" version of the preformation model presented the "ovaria" as tiny bunches of grapes, each little berry supposedly containing "a child sketched out in miniature in all its parts". (At this point, the ovarian follicles had been mistakenly assumed to be female eggs.) The "subtile penetrating vapour of male fluid" was somehow supposed to spark off its growth in the womb.

But when in 1677 sperm was identified in semen by an amateur Dutch microscope-maker, Antoine de Leeuwenhoek, the ground shifted again. As Graham put it, after he had "by means of his glasses, discovered certain opaque particles... so many *animalcula* floating and skipping about in the male seed", some theorists instead began to credit sperm with the lively role of providing multitudes of perfectly formed little people. Leeuwenhoek himself conjured up a picture of male spermatozoa as intrepid sailors in the vast and inhospitable womb of the female species, turning fertilization into a maritime drama: "The Womb being so large in Comparison of so small a Creature, and there being so few *Vessels* and places fit to feed it, and bring it up to a *Foetus*, there cannot be too great a number of Adventurers, when there is so great a likelihood to miscarry."

Procreation was a subject which, in the absence of sufficient visible evidence, seemed to bring out the poetic even in the most scientific investigators. Leeuwenhoek's drawings of his discovery lined up bulbous-eyed, tadpole-like creatures, sporting extraordinarily long tails. A confusing but influential forgery of these pictures published in the Royal Society's *Philosophical Transactions* showed a pair of shadowy miniscule men, suspended from their heads like a couple of creepy Christmas-tree decorations. In the eighteenth-century imagination these quickly evolved into *homunculi*, whose existence was taken seriously enough to be mocked heartily by Laurence Sterne in *Tristram Shandy* in 1760, a novel ostensibly narrated by just such an unborn creature. Graham was unconvinced by what has since become known as the spermist version of preformation. To him, as to many, it seemed too ludicrously wasteful for God to have designed. Why would he have bothered to create so many millions of tiny people, if only one was needed each time? It was "whimsical, or even ridiculous, to suppose, that all those animalcula are *homunculi*, little men and little ladies, striking and playing about in the male seed, each of them endeavouring to get first into the ovarium, and from thence into the womb, so that in time they may become fine ladies and gentlemen, princes, prime ministers, lawyers, heroes... and even... electrical quack-doctors."

So what was Graham's explanation? It was slightly confused, a characteristically contradictory blend of dry science and spirituality. "There is the greatest reason to believe, that an impregnation of the ovum by the influence of the male sperm is essential to generation," he concluded. Without committing himself to complete certainty, Graham thought the principle that the complete future child was already there in its mother's "ovarium", like "the plant with its leaves, flowers, fruit and seeds, wrapped up to us invisibly in the seed" was most likely to be correct. Conception was the act of setting "the little animal machine agoing – or in motion". This would explain two significant observations. Firstly, the Russian-doll-in-Eve's-ovaries idea could be one reason why the human race was becoming ever more feeble and degenerate. ("We may by and by perhaps realize the stories of fairies, imps and pigmies.") Secondly, semen, that "prolific liquor", had to be so copious because it was the first foetal food, the "exquisitely penetrating" substance that also rouses the female seed to life itself (or, LIFE!, as Graham prefers), through a process the Doctor described as "absorption".

Graham described the whole process of reproduction in astonishing detail. He had a persuasively medical explanation for female pleasure: "during the connection of the sexes, [the vagina and the womb] seem to be endowed with a ten-fold portion of sensibility. The state of the nerves which occasions this increased sensibility is no doubt communicated to the fallopian tubes, by which their ragged ends are erected, and applied to the germ [i.e. ova] in the *ovarium* in such a manner as to facilitate its escape." However inaccurate, this was a significant statement in a period when women's rights to sexual pleasure were being increasingly undermined by more sophisticated understandings of male and female anatomy. Previously, it had been assumed that women were just inside-out versions of men. If the ovaries were internal versions of seed-producing testicles, then to conceive, women needed to be aroused to ejaculate and release the all-important seed just like men. The new "two-sex" model seemed to make female stimulation an irrelevance. It was ultimately the reason why all those passive Victorian mothers-to-be had to lie back and think of England.

Graham went on to describe how the "germ" passes through the tube, finding its way to the womb, where it sticks, to be nourished for nine months by the mother's blood. Much though he would have liked to trace every moment of that gestation, it was time at this point in the lecture to move away from dry philosophy, discussion of the *corpora lutea* and the like, and on to "more delightful matters... the richest, the merriest, the most useful, and most interesting parts of the subject".

In late November 1783, when James Graham finally published the full text of his *Lecture on Generation*, he felt able to include details which even he had shied away from uttering out loud, though he doesn't specify which these were. He had been stung into action by several acts of piracy. A Scottish publisher had produced quite a convincing edition, claiming Graham's authorization, while a new erotic gossip magazine, *The Rambler's Magazine: or the Annals of Gallantry*, had launched itself by serializing a fairly similar version with much fanfare, strung out over many months. These Lectures read like notes taken in haste from the back of an audience, a rather pale and lifeless imitation of Graham's metaphorical excesses and circumlocutions, less convincing even than the numerous parodies of the Doctor's style of speech. Both leave out or abbreviate most of the science, and concentrate on the final, raciest section of the lecture.

Graham's daring – or impudence as it was usually described at the time – lay in putting on stage what was still barely acceptable on the page. When a Church of Scotland minister, Robert Wallace, had written a serious consideration of sex and marriage twenty years earlier, he had not even tried to get his ideas into the bookshops: "The many good hints... are so contrary to our present notions & manners, that it will be needless & by no means proper to publish them at least at present." Graham's *Lecture on the Generation, Increase, and Improvement of the Human Species* burst onto the scene at exactly the point at which reproduction was being transformed from a private, domestic concern to a public topic. Knowledge and power over the process was well on the way to passing from women to natural philosophers and man-midwives. In 1776, John Hunter had overseen the first successful attempt at human artificial insemination. He advised a draper whose deformed urethra and penis prevented him from delivering sperm into the uterus in the usual way to impregnate his wife with a warm syringe instead. (Aware of his morally ambivalent position, Hunter suppressed records of this treatment, and it was only reported after his death.)

Echoing the medical lessons of his former mentor William Buchan, James Graham sought to use the discoveries of the Enlightenment to return sexual knowledge to ordinary people. One day, he declared, every "good sensible couple" of middling means in the land would be able to have a celestial bed in their own house if they needed one. Meanwhile, his explanations of the causes of infertility in men and women, his advice about both regimen and, significantly, conduct, would "exalt and prolong the temperate and serene pleasures of the marriage-bed", while "heightening... personal beauty and loveliness", and "prolonging human life to the longest possible period of human existence".

Graham's audience sat like a congregation of sinners waiting to be saved. They turned out each evening in all their finery to mingle in one of London's most luxuriously decorated public spaces, only to be lectured on the dangers of wearing themselves down by doing just that. Graham repeatedly condemned "the mad, irrational, expensive, health destroying, and unsatisfactory attendance upon public places, with the agitations of play, with midnight racketing, with amorous indulgences, and… the consequent hysterical and other nervous diseases."

But the Doctor was dealing with an even more complicated conundrum. He clearly loved sex. His poetic descriptions of orgasm were both inspired and inspiring. He conveyed true sexual pleasure as an out-of-body experience, something that lifts men and women together to higher realms of existence. That "convulsive and extatic spasm, – that temporary dissolution, ejection, or going out of all the faculties of body and of soul!" which takes place during an act of conception is "the means employed by nature to animate the germ, or embryo". He portrayed the creation of life as so utterly momentous that it had to be accompanied by momentous sensations.

How, then, to persuade his audiences to exercise restraint? It all comes down to semen. Graham was convinced that semen was the life force within, crucial for good health and "celestial tranquillity of mind", as essential as oxygen. On no account should it be squandered. Procreation was actually a secondary function: "The chief use of this balmy – spirituous – vivifying essence, is after it has been thoroughly concocted and exaled into the general system, and intimately blended and churned as it were, with the blood and all the juices, bedewing every fibre, bracing and sheathing every nerve, – and animating with light, strength, and serenity the whole frame!" Neither men nor women could apparently enjoy health or happiness without "a full and genial tide of this rich, vivifying, luminous principle, continually circulating in every part of the system". This, of course, rather raised the question as to how a virtuous unmarried woman was supposed to acquire it. No matter. Graham was so swept away by the remarkable attributes of semen that he rushed on regardless. He simply couldn't find words expressive enough to describe it. "I ought to have called it the breath of beauty! condensed light! the life of the body! the soul of the soul! the magnet of love! the essence of ages! the liquor of life! and the true *pabulum* or food of all pleasure! ! !"

It is hardly surprising then to find a vigorous diatribe against masturbation at this point in the *Lecture*. According to the Doctor, solitary sexual activity was even more unhealthy than racketing the night away in public. "O my Son," the Doctor's favourite poet, John Armstrong, had written in a notorious versified sex manual nearly half a century earlier:

Banish from thy Shades
Th'ungenerous, selfish, solitary Joy.

Hold, Parricide, thy hand! For thee alone
Did Nature form thee?

General anxiety about onanism was hardly abating. Perhaps it fed
off parallel uncertainties about the confusingly contradictory values
linked to shamefully immoderate consumer spending. Graham's
frankly terrifying animadversions followed Tissot and others.
Wasting semen led directly to debility of body and mind: "infecundity
– epilepsy – loss of memory, sight, and hearing; – distortions of the
eyes, mouth, and face, – feeble, harsh and squeaking voice, – pale,
sallow and bluish black complexion, – wasting and tottering of the
limbs, – idiotism, – horrors …extreme wretchedness – and even
death itself."

Nothing could be more urgent than Graham's exhortations on
this subject. "[E]very seminal emission out of nature's road – I must
speak plainly, gentlemen! – every act of self-pollution, – and even
every repetition of natural venery, with even the loveliest of the sex,
to which appalled or exhausted nature is whipped and spurred by
lust, habit, or firey unnatural provocations; – but especially every act
of self-pollution, – is an earthquake – a blast – a deadly paralytic
stroke." Graham conjures up a world populated by stunted, skinny-
limbed wankers – "creeping, tremulous, pale spindle-shanked creatures, who crawl upon the earth, spirting, dribling, and draining off,
alone, or with their vile unfortunate street-trulls" – alongside those
(rather fewer) chaste heroes – Hercules, Angels, Gods – who have
managed to reach their twenty-first or even twenty-fifth birthdays
without having ejaculated "in their whole life, asleep or awake,
voluntarily or involuntarily".

The consequences of early or excessive venery were equally alarming. "As to my own part, gentlemen!" Graham would confide, "if
you will pardon this breach of politeness, I seriously declare, that
had I my time to live over again, and were I possessed of the same
knowledge I now have, I would be, I believe, thirty or forty years
of age, before I would know any at all, from personal experience,
about these matters." As a physician and a specialist in the cure
of venereal diseases, he reminded his listeners, he had seen the full
spectrum of self-inflicted horrors resulting from indiscriminate
sex. Without knowing that gonorrhoea and syphilis were separate
diseases, Graham was all too familiar with the discharges, "buboes",
"chancres", facial disfigurements, suppurating sores and swollen
bones presented by infected patients. He knew from the evidence of

hundreds that advanced sexually transmitted diseases and infertility were closely related. Rejecting the traditional and often deadly cure of mercury, he offered his own medicines and advice to deal with what had long been known as "the foul disease".

Graham was passionate about the importance of choosing the right kind of spouse in the first place. Anyone who wanted children should forget the attractions of "beauty, family or riches" and look instead for a wife in physical good health. Such a marriage, built on a foundation of mutual love and esteem, would be bound to produce healthy offspring. Graham's prescriptions for marital happiness were precise, liberal and rational. Bad habits to be avoided included tight lacing and high heels, both condemned as hurtful and unnatural, and most unfavourable to child-bearing. Good habits to be encouraged were temperance and moderation in all things, particularly sex and alcohol. (The joys of Bacchus never enhance the rites of Venus, according to the Doctor of Love.) Regular exercise in fresh air was recommended, alongside open windows, early hours and a diet of fresh green raw salads, succulent vegetables, sweet fruits, "the mild farinaceous grains", with plenty of pure water or milk. Graham did not regard breast milk with quite the awe with which he viewed semen, but he correctly, if metaphorically, ascribed it a very important role in child-rearing: the Duchess of Devonshire, unnamed but clearly identifiable, was praised to the heavens for setting the excellent example to her countrywomen of suckling her own baby when it was finally born on 12th July 1783, thereby imbuing her offspring "with the celestial sweetness of [her] own angelical nature".

In Graham's *Lecture on Generation*, he articulated the ideal of companionate marriage in the most appealing detail. He elevated a long-established genre of written conduct manuals into the dramatic performance of a lifestyle-coach-cum-sexual-guru. Music still a favourite model, Graham moved from explaining the importance of "tuning" both body and soul to inspirational recommendations of how this should be done, and the results that would follow. Everything was foreplay. His perfect spouses would talk together, play instruments together, pray together and be supportively attentive to each other in every way, ending the day harmoniously engaged in mutually satisfying sex. Finally they would retire to their separate beds or even bedchambers, since "pigging" it together 365 nights a year was tantamount to "matrimonial whoredom". Such ideal partners would be so happy together in their sexual sublime that neither would ever be tempted to stray.

"Domestic music, gentlemen! little family concerts, and especially singing together, or in turn, trifling as these may appear to some, I strongly recommend; and still more strongly regular family worship, and sentimental, philosophical, and religious conversations and intercourses. For, gentlemen, after the souls of an amiable couple have been softened, harmonized, illumined and filled with approving peace, by duties and amusements, so rational and delightful, when they return to an early bed, sober, serene, and healthful! their bodies and souls rush sweetly together! With the fullest, purest, intensest, and most celestial transports! and feeling themselves no longer inhabitants of this lower world they wing their soft long-waving way, through the flowery fields of Elysium! their souls float undulating, melting, and finally launching forth upon oceans of extatic bliss!"

As one visitor observed on his second visit to the temple, "Among much commonplace, there were some good observations." Far from commonplace were Graham's hygiene recommendations. "Gentlemen!" he would declare, night after night, "Were an angel arrayed in celestial glory to descend from heaven visibly on earth, and to declare to me, commissioned by the MOST HIGHEST!!! that I was to die this night, and that the welfare of my family, and the eternal happiness of my soul, depended on leaving to the world the most useful precept that could be given for the preservation of the health and strength of mankind; or even were I permitted to remain on the earth, to deliberate on the matter for a whole year, I would then proclaim to my fellow-creatures, with a loud and affectionate voice, that next to abstaining totally from animal food and strong liquors, from frequent venery, from warm meat and drink of any kind, and from close rooms and feather beds, BATHING THEIR PRIVATE PARTS WITH COLD WATER THOROUGHLY! AND FOR A LONG WHILE, EVERY NIGHT AND MORNING, FROM THE FIRST MOMENT OF THEIR LIFE TO THE LAST HOUR OF THEIR EXISTENCE, was in my opinion of the highest importance to the preservation of their health, strength, beauty and brilliancy, bodily and intellectual, of any thing that can be recommended or observed."

This suggestion was far more radical than it might today appear. A Quaker physician and dermatologist, Robert Willan, observed twenty years later that "most men resident in London, and very many ladies, though accustomed to wash their hands and face daily, neglect washing their bodies from year to year". In many people's minds, contact with water was likely to lead to ill health, or sunburn at best. Here was Graham, in contrast, recommending thorough washing to men and women, particularly of the genitals, not only morning and night, but immediately after every sexual act. He even suggested sparkling water as the most appropriate liquid to "crimp and cabbage up afresh the rich purse of Venus" or brace "the manly standard of love". Not only would this enable husband and wife "to renew the tender combat" as often as they wished, but each would become so addicted to the sweetness of genital hygiene that should they be tempted to wander from the marriage bed, they would only be revolted by any lover less clean, and instantly "spring back to their former love". Neglecting to wash after sex was as ludicrous as leaving a tap dripping. Cold vivifying water "effectually locks the cock, and secures all for the next rencontre", ensuring that not a drop of precious, life-renewing semen can escape. "Indeed, certain parts which next morning after a laborious night would be relaxed, lank, and pendulous, like the two eyes of a dead sheep dangling in a wet empty calf's bladder, by the frequent and judicious use of the icy cold water, would be like a couple of steel balls, of a pound a piece, inclosed in a firm purse of uncut Manchester velvet!"

He dismissed his audiences with the rousing cry that was echoed at the head of the Grand State Celestial Bed: "Go home, therefore, gentlemen! to the beloved wives of your bosom... Go!... In the name of health and happiness! In the name of posterity! – in the name of God!!! join delicacy with your ardour, in all amorous and conjugal pursuits, let moderation at all times controul your power! and obeying the first and greatest commandment of God! BE FRUIT-FUL, MULTIPLY, AND REPLENISH THE EARTH!"

According to Graham's own statistics, he delivered his *Lecture on Generation* on 167 successive nights, though its format soon began to vary. Even for his sexually adept and liberal audiences, Graham quickly felt he may have overstepped the mark. Within a fortnight, he announced that his lecture "on the art of propagating a numerous, healthy and beautiful Offspring..." was "calculated for Gentlemen", and that those suited "to the Delicacy of the Female Ear" would shortly be announced in the "Public Papers". For this alternative version, the focus shifted "to the beauty and importance of the female sex", and the audience was smaller, but nonetheless respectable. About thirty ladies "of rank and fashion" attended its first performance, most of them concealed behind masks. They were outnumbered by some fifty "genteel women", "who, without masks or affected delicacy, applauded, and seemed highly satisfied, and

delighted by this new and extraordinary species of entertainment".
Here they learnt how to build themselves speedily up into rocks of
"snowy blooming health, studded as it were with roses, and streaked
with celestial blue: becoming daily a sweeter, lovelier and more
intensely desirable companion; and in due time, the amiable and
happy mother of a healthy and virtuous offspring." A paraphrase of
Proverbs 31:28 was Graham's guiding text: "Her husband praising
her, and her children rising up, and calling her BLESSED!"

One anonymous visitor reported that "He uses the plainest language in dealing with the parts concerned in generation; yet ladies as
well as men crowd to hear him without scruple." When Sylas Neville
went to hear him later in the year, he applauded Graham's decision
to segregate his audiences: "Heard the King of *Quacks* deliver his
curious lecture on *Generation*, and indeed – he may well say to
Gentlemen only; few ladies, not of the Town, would come to hear
him."

Graham had a solution for those too shy to come to see him in
person. For the fat price of a guinea (theoretically to prevent it
"being publicly prostituted among the vulgar and licentious"), *A
Private Advice* could be bought. This little manual, aimed primarily
at a female readership, reaffirmed much of the practical information
which could by now only be heard at the gentlemen's lectures.
Chocolate was added to the banned list of alcohol, tea and coffee,
and husbands and wives advised not simply to be kind and attentive
to one another, and keep themselves scrupulously clean, but ensure
that "sweet and aromatic scents be for ever ascending, day and night,
from the body and garments of both husband and wife". This was on
the basis that "the happy influence of delicate scents is astonishing
in forwarding conception". Of more practical use was Graham's
recommendation in *A Private Advice* that the conjugal pleasures
should "be chiefly celebrated after certain periods". Inviting couples
to pay their fifty pounds to use the Celestial Bed when they were
at their most fertile must have hugely increased its success rate.
He applied the same principle as he had used in constructing the
Celestial Bed's tilting mechanism to his general advice: "After those
mysteries the lady should rest for an hour in the posture in which she
received the blissful effusion of luscious love, or on one side with her
head rather low, and knees and feet bent, so as to be perfectly easy."

The borders between erotica and medical texts in the eighteenth
century were rarely impermeable. Even the most rabid rant against
the evils of onanism could function equally well as masturbatory

material for a private reader. At least one modern commentator sees
A Private Advice as a deliberately titillating pornographic promotion,
disguised as social concern. But most pioneering attempts to discuss
sexual matters openly in a genuinely accessible way have met with the
same charge. Even in the twentieth century, Marie Stopes – who had
a surprising amount in common with Graham, sharing his litigious
disposition, extravagant sense of self-worth and belief in his own
longevity – had difficulties just in finding a publisher for *Married
Love*. When it came out in 1918, it was reviled as obscene by the
church, the medical profession and the press, and it was banned in
America. A gently mocking letter in *The Rambler's Magazine* shows
how unusual Graham's approach was:

> Your Private Advice to Ladies and Gentlemen (*sealed up*) cost
> me a golden guinea: had the price of it been twenty guineas I
> should have purchased it, and should have thought it dog cheap.
> It contains more real information than all the three folio volumes
> of Doctor James's Medicinal Dictionary: besides, Sir, you are so
> plain and intelligible – you never *mince matters* as some physicians
> do, but talk as familiarly and distinctly about generative matters,
> as others do about a hand or finger. I commend you highly for
> so doing, for when you address the public, respecting their health
> and vigour, you cannot be too plain, open, and ingenuous. It is the
> height of absurdity to call any part of the human body by a Greek
> name, when we have got an English name for it that every body
> understands.

Of course Graham used his publications to increase sales of
his medicines, and to publicize both his lectures and his medical
practices, but context makes it clear that the prime function of most
of his work was not to serve as erotica. Undated pirated editions
of his lecture on generation have helped confuse the issue: one
was labelled as "a genuine libidinous lecture" and published with
a titillating frontispiece showing a glamorous lady in a fashionably
large hat reading *A Private Advice* while sitting on a gentleman's
lap. Before Freud, the word "libidinous" simply meant "lustful",
and would hardly have been welcomed by Graham. Today it seems
a more appropriate adjective, conjuring as it does the Grahamesque
notions of psychic sexual energies. Graham's own emphasis on the
part played by the imagination in sexual arousal has undoubtedly
encouraged simplistic interpretations of his work as pornography.

Even his dietary recommendations were suggestive: ripe fruits, new-laid eggs and particularly whipped-up egg whites. Satirists became curiously fixated on the mealy potatoes he prescribed, perhaps because of their resemblance to testicles.

But the self-proclaimed "physician of the soul" had a very practical interest in the relationship between mind and body. He believed that the greater the intensity of sexual pleasure, the greater the chance of conception taking place. Not everyone could achieve these peaks of sexual ecstasy unassisted. "That *extraordinary Physician* and *natural Philosopher,* Dr. GRAHAM, in his sublime theories of generation, was perhaps the first who informed mankind that *certain aids* were necessary, even in the most athletic and vigorous constitutions, to enlarge and enrapture the practice," wrote the anonymous author of a 1791 tract about auto-asphyxiation.

The function of the Celestial Bed was to stimulate the imagination by "ravishing" every bodily sense. "In sweet assemblage are found all that is delightful or supremely beautiful to the eye, to the ear, to the taste, to the smell, and to the touch... Thus regaled with love and beauty... the entranced pair! no longer inhabitants of this world, *but* dissolved in the soft gushing tides! are launched forth upon oceans of extacy!" The same philosophy underpinned Graham's suggestion that anyone past their prime could be usefully fired up with erotica, which could hardly have helped interpretations of his own writings. By implication, some men and women "ought... at certain critical and important times, to have their minds stimulated, and their passions roused and excited, by the sight of rich, warm, or of what are called lascivious prints, paintings, and statues; by amorous stories or dalliances, and by every possible and natural means: for it is not to be imagined how very much the venereal appetite may be whetted by artificial means, or by accidental causes". How much safer these kinds of "artificial" means were than popular aphrodisiacs such as Spanish fly. (A decade earlier, the Marquis de Sade had been sentenced to death *in absentia* in Marseilles for poisoning prostitutes with aniseed sweets laced with cantharides.)

The closest Graham himself edges towards actual pornography is in a short series of anecdotes in the *Lecture*. These seem more comic than stimulating. He tells of a Scottish hairdresser so "maddened" by desire after ten minutes of combing the hair of a particularly beautiful new client that he made up an apology about forgetting his curling tongs, rushed home to spring "aboard his astonished wife", and they immediately conceived triplets. He suggests different positions for intercourse might suit some couples better than others, referring to "a certain lady of quality of this country, still beautiful and lively" (perhaps Lady Tollemache?), who "has frequently been heard to say, that for her part, she never could be got with child, till like St. George of Old, she had subdued the dragon". Graham also mentions a common peasant practice of encouraging women to conceive by taking them to watch horses and bulls copulating. Some other mildly titillating examples of the forces of the imagination follow: a threesome and a toothless old lady who nonetheless involuntarily bit a coin in two at the sight of the "turgid plenitude of vigour" of a noble stallion in action in the marketplace of Norwich.

As he sped in his conspicuous carriage from Temple to Temple, Graham was still treating patients put in his care by Lady Spencer. She seems to have maintained a decorous silence about his antics up to this point, despite her daughters' rumoured involvement. On 8th July, having finally cleared his Adelphi apartments, Dr Graham wrote from Pall Mall to apologize for the delay in thanking his patron for her latest sixteen-guinea payment, and described the difficulties he was having with the drunken mother of one young boy undergoing treatment. (He was concerned to set the record straight in case she complained to her benefactor of being dismissed from her son's bedside.) A few weeks later in a dawn-lit letter to her son, Lady Spencer complained of having been woken at five by the tumult of an express postal coach: "I never like the hurry of an express, but I begin to be enough acquainted with the Zeal of Doctor G and G's friends, to suppose it was about him which it proves – he will certainly be ruin'd by mere postage or letter carriage."

Her offhand comment about the form of Dr Graham's extravagances is extremely revealing. His mounting debts were clearly not just due to excessive spending on the contents of the Temple of Health, arguably a speculative investment which at least had the potential to generate an income. The Doctor seems to have had a complete disregard for the kind of minor economies even the wealthiest of his generation were happy to make. Members of Parliament were allowed to frank letters, sending them free of charge; their wives, daughters and friends regularly took advantage of this privilege. One explanation for Graham's ostentatious behaviour could be the need to keep up appearances – always an expensive business. An air of impoverishment was, after all, a sure way to attract the attention of creditors. And despite the excitement surrounding the opening of the new Temple, the Doctor's financial problems were showing no signs of going away.

Graham featured in one newspaper after another that summer. "The Temple… is now fitted up with a degree of elegance and magnificence far superior to most royal palaces in the world," his own advertisement declared at the end of July 1781, announcing the "Grand Illuminations" to accompany the lecture on "the Art of exalting and rendering permanent the joys of the Marriage Bed". Bottled spa water had by this time doubled in price, thanks to the Doctor's douching prescriptions to "the *steril* ladies of this kingdom". It was suggested that another Dr Graham, a wealthy Cumberland clergyman, should henceforth be called "the *Non*-Electric" Doctor, "for the better preservation of identity". Over in Islington, a new song and scene had meanwhile been incorporated into a well-received satirical entertainment at Saddler's Wells theatre. Here Gog and Magog made yet another stage appearance: the actor Mr Doyle, "in the character of the Doctor's porter", premiered a song which remained popular years after the show had closed:

> A bed that's celestial to bodies terrestial
> Will warmly inculcate its wonderful use,
> Bring children like giants, that set at defiance
> The pigmies that Nature alone can produce;
> > Your feelings are such,
> > From its delicate touch,
> With pleasure and charms universal ye glow,
> > Come see,
> > Where electricity
> Tickles ye all from the top to the toe.

Graham's ubiquity as a vehicle for as much as an object of satire was the subject of one of the many chapters of a whimsical topical serial in the *Morning Herald*: 'A Sentimental Excursion to Windsor'. A series of scenes spoof the Doctor's periphrastic rhetoric, his love of mythological symbolism, theories about medical music, and of course the mono-thematic inclinations and increasingly elaborate mechanics of London's theatre world. A fictional dramatist, Miss Verjuice, explains the term *"medium"*: "I mean, my dear, …the *machinery* by which I convey my satire to the audience. I have fixed upon the *Temple of Hymen* and the *celestial beds*." In one scene from her play an Ambassador seeks treatment from the Doctor after an overturned carriage has caused him and his fashionably phoney body parts to disintegrate. His dormouse eyebrows, Parisian artificial eye, cheek plumpers and the rest are scattered to the winds. A medical consultation with General Lightfoot betrays the cowardly character of British generals happily battling rhetorically about the American war on the safe side of the Atlantic, while keeping well out of combat themselves. He is delighted to learn that the Doctor's treatment depends on fire. "An apprehension of fire is the cause of my complaint," he confesses, "and a deafness which always seizes me previous to action, and prevents me from understanding orders."

Fleeting references to Graham appeared in numerous plays and poems over the next few years. A couple of writers were storing up more substantial material for future novels. Thirteen years after it opened, Robert Jephson set a section of a satire on revolutionary politics at the Temple of Hymen in Pall Mall. *The Confessions of James Baptiste Couteau, Citizen of France* told the tale of a fictional revolutionary who, like Brissot, had spent the early 1780s struggling to make a living in London. Coming across one of Dr Graham's manifestos, the hero decided to present himself at the Temple to offer his services: "The Lectures of this worthy Professor were well attended, but the Experiments much better." Thanks to his Herculean physique, Couteau was taken on as a sperm donor. "[Y]ou see, we assist Nature," explained Jephson's fictional doctor, "We conceal where she has played the stepmother, and all is displayed to the best advantage where she has been bountiful." Couteau was surprised to be equipped with a "beautiful masque" painted on a material lighter than gauze, with openings for eyes, mouth and nose. With the help of this and his own muscles, he "assisted at an infinite number of Experiments", and became one of the favourites of the Temple:

> How many families at both ends of the town may have been obliged to me for those pretty little pratling cherubs always so endearing to their supposed fathers, I can't pretend exactly to determine; the number certainly must be considerable.

Jephson's gigolo joke fleshed out hints that had long circulated about the exact nature of Graham's fertility treatments. His approach is light-hearted but the suggestion that something altogether more sinister was going on at the Temple of Hymen is nonetheless quite shocking. For all his talk of marriage certificates, was it really possible that Graham's "priests" were more than mere acolytes? Far more likely, this was a dig at the Doctor's own rhetoric. In *A Private Advice*, he declared how delighted he would be to become "the moral *father* of many an heir to *noble* honours and ample estates, which but for me might be been dissolved in chaos".

Mary "Perdita" Robinson waited for Graham to die before introducing him in print as Doctor Pimpernel in her fifth novel, *Walsingham*, published in 1797. She seems to have known Graham pretty well in her youth, and continued to be linked with him in prints during the early 1780s, together with Charles James Fox, who had briefly become her lover in 1782. Bowing and hemming and name-dropping in a "strange farago of incoherent nonsense", Pimpernel and his speeches perfectly reproduce Graham's style and rhetoric. Robinson echoes Lady Spencer's allusion to Graham's modus operandi: her fictional version of the Doctor enters Walsingham's chamber "with a boisterous tone and a thundering knock", and charges down the stairs just as energetically as he leaves.

But Robinson's caricature of Graham is cruelly at odds with the Doctor's own print persona. When she wrote *Walsingham*, Robinson was a professional writer approaching forty, in a painfully debilitated state of health. She had long ceased to trade on her exquisite looks, and successfully remodelled herself as "the English Sappho". Her interpretation of Graham's obsession with young women's looks reveals as much about her own experience of life as a fading beauty as it does about the Doctor's true character. Every time Pimpernel speaks, he betrays a loathing for any woman past her mid-teens, and a cruel delight in the imminent deaths of the elderly dowagers on whose wealth he depends. "I left the old Duchess of Bloomingdell in hysterics. Well, no matter – she has lived long enough; d—n old women – they are only fit to see physicians, and to propagate false politics." After listing all the ladies of fashion who can't live without him, a character called Mrs Woodford declares with ardour: "Never was there a man so universally beloved by the women!"

"Pardon me, Madam" interrupted her daughter, "if I beg leave to mention myself as an exception: Doctor Pimpernel is my aversion: his hypocrisy would, alone, teach me to despise him, even if his licentious conversation afforded no plea for my abhorrence. He has often soothed your ear with fulsome praise, one moment; and the very next ridiculed the weakness of our sex, for crediting his duplicity."

Dr Pimpernel's fawning but mercenary attitude to nobility vastly exaggerates Graham's obsequious tendencies. Robinson targets Graham's literary and professional ambitions just as harshly.

"I am the phoenix of physic!" declares Pimpernel. "The only Being on the face of the earth who has really dived into the arcanum of medicine! I have done more in the experimental way than all the gossips of our fraternity. Did you never read my book upon Barley-water? – Five volumes quarto! with notes medical, critical, botanical and methodical! – The first work that ever was published!"

"Of the kind," said Mr. Optic gravely.

"The game is up!" is Pimpernel's catchphrase in *Walsingham*. So it certainly seemed for Graham by mid-September 1781. The Doctor's life was at a turning point. He had achieved his ambition of national fame, and come close to realizing his most exuberant fantasies. But its cost would not simply be financial. From this moment on Graham's survival could only be at the expense of his original vision. The natural philosopher had to step aside for the showman, and the showman desperately needed the crowds to roll up. His financial embarrassment had become so acute that he was in danger of losing everything he had worked for. At Essex Street, off The Strand, a Mr Benge was printing the catalogue for his auction of the Doctor's effects, to take place within the week. Lot 36 would be "The Grand Celestial Bed… covered with rich silk damask, supported by 28 Glass pillars, covered with a rich carved & gilt canopy, with crimson silk curtains fringed, and tassel'd, with a conducting glass tube & chain to ditto".

Isolated and misconstrued, "the Prince of Electrical Joys" composed a candid new handbill setting the record straight, and threw himself on the public's mercy. "Dr Graham is oppressed with shame and mortification" at having been forced to open the Temple of Health "with arrangements so many thousand degrees inferior" to his original scheme. He now admitted that he had not even managed to pay off "all the enormous expences incurred at the Adelphi", before launching the scheme for "the Temple of Prolific Hymen". Workmen were refusing to go on with his plans, the great room of the temple remained incomplete, and now it was revealed that the Celestial State Bed itself was not yet finished or erected. All that Dr Graham could depend on was his own consciousness of "the integrity and usefulness of his views and intentions". He announced that he was

to throw himself and his great undertaking on the candour, good sense, and liberal benevolence of the public at large for countenance, protection, and support – that he may be enabled to go on with and complete, and render diffusively useful THESE his most arduous undertakings...

Graham protested that his purposes had been misinterpreted. "The chief object of his ambition," he argued, as he always had, was "to promote the happiness of private families, and to prevent chagrin, adultery, and divorces, which frequently arise from the want of children in illustrious and noble families".

The Pall Mall premises, now renamed the Temple of Health and Hymen, seemed on the brink of closure, and the entry charge was reduced to just one shilling. And, as proof of the certainty of his methods of treating barrenness, Dr Graham was prepared to give advice to "any decent poor married couple of character" at no expense whatever.

His charms prevailed. He was indeed the "phoenix of physic", and this would not be the last time he rose from the ashes. Over the next few days, ladies "of Reputation, Rank and Fortune" turned up in their hundreds in support of Graham's cause, while the gentlemen were only slightly less numerous. They raised between them "so many hundred pounds, that Dr. Graham's creditors, with the consent of the Sheriff of Middlesex... agreed to postpone the sale for a few days longer, in order to serve Dr. Graham, and to give every individual of the public, an opportunity of viewing this stupendous undertaking, and of hearing, at a very low price, the Lecture on Generation, which has been attended, and highly approved of, by the first personages both in church and state in this kingdom." Graham was apparently then pressed by his female admirers to open the Temple, not for a lecture, but for a mixed-sex "Elysian Promenade", lit up by hundreds of wax candles.

The enchanting glory of these seemingly magical scenes, will break forth about seven, and die away about ten o'clock; during which time oriental odours and aetherial essences will perfume the air, while the hymeneal sopha blazes forth with the plenitude of the same lambent celestial fire.

In the following months, the Doctor introduced new lecture themes, abandoning "masculine health, vigour, and serenity of body and mind", in favour of "Love, Friendship, and Domestic Happiness". He announced a lecture on "the State and influence of Women in

Society, and on the mutual duties and obligations of both sexes". Whether these "glowing... enchantingly lovely, yet delicately chaste descriptions of personal beauty, and... moral excellence" were produced in language or in the flesh is ambiguous. The Doctor himself became the subject of a one-shilling lecture and discussion. London's debating societies had been heatedly discussing marriage, bachelordom, gallantry, coquetry and mental and physical charms for the past year and more. In October, at the Three Tuns in Fleet Street the Revd E.B., MD took as his subject "Dr Graham's Efforts to improve the Works of Nature; with a few remarks on the CELESTIAL BED".

Still open at half-price, the Temple was flooded with visitors – over 11,000 during the next three months, according to its proprietor. These cut-price audiences just about shielded Graham from his creditors, but did little to improve his reputation. One man-midwife was said to have been shocked at "the slow dances of half-naked wretches" at the Temple, and supposedly attended a number of women worn out by their exertions on the bed.

Whether or not this was true, Graham's integrity was beginning to fray. His high moral tone was proving ever harder to maintain. Finding "the majority of the world... still prejudiced against" his Celestial Bed, as ruinously expensive to its operator as to its occupants, the Doctor publicly determined "no longer to solicit the attention of the public to that grand discovery".

It was a resolution which, unsurprisingly, "His Highness the Hymenical Doctor of Pall-Mall" found difficult to keep. Over the next few years he repeatedly threatened closure, only to be tempted back into the limelight by the possibility of new clients. Declarations of peace and defeats abroad brought the Army and Navy slowly trickling back from overseas duties, ready to be entertained with delights which they had previously only been able to imagine. "Where can our sailors and soldiers more elegantly relax from the fatigues of war?" wondered a letter-writer in the *Morning Post*.

They were attracted by a distinct shift in emphasis. Graham no longer even tried to promote the Temple as a sanctuary of science, or a medical museum, but as an unabashedly commercial venture, which vied with grand assembly rooms the world over. "It is needless to say any thing with respect to the pre-eminence which these apartments have, in point of richness, elegance, and brilliancy, over every other suite of public rooms in Europe; as their superiority is unanimously allowed by upwards of 20,000 persons of taste and fashion, who have already viewed them, the greatest number of which have visited the principal courts in Europe, and have given a decided opinion in favour of the Temple of Health [and Hymen]." When he did perform his lectures, Graham began to introduce tone-lowering fairground tactics: "The Rosy Herald of Health", was a gigantic woman over seven feet tall, who was accompanied by "a Dwarf Lady". Together they were meant to exhibit "the strength and stature of that race of beings which would spring from the Celestial Bed, and... the present puny degeneracy of mankind, which due attention to the precepts inculcated in that extraordinary Lecture, would effectually improve". Singers were employed for evening promenades, and gentlemen tempted in with the promise of a fifty-guinea prize for the raffle tickets given out free at lectures.

But even with all these efforts, Graham was left with outstanding debts. Fatally, he began to sublet the new Grand Apollo Apartment and other public rooms at Schomberg House. The gamblers moved in. "Society in those days was one vast casino," as Charles James Fox's Victorian biographer, George Trevelyan put it. "On whatever pretext, and under whatever circumstances, half-a-dozen people of fashion found themselves together, whether for music, or dancing, or politics, or for drinking the waters, or each other's wine, the box was sure to be rattling, and the cards were being cut and shuffled." Earlier in the century gambling legislation was put in place principally to prevent addicted aristocrats from betting away their family fortunes. But as soon as one type of game was outlawed, another would be invented in its stead. Fantastic sums of money went on changing hands as rapidly as ever. Many of the highest-stake games were played in gentlemen's clubs such as the exclusive Brooks's, the Whig headquarters, or White's, its Tory equivalent. "Deep play" of this kind was a luxury which did not simply display one's wealth, but showed how little one cared about losing it. Its elite participants were clearly visible to passers-by through ground-floor windows in St James's, theatrically dressed in embroidered coats turned inside out, or wearing coarse protective overcoats or leather cuffs to keep their fine lace clean. Some sported broad-brimmed, high-crowned hats decorated with flowers. Women – including many of those linked to the Temple of Health – were meanwhile winning and losing huge amounts more privately at late-night soirées at each other's homes, playing faro, quinze, whist, loo and the aptly named hazard.

Illegal fly-by-night gambling clubs were also springing up all around the West End, rather like Nathan Detroit's floating-crap games in *Guys and Dolls*. E.O. was the favourite here. A game of chance similar to Roulette, it was played on circular tables divided into "Evens" and "Odds" around their perimeters, with a revolving central section into which a ball was thrown. In 1781, it was reported that the venues which housed these clubs were closely guarded, secured against any unbribable constables with multiple lookouts and early-warning systems. "When this bell is rung the E.O Table is instantly dismissed through a trapdoor, and a pantomimical shifting brings up a table, bottles, and glasses in its place; round which the company sit in seeming conviviality. This device was the invention of a Bow-street runner, who is a rider on the profits of the cheat." Exposures of "these infamous places of nocturnal rendezvous" were newspaper staples that summer.

By June 1782 the Temple of Health had become notorious for its E.O. tables. It was referred to as the *Temple of Thieves*, and one night a Lord G— walked away with winnings of £15,000. Brawls began to break out with alarming frequency, as Horace Walpole reported to a friend: "As Lady Chewton and her sisters came from the Opera, they saw two officers fighting in Pall Mall next to Dr. Graham's, and the mob trying to part them. Lord Chewton and some other young men went into the house and found a Captain Lucas of the Guards bleeding on a couch. It was a quarrel about an EO table, I don't know what: this officer had been struck in the face with a red-hot poker by a drawer, and this morning is dead." The newspapers could add nothing to the origins of this "violent *fracas*" but reported that "all the windows in the *Temple of Hymen* were destroyed". At the end of July there was a "riot and robbery" at the Temple. Graham's house was "burglariously" broken into by a number of "idle and disorderly Persons, Burglars, Felons and Thieves" who made off with some furniture and smashed up several large chandeliers and girandoles as they escaped. They pretended to be acting on official authority. A few days later the Justices Hyde, Wright and Addington really did set off on a mission to destroy every E.O. table in the city of Westminster, starting at Dr Graham's. In the course of breaking two tables at the Temple, Addington sustained a blow to his head, which "would have finished off an ox". Rumours of his death brought a huge crowd to the house, and the incident was immortalized in a caricature by Gillray.

Graham must have been a little encouraged by mounting public anger about these authorized raids – they were perceived in some quarters as violations of liberty. But these incidents still amounted to a series of public-relations disasters for the Doctor. As usual, he defended himself in the newspapers in which he'd been pilloried. His story was that he had been "importuned and tempted" for months with lucrative offers to hire out his rooms for "the wretched and deadly purposes of gaming", but that his soul had revolted at the suggestion "with indignation and horror". In April though, still owing two of the twelve thousand pounds spent on fitting out the Temples in the Adelphi and Pall Mall, he had succumbed at last. "A handsome weekly rent for the rooms", together with every half-crown taken at the door was impossible to resist. Six months later only about four hundred pounds was owing to his creditors, which he intended to pay off by January. He assured the public that he had now reclaimed the reins, and was back in place running the show himself with "decency and decorum".

Undeterred by his remaining debts, he had even sunk another thousand pounds on still more decorations to impress "the Peasant, the Philosopher, and the Prince", including a superb new piece of "Musical Machinery" displaying the "various powers and beauties of Nature in her four elements, and in her most pleasing scenes". When Charles Byrne, "the surprising Irish Giant... the tallest man in the world" arrived in town, Graham fanned newspaper speculation on the latest celebrity's love life and his oversized physical endowments by offering him a trial of the Celestial Bed. It was politely rejected, with the assurance that Byrne was "a perfect stranger to the rites and mysteries of the Goddess Venus". Graham turned to promoting "new and eccentric" Lectures on Venereal diseases, and then threw himself into composing a fresh extravaganza for the Temple. Never before had he strayed so far from his original purpose.

The new entertainment was emphatically "NOT A SATIRE", but "A serio-comic philosophical Lecture, to be delivered by Vestina, the Rosy Goddess of Health", called *Il Convito Amoroso* – or "The Amorous Banquet". Its subject was love. Its inspiration was either Dante, a favourite for English translation that year, or perhaps a new Italian opera in rehearsal at the Haymarket. Advertisements for Graham's short-lived show even carried a health warning in poor French. It was designed only for "Adepts Hibernian and British, for the Cognoscenti, et pour les Amateurs ardens des delices exquise de Venus [the ardent lovers of the exquisite delights of Venus]" Any Lady or Gentleman with a weak or squeamish stomach was advised to stay away from such a "rich Banquet". The "Grand Feast of very Fat Things" took place on Monday 25th November 1782 in the company of a mixed but apparently "glowing" audience of three hundred. Graham's latest Vestina (the third woman to be employed in the role) ascended to the Electrical Throne to cries of "Bravo! Hebe! Bravissimo! Vestina! Fat, fat and more fat!"

The published version of Vestina's lecture was already in its second edition barely a fortnight after the bizarre party took place. It made the Gothic claim that this lecture on her new "Philosophy of the Universal Passion" was actually a "ludicrous yet philosophical parody" of "a little old Book" thrown her way by Chance, or perhaps the Junior Priest of the Temple. For all the theatrical window dressing, the message of *Il Convito Amoroso* was essentially a heavily eroticized version of the theories Graham had been promoting for years: the "invisible magnetico-electrical fire or effluvium, constantly circulating in, and exhaling from human bodies", was the life force which could allow body and soul to dissolve into one in the sexual act. From Vestina's lovely lips emerged Graham's undoubtedly eccentric explanation of the science of sexual pleasure. She hailed this "grand animating principle, the all-mighty agent" in terms that recalled Graham's inadequate epithets for semen: it was the "*real, the EVER-LIVING* cause of what we call LOVE!"

The lecture swept through Plato, Aristotle, Descartes and their varied philosophies of love, erupting from time to time into fervent supplications to "THE GUARDIAN GENIUS OF THE HYMENEAL TEMPLE, AND OF THE CELESTIAL BED". Compelling images of the misty mark made by a warm hand placed on a cold mirror were brought forth as evidence of the existence of "animal electricity": the very pores of the skin (discovered, like sperm, by Leeuwenhoek with his microscope) were said to exist so that these subtle particles of "odorous or luminous matter" can continually escape. Love strikes not when a naked cupid lets fly his dart, but when these "insensible transpirations" are borne through the air and strike another's "bodily organs" (i.e. senses), especially those of sight and smell. "It is pretty well known how they act upon the taste; – that *suction* most powerfully attracts them; – that *kisses* dissolve them; – that pleasure spirts them from the papillae of the tongue; – that they gush from the rich pulp of the lips; – and that by the touch of collision of *certain parts*, they undulate and thrill from the *magical centre*! With electrical swiftness – with harmonious vibrations! – and with extatic soul-dissolving delight! – thro' every, even the most distant nerve!" The romantic hand-squeezing and subtle pressures of happy young lovers are dictated "by nature herself", so that a greater flow of animal electricity can get to work on their hearts, and thus circulate around the lovers' entire bodies. But age and overuse inevitably bring a decline in these electrical emanations: "As we decline into the vale of years, the organs of life, and *the Cyprian apparatus of pleasure* harden and shrivel; THE MANLY STANDARD OF LOVE almost disappears." Graham's forthcoming obsession with preserving youth was beginning to surface.

Lavish and titillating descriptions of sexual love punctuated the feast. Human sexual intercourse was equated with the workings of electrical machinery more clearly than ever: "The electrical effects and phenomena that are produced by the vivid flashings of the eyes, the attritions and balmy suctions of the lips, the touch or squeeze of the hand, and finally, *by the soft, firm pressure of a tight-new virgin elastic cushion, well amalgamated*, all, all, demonstrate that my theory is founded on nature and on facts," Vestina declares, apparently without a blush.

Il Convito Amoroso is not in the same category as *A Private Advice*. It is a far more slippery piece of writing. Self-consciously both parodic and philosophical, the printed lecture slides between performance and private reading matter, between the sensual and the scientific. Graham's characteristic breathlessness echoes "the dashes and drifts of language – the sighs and caesuras so typical of passages describing sex in the eighteenth century". But these pauses also point towards the enormous difficulties Graham constantly faced in getting his audiences to take pleasure seriously. How could he ever address the subject of sex in a manner which did not admit misinterpretation?

Il Convito Amoroso is clearly addressed to both men and women. It acknowledges male and female desire with almost equal attention. In a period when solitary novel-reading was often regarded as a dangerous activity for women and erotica generally aimed squarely at male audiences, this was liberating. Vestina's sisterly attitudes suggest that Graham's views about women were far more admirable than Mary Robinson later bitterly implied in *Walsingham*. The Temple Goddess condemns overly ardent romantic male lovers, thoughtlessly caught up in their own passions and desire to possess their object. She also damns those men who "from a natural frigidity of constitution, (or from certain early unnatural practices… [i.e. masturbation]) consider the ladies as only beautiful figures placed in the world by way of ornament, or as delightful flowers, formed merely to variegate and enrich the colouring of the universe". Equally reviled are frivolous men who treat women like "agreeable nonsensical toys, *pour passer le temps*". Finally, Vestina declared that it is "degrading" to regard women only as vessels for procreation.

Graham's goddess may not have got to the end of her performance. It seems that the Middlesex justices were once again on the moral rampage, and "his Worship, MIDAS NEUTERSEX, Esq; and his Bum-Possé" burst in just as "Dessert" was about to be served.

Yet again, the end threatened. Within a couple of weeks of this intrusion, Dr Graham announced that he was retiring to the continent. (He had always predicted he would after three years.) The contents of the Temple of Hymen were to be "peremptorily sold". His property could be viewed at the cost of a shilling's admittance, before its "final close and dissolution" on Thursday 19th December. Ladies and gentlemen flocked for their last chance to see "all the elegant Household Furniture, a capital Electrical Apparatus, the Celestial Bed, large and beautiful Pier Glasses, brilliant cut Glass Lustres, Statues... Pictures" and other splendid decorations.

So many came that Graham's creditors let him keep his former possessions on display, and allowed a weekend of celestial sociability before the place was cleared on Monday morning. The Doctor was allowed to pocket the profits. For three evenings, Dr Graham performed his world-famous lecture, complete "with many new strokes", pouring out, he promised, "unreservedly, his WHOLE SOUL". The apartments were dazzlingly illuminated and ladies as well as gentlemen admitted for what the Doctor described as "very merry meetings, or rather rich sentimental love feasts, the three last nights of this most sublime and extraordinary institution". Thousands more turned up, according to the Doctor. Once again, in his phoenix fashion, Graham rose triumphantly from the absolute brink of ruin. His profits from the latest wave of admirers were enough for him to buy back his property, and the show went on.

"Now or never!" was the cry through the first half of 1783. Thanks largely to the constant stream of new arrivals from abroad, "Gentlemen of the Navy and Army" earnestly begging, according to Graham, to hear his celebrated lecture, the Temple seemed to go from strength to strength, financially if not philosophically. But all these triumphant comebacks were actually no more than short-lived postponements of the inevitable. Debts on the scale he must have racked up could never be cleared simply by knock-down admission fees, private lotteries and increasingly hollow-looking promotional campaigns. He could only keep the creditors at bay for so long. Despite Graham's best efforts, his dream was dying.

Some new audiences were drawn in, believing it really might be their final opportunity. Samuel Curwen, who had bumped into Gog and Magog three years earlier, was tempted at last to pass an evening there and found Graham "a most curious character and speaker, who for 2 long hours in an extempore address to his hearers in numbers about 200, male except 6 females, 4 of whom left the room when modesty required the absence of all, but 2 resolutely staid it out and heard such luscious descriptions of the facts of generation in both sexes; the arts of getting and bearing fine healthy offspring; mode of conception; maladies to which both are liable, cures, preventives of infection from foul diseases, &c &c. as would, I should have thought, shocked female ears, but curiosity is as insatiable as the desire of material intercourse, and to that these females sacrificed decency."

Curwen considered the Doctor himself as more of a draw than his slightly tawdry decor: "The first room we entered was properly a vestibule from whence through a pair of folding doors one passed into the apartment holding the electric bed, being about 7 foot square raised about 3 feet from floor on 6 posts. The bed a matress of hair from stallions tails, as the Doctor told us, the covering red damask flowered, over the frame at the head is fixed 2 balls gilded at 4 inches diameter, at one inch apart to receive the electric spark from the machine above, continued down in a glass tube through the floor. Passing this you enter the room of Apollo through a narrow entry, having on each hand 2 or 3 niches containing statues gilded, about 1/2 the natural size. The first object that meets the eye is the temple of Apollo, being a round Cupolo 5 feet in diameter, supported by 6 fluted pillars of the Corinthian order 8 feet high in imitation of Scagliola [fake marble]." Curwen describes the glass and gilt and "decorations of the fripery kind... in great profusion", the paintings, statues, tripods, branched sconces, candelabra and chandeliers, all dripping with shimmering crystals, set into even more brilliant "tremulous motion" by the footsteps of each visitor. The "Master's performance" did not disappoint. Curwen thought Graham possessed "a most ready elocution, great medical knowledge" and believed him "excellently qualified in every respect for supporting the character he assumes". He left Pall Mall at ten that night, "amidst crouds of a less respectable quality than [he] expected to have met there, though there were not wanting some gentlemen".

The *Morning Herald* had given Graham a hard time for a few years. When *The Rambler's Magazine* launched itself on the back of the Doctor's fame at the beginning of 1783, it was merciless. A late Georgian "Rambler" could hardly have been more different from his hedgerow-surveying modern counterpart. This magazine was devised for an audience of dissolute metropolitan gentlemen, idly wandering from one luxuriously debauched scene to another. It described itself as "the annals of Gallantry, Glee, Pleasure and the Bon Ton: Calculated for the entertainment of the Polite World; and to furnish the Man of Pleasure with a most delicious banquet of Amorous, Bacchanalian, Whimsical, Humorous, theatrical and polite entertainment". It was scurrilous, gossipy, obscene, pitiless, and deeply misogynistic. Free of the "restraint of prudish squeamishness", and full of warnings against female wiles, the first issue promised to take down in shorthand and serve up to the public the highlights of all "crim. con." court cases, and any Old Bailey trials that might supply suitably pornographic material ("Rapes... &c."). By early February, the first edition was on its third reprint.

Graham was its twofold victim. *The Rambler's Magazine* stole "mutilated" sections of his *Lecture*, his *A Private Advice* and *Il Convito Amoroso*, and promoted them with relentless strung-out campaigns worthy of the Doctor himself. Month after month it also published prints, poems, dialogues and parodic letters closely mocking Graham's style and advice. Images of the bed, the Doctor and his putative patients appeared with no remittance. The themes were predictable, dominated by lecherous old women obsessively feeding eggs and mealy potatoes to their flat-as-flounders husbands to stir them into action. One planned to name her baby "Graham" after his "artificial father".

So it is quite a surprise to find in *The Rambler's Magazine* a pirated version of one of Graham's most serious and radical lectures. At least this time the Doctor managed to beat his rivals into print. In March he published Vestina's latest lecture, composed "chiefly for the ladies". Equality between the sheets was always implicit in Graham's earlier performances. *The Blazing Star;... a complete defence of the fair sex*, delivered by the High Priestess of the Temple, takes relations between the sexes into the wider world. An astonishing protofeminist text, it crudely pre-empted some of the arguments Mary Wollstonecraft advanced in the *Vindication of the Rights of Woman* nearly ten years later. Ideas that shimmered beneath the surface of *Il Convito* were clarified with un-Graham-like directness:

The ladies ought not, therefore, to suffer themselves to be imposed upon by poetical metaphors and flimsy flourishes. No... women ought to know that they are formed for *far* different purposes; that they are formed for much NOBLER ends, than for empty show, or merely *sensual* delights. – Yes, their various charms and beauties are indications of higher and more *interesting* qualities. To confine the sex, therefore, to external attractions, would be *degrading* them; it would be to reduce them to the level with their bust or portraits.

Graham even uses the term "conditioning" to refer to the way society prevents women from cultivating their "mental qualities". He sees the two sexes as inseparably connected, "reciprocal instruments of each other's improvement", and regards "wranglings about superiority" as ridiculous:

> Gentlemen, ye are born the friends of women, not their rivals, and still less their tyrants. To make slaves of them, therefore, by shewing your authority, and secluding them from your society or amusements, would be contradictory to reason, and a savage and unnatural abuse of that strength which was given you to protect them.

Women should be better educated and men's manners improved. Then ladies could be excited "to truly noble pursuits, and to a due regard for the dignity of their rational nature". Dr Graham's soul was said to pant

> to promote the happiness, bodily and intellectual, of MANKIND AT LARGE... and to rouse them from their lethargy – to usher them from chains and darkness, into liberty and light – to excite in them a proper sense of their natural freedom... he will not, I am persuaded, rest day nor night, but do everything in his power, to the last *moment* of his life, to advance these most important matters.

The more Graham strove to impress on the world the seriousness of his intentions, the more the world mocked him. "Largest in the world" was inscribed on the vast phallic prime conductor rising from between his legs in a print called *The Quacks*. The caricature showed him electrically duelling with his perceived rival, Dr Katterfelto, whose advertisements often appeared opposite Graham's on the front pages of the daily newspapers. A less ambiguous charlatan, Katterfelto was by this time promoting his solar microscope. He had spent the previous year's flu epidemic alarming audiences by projecting the vastly magnified writhing bodies of 50,000 death-dealing "insects". His patent medicine sales soared. Now he was said to be ordering a swanky new coach and nurturing aspirations to become Lord Mayor of London.

"Away thou German Maggot killer, thy Fame is not to be Compar'd to mine!" declared the cartoon Graham. But Katterfelto's financial success seems to have pushed the real Graham to greater extravagances. No longer content simply to compare his Temple with European Royal Palaces, Graham tried to cash in on the growing vogue for oriental tales of enchantment. English versions of an early-eighteenth-century French translation of *The Book of the Thousand and One Nights* were multiplying and Graham designed his latest redecorations to evoke the splendours of the Persian King's palace, Scheherazade's story-weaving backdrop. "The suite of apartments in this Elysian Palace... will now be found to realize the Celestial Soul-transporting and dissolving descriptions that are given in the Fairy Tales, – in the Tales of the Genii – and in the Arabian Nights Entertainments." These tantalizing allusions summon up the voluptuous sensuality of Scheherazade's tales, with all their conflicting excesses and constraints. At the same time they evoke the moral restraint promoted by James Ridley's reimagined versions of the orient in his recent *Tales of the Genii*.

"In the course of the Lecture, Dr Graham will unlock, with delicacy and respect, the inmost and sweetest cabinets of Nature, and he promises that the souls of his Auditors, male, mulish and female, according to their several capacities, and degrees of spring and sensibility, shall expand, and float, and undulate, through the flowery and airy fields of Elysium, or swim upon ambrosial oceans of love and extacy to orbs and regions of ineffable bliss!" Perhaps discreetly released nitrous oxide did more to achieve this bliss than either the Doctor's lecture or his newly unveiled spectacular decor. Ladies were advised to come early, to be sure of a seat. The "remarkably tall" Goddess of Health seems to have adopted those loose, informal muslin dresses popularized by Marie-Antoinette and the Duchess of Devonshire. She was transformed by the press into "the Goddess of Fashion", as her sash became the latest must-have accessory. Graham continued to pour out his soul.

As he announced his absolutely final performance, an accomplished valedictory "poetical epistle" was anonymously published. Graham's penchant for quoting Horace was mocked in an appropriately ambiguous heading: *Valeat Res Ludicra*. "Farewell to the drama", or "Farewell to the ridiculous"?

> O delicate, respectful King
> Of Science! Ope my warmest Spring
> Of tickling Sensibility.
> Thy firmest Friendship let me prove,
> Brilliant – elastic – let me move,
> Transcendent in Agility.
> I feel – I feel th'enchanting *Touch*,
> A Rapture, that's almost too much,
> For Human Nerves to bear.
> Ah me – I pant – I faint – I die –
> But now I glow – burn – vivify –
> And range the Realm of Air.

This frank, erotic poem, though packed with innuendo from beginning to end, also incorporates reflections on taste, novelty and commerce, as well as addressing the fleeting nature of medical fashions:

> Your system, as it's somewhat New,
> Awhile may please the gaping Crew,
> But titillates not all.
> Systems of Physic fluctuate,
> And, never in one settl'd State,
> Like Stocks, they rise and fall.

On 19th July, after a morning spent shooting the rapids at London Bridge, Sylas Neville went to Graham's last London lecture of the year. He found it crowded, mostly with gentlemen, though there were "a few <u>impures</u> intermixed". He admitted to his diary that Graham was a "strange fellow... sometimes not without humour". Immediately afterwards, the Doctor set off for Edinburgh.

8

The End

James Graham spent the rest of his life getting in and out of trouble.
En route for Scotland, he stopped off at Norwich, introducing himself "with his usual ceremonial of florid advertisements". But for the
first time the authorities intervened. "He was very early informed
by the Mayor, that he must be silent or he would be sent to Lecture
'to the spirits that were in prison'." Hurrying on to Edinburgh, he
returned to a city in a state of transformation. George Street was
surging westwards, the civilized suburbs of the New Town rising on
either side of it, while even the Old Town, where the Doctor based
himself, was changing fast.

Graham's Freemason connections probably secured him an airy
lecture venue in Mary's Chapel, in Niddry's Wynd, just off the
High Street. There he survived for just three nights before the city's
magistrates banned him from public lecturing. He was forced to
retreat to private performances at his lodgings, in the coffeehouse
quarter of the Exchange. Walter Scott remembered handbill after
handbill appearing on the city streets, arrogantly denouncing the
magistrates: Graham looked "down upon them as the sun in his
meridian glory looks down on the poor, feeble, stinking glimmer
of an expiring farthing candle, or as God himself... may regard the
insolent bouncings of a few refractory maggots in a rotten cheese".

The electric Doctor was convinced he had been betrayed by the
envious rumour-mongers of the medical faculty. But one, at least,
appeared to be publicly on his side. "I never heard more practical
excellent rules than you there delivered," declared his brother-in-
law's former Botany professor, John Hope, in a letter printed in the
Edinburgh Advertiser. Except that he didn't. Graham, or possibly
some practical joker, had forged Hope's letter of praise for the Doctor.
Within a week of its publication, Graham found himself being led
through the carved-stone gateway at the base of Edinburgh's massive

Tolbooth turret. He was charged with "publishing Lascivious and Indecent Advertisements & delivering wanton and Improper lectures within the city".

Passing through another two doors, he entered a hall filled with shabby prisoners, where a rusty-coated town guard marched back and forth with his bayonet. Graham was greeted by a dispiriting gilt-framed board:

> A prison is a house of care,
> A place where none can thrive;
> A touchstone true to try a friend,
> A grave for men alive.
> Sometimes a place of right,
> Sometimes a place of wrong,
> Sometimes a place for jades and thieves,
> And honest men among.

The gauntlet had been thrown down, and the Doctor picked it up with relish. On 12th August, Graham brought out a sixpenny pamphlet giving an account of "proceedings, persecutions, and imprisonments, more cruel and more shocking to the laws both of God and man than any of those on record of the PORTUGUESE INQUISITIONS". The following Sunday, he mounted the imposing old pulpit towering over the central hall-cum-chapel-cum-taproom of the Tolbooth. To the right, a door lead up to the criminals' floor above, where the condemned were permanently chained to an iron bar and the most unfortunate felons were kept in a plate-iron central cage. In front of the pulpit the better-off prisoners and debtors enjoyed ale and porter sold under licence by the jailer himself, as much as they could pay for. They were usually joined in their drinking by Edinburgh's less salubrious townsmen.

Graham stood up before his fellow prisoners in this "loathsome filthy jail" like a new messiah. To an audience who had less choice than most about what they ate or did, he preached on vegetarianism, moderation and love. His text was "All Flesh is Grass" (Isaiah 40:6). He had already touched on these ideas in lectures at the Temple of Hymen. Meat-eating was part of the Fall of Man, alongside carnal knowledge, and the Doctor delivered his anti-*carne* polemic with as much force as the best fire-and-brimstone revivalist preacher. In an invigorating outpouring, he stirred together the literal and the metaphorical, seasoning scriptural interpretation and ideas from his seventeenth-century Pythagorean predecessors with evidence supplied by Enlightenment anatomy. Violent images of slaughter, gorging, cramming the flesh, spilling blood and dashing out brains dominated his *Discourse*. To eat meat, Graham argued, was to sow "the seeds of horrors, of diseases, of corruptions, and of premature, painful, and inevitable death, making a charnel-house, a Pandora's box – a corruption bag of your body... adding flesh to flesh, is... a kind of incest".

With an eye on the actual iron chains clanking around him, Graham explained to his involuntary audience the connections and circulations that take place through the linked chains of universal life and the afterlife. Graham enthusiastically explored the relationship between the "vile perishable body" we inhabit on earth and the "invisible, spiritual, staminal and incorruptible body" which, under the right circumstances, takes ecstatic flight to heaven. Through perfect bodily health, or ideal conjugal union, "we live in heaven while yet on earth, as it were". The body may be a mere husk, the "outergarment of that glorious and immortal body" which will ultimately be revealed, but it too is perpetually and literally resurrected through the cycles of nature: "every part and particle of our bodies, that has not the THINKING POWER... was once floating in the air, running in the waters, or growing like the grass and green herb of the field; and... in time, sooner or later, they will most assuredly revert into the like states again... our very bones, in various ways, shapes, and characters, will be, by and bye, flying about in the open air; and our flesh and blood at some period or another, (although unconscious of our present existence) may be preaching or hearing in a church; cringing, wretched, and smiling at court; bowing behind a counter, or languishing in a loathsome jail under the persecution of tyranny and ignorance, and under those inhuman stretches of power which are every day exercised even in Britain."

This unofficial sermon and political critique was concluded by a hearty dinner and a cheering glass at Graham's expense. When it was published (one edition following after another in rapid succession), he recommended it should be read alone – or with an intelligent friend – on the top of a high mountain, or in the wide openness of a plain, on a "clear, sun-shining day", or a bright serene night, with all the celestial bodies twinkling and revolving high above. Around this time the doctor-turned-preacher sought permission to build a house on the top of Arthur's Seat, the rocky, windswept hill overlooking Edinburgh. He presumably planned it to be the literal

"Ark of Separation from the follies, vanities, and sensual indulgences of this world", for which he prayed to God for strength to build.

Two days after this extraordinary performance, charges were suspended, and Graham was liberated. Fired with fury at his treatment, he dared not risk further forgeries. Instead he pursued his well-worn path of taking refuge in invented identities. His abiding image of the human state was of a soul enveloped in garments, layers of clothing. Under pressure, he always resorted to print, often in borrowed robes. The fictional personalities he adopted were generally committed to conveying an unwavering message: that he was a misunderstood visionary, who deserved praise and understanding rather than scorn for his selfless efforts to save the world.

He began to write a letter in the guise of his own lawyer, addressing himself to the editors of the *Edinburgh Evening Post*. Graham felt himself triply persecuted – by the medical faculty, the law-enforcers and the newspapers – and wondered, with some reason, of what crime he was actually guilty. Was it his "stile of writing... too florid, hybobolical" and savouring of "Quackery"? Was it that he had dared – like John Brown, the laudanum-addicted founder of a controversial alternative therapeutic system known as Brunonianism, with whom Graham evidently identified – to confront Edinburgh's medical orthodoxies? Or was it simply that by advocating virtue and temperance, he was robbing conventional doctors of their livelihoods, which largely depended on treating the results of "vice and Irregularities"?

Graham re-established himself in a large room in Baillie Fyfe's Close, stocked up on wax candles, and took to the podium again – always, of course, for positively the last time. A contemporary print shows an audience as crowded as the Doctor claimed, entirely made up of men. Further dramas followed at the end of the week, when the Magistrates gave their judgement. Just as he was about to start his lecture, he was arrested again, having now been found guilty of "publishing a scandalous and malicious libel against the Lord Provost and Magistrates" of Edinburgh, and fined twenty pounds. Glorious vindication for Graham followed immediately. One of his admirers instantly produced the sum required, and the Doctor proceeded in triumph to the lecturing room.

A letter written the next day reads like a trial staging of his own forthcoming repentance. Headed with the ambiguous quotation "– There shall come in the last Days Scoffers, walking after their own Lusts!", this pre-enactment appeared in the guise of a missive from

"A Minister in Edinburgh to the Celebrated Dr. Graham, President of the Council of Health, &c.". It was signed "Theophilus" and issued in the form of a handbill. It could conceivably be genuine, but it seems more likely that the Doctor himself was using yet another borrowed persona to put a first tentative foot onto the path of penitence. He accused himself of using language so blush-worthy, it gives "a vermilion tincture to the cheek of youthful modesty... the hoary head of age shrinks at [his] indelicate expressions; expressions which might well suit the keeper of a bagnio, but by far too indelicate to proceed from the pen of a physician." Dreadful warnings and "awful [Biblical] texts" followed. "Know, Sir, *the end of these things is death!*" The pseudonymous letter-writer concluded with the words: "My intention is to reform, not drive you to despair."

Despite this, another week of lectures followed. The price of admission steadily dropped, and free copies of his new lifestyle guide, *The Guardian of Health, Happiness and Long Life*, were offered as presents "far more precious than the purest gold" to everyone who came. Graham then contemptuously "shook the dust off his feet" onto Edinburgh, and set off back to London. On an extended tour he passed through Dublin, Leith, Glasgow, Dumfries, Kelso, Gateshead, Newcastle, Chester, Liverpool and Manchester, pouring out his soul all the way. At least he tried to. In at least five places – all "vile, gutling, and guzzling corporation towns" in Graham's words – "liberality and science" were suppressed, and he was quickly banned from lecturing.

Returning to Pall Mall in November, the embattled Doctor immediately embarked on a publishing and bookselling frenzy. Cobbling together many of his early productions, he cannily repackaged them in the form of *Travels and Voyages*, a genre flourishing then as never before. His Edinburgh sermon and appeal were both reprinted in London, his *Private Medical Advice* knocked down to half a guinea, and a new *Discourse on the Duty of Praying*, with a short sketch of the doctor's *Religious Principles and Moral Sentiments*, came out to accompany an expanded *Christian's Universal Prayer*.

Graham meanwhile took on his enemies in a new and authorized edition of his *Lecture on Generation*, clearly distinguished from its fakes by its footnotes and preface. On the opening page he slightly misquoted Laurence Sterne speaking through his fictionalized self, Parson Yorick, in *Tristram Shandy*: "I think... that the procreation of healthy children is as beneficial to the world, as finding out the longitude." Dr James Graham could not have said it better himself. The clockmaker John Harrison had enjoyed all the glories of worldly recognition for his discovery. Why, wondered Graham, had his own efforts to improve the nation been so little rewarded? Surely he deserved a government pension for his services to his species, at the very least? Where were the statues in gold of his handsome features which should have been commemorating his life's work in every town in Britain? How had the world misunderstood him so utterly?

The Doctor was now a long way from basking in the admiration which Harrison had earned for himself. Instead, Graham was being hounded from place to place, the object of mockery rather than respect. There was no "Board of Generation" awarding prizes for discoveries in the field of conception. Graham's visionary experiments in fertility had backfired on him. Instead of retiring on the fruits of his labour, the doctor was facing financial and professional ruin. Far from being hailed as a genius, he was called the King of Quacks.

The injustices of the past few months and their loathsome per-petrators were dissected in this edition of the *Lecture* in self-justifying fury. To Graham's utter disgust, virtually every newspaper in the country had "eagerly inserted the news of... what they thought were [the] disappointments and disgraces" of his tour, "readily printing every cruel and sarcastical paragraph that envy or malevolence could suggest". His successes on the other hand, such as they were, "were passed over in sullen silence, by ...those carrion flies; who, when they cannot find sores to feast on, and to blow on, will make them." His feelings were those of any modern celebrity betrayed by a faithless gutter press. After "so many years" of "sweating and slaving" – providing the newspapers with advertising revenue and copy month after month – he was naively astonished to have been rewarded with such cruelty.

As for the lecture itself, he recommended it should be read very slowly, a line a minute, once a month, so that not a nuance should escape. Applauding his own professional survival, he swept aside his medical origins and invited only theatrical comparisons: "What play, concert, or any other public discourse, entertainment or spectacle, even with all the advantages of a great number of performers, male, female, and *demi charactère,* superb dresses, and of new and magnificent scenery, could have run on so long, or been so often and so well attended as this same unvaried Lecture, spoken by one and the same person, in the same room, and with, I may say, the same set of scenery!"

Despite his bluster, Graham recognized all too well that his glory years were coming to an end. No novelty could endure, by definition. London's attention had now been thoroughly distracted by a new craze for ballooning. As one cartoon succinctly expressed it, the previous years' fashionable and political follies were poised to take flight like so much hot air: the *Aerostatick Stage Balloon* showed Graham and his Vestina about to ascend to the heavens along with Katterfelto and his cat, Mary Robinson, and other assorted social and political has-beens. They took with them all a tub of froth.

Graham reiterated his intention of retiring peacefully to Edinburgh's New Town, but couldn't resist a further appeal to the public. "I beg that some rich, liberal, benevolent-minded lady or gentleman will have the goodness to leave me when they die without worthy heirs, or near relations, four hundred pounds *per annum*, for my life... I have not the smallest doubt, but that some good soul will do this, and I promise to erect an eternal monument in my heart and in my writings, to the honour of their memory and singular liberality." This "odd request" was not of course for his own gratification. The Doctor simply wanted to be able to pursue his studies for the greater good of mankind, and ensure that his "worthy wife and three amiable children" were decently provided for. Above all, he hoped to "prove indisputably" to present and future generations that he was not merely a doctor of medicine, but "a physician also of the soul!"

By this point he genuinely seems to have been living his life according to the tenets he preached, by design not merely necessity. Graham claimed never to eat or drink more than a sixpence-worth a day, or ever indulge in any kind of luxury. Six months later he was putting into practice "that plain and simple diet, by which according to his own Hypothesis, he is to live to extreme old age" in Newgate, London's most infamous prison. Sniggering puns about the Doctor's discharges (electric, financial and biological) were inevitable. *The Rambler's Magazine* claimed that when the bailiffs turned up, Graham had been about to crank up his bed for the Chevalier d'Éon, an infamous transvestite recently returned to London from Paris, now said to be "standing for *Middlesex*". The Doctor's Pall Mall landlord then sold all his furniture and apparatus at giveaway prices to cover outstanding rent, taxes and other expenses, allowing for Graham's release. Without the electrical apparatus, Graham could not see even how to feed his family. He immediately bought most of it back, but still couldn't actually raise the money to pay for it. Again it was seized and the threat of its sale hung over Graham. He had until ten o'clock on the morning of Monday 29th March to save his life's work.

Graham wrote a final, pitiful letter to his former patron, Lady Spencer. He explained his embarrassment. For the sake of one hundred pounds, he now stood to lose for ever possessions which had cost him thousands. Could he prevail upon her Ladyship to advance the sum for six months? "God knows!" he declared with convincing and desperate candour, "I mean fairly, honestly, and even generously by the whole world – and whatever expences and difficulties indulging a too eccentric and too expensive imagination has led me into – yet the health – the happiness – the elevation of the minds of my fellow creatures, and strict honour and honesty to all mankind, were at the top and bottom of my heart, and were the chief objects which my whole soul ever panted to promote."

Lady Spencer replied instantly, then filed his letter with a brief note. "Told him I could not do it & added that the character he had acquired prevented me from doing any thing for him by way of recommendation."

Graham limped back to Edinburgh with what equipment he had managed to reclaim from his landlord. Licking his wounds, he re-opened a vastly inferior new Temple of Health on South Bridge Street, claiming to charge for admission only under pressure from his friends. He was "mortified" at the thought of people of taste "viewing these broken fragments and ruins of former elegance and magnificence in their present very mutilated and miserable state". Nearly all the best furniture and "magnificently brilliant ornaments" had been sold when the Temple in Pall Mall had closed. A third of the rest was lost or stolen in transit, and another third "broken to useless pieces". Graham made no mention of the Celestial Bed, which was rumoured to have been bought by the sexually adventurous artist Richard Cosway, an aficionado of Swedenborg's tantric techniques. Cosway and his wife had moved into the doctor's former apartments in Schomberg House, and were noticeably slow to remove the Temple's insignia.

Graham said he was resurrecting "the remaining part of the general wreck" in Scotland only in order to dispose of it. He had finally resolved to "relinquish the gewgaws, and the public scenes of this life for ever". Unable to find a tall enough room in Edinburgh to do even these sad remains justice, Graham was left torn between a yearning to recreate the original magnificence of his Grand Electrical Temple and the contradictory urge to use its broken relics to convey a poignant moral message. Shorn of its pyramid of gigantic golden globes, bereft of Jupiter thundering on his Eagle at the top, the vastly diminished glories of the Adelphi Temple of Apollo offered a *sic transit gloria mundi* lesson to benefit a "judicious Public". Such departures from simplicity, nature and God would, the Doctor argued, always prove sinful, transient and unsatisfactory, "dangerous to our temporal, and fatal to our eternal happiness".

Before relinquishing his apparatus for ever, Graham concocted one last medicine, and went to Manchester to promote it. He may have given up the world's "gewgaws", but his addiction to "the public scenes of life" proved harder to conquer. In an extended advertisement for his new product Graham surpassed himself: he transformed the sales pitch into an art form of its own. The "Aetherial Ambrosial Quintessence of Gold, Honey and Rosa Solis" was supposed to rejuvenate the body, cheer the mind and prevent and remedy the decays and evils of old age. It was brewed in the "Adelphi Al-chymical and Medico-electrical and Philosophical Apparatus... so curiously contrived, that the same wheels that turn the enormous cylinders, which excite the electrical fire, set in regular and continual motion the heavy glass flint pestles of the close glass mortars, which contain the precious substances from which the Quint-Essence is exalted!" Coming forth "from the tremendous pyramid of great Metallic Globes on the Dome of the Electrical Temple of Health", Graham described his new potion as "Potable Gold! Condensed Light! A Macrocosmic Essence!... or Quint-Essential Spirit of the Universe", as friendly to the human frame as milk from the breast of the Virgin. It turned your urine golden yellow – with, in certain lights, the rosy tint of the sundew flower from which it was made – and made your breath smell of nectar. Being Graham, he could not resist slipping a radical political digression into all this hyperbole: his discussion of the properties of gold rushed headlong into a diatribe against slavery in the Atlantic triangle. (The Abolition movement was in its infancy, and had signally failed to persuade the Anglican Church to take up its cause.) God could not have created gold to be a medium for the traffic of human carcasses, Graham argued, "to glut the insatiable appetites of infernal avarice and mad ambition". Gold was never designed for "buying and selling the souls, bodies, and natural liberty of our fellow-creatures, by the Christian, British and other European merchants on the African and American coasts".

This handbill, with its references to "the true principles of the Hermetic and Rosi-crucian Philosophers" is the only direct evidence that Graham ever came close to dabbling in the alchemical mysticism

of that occult fringe frequented by a number of his Masonic contemporaries. The route of theosophical enlightenment seemed to
appeal particularly to émigrés: Count Cagliostro and Dr John de
Mainauduc (Britain's answer to Mesmer) embraced these arcane
cosmologies with fervour. Richard and Maria Cosway were equally
keen. Under their influence Philippe de Loutherbourg and his wife
Lucy took up faith-healing in Hammersmith only a few years later,
and in one print were linked in an eternal triangle with Graham and
Katterfelto.

But the Scottish Doctor was heading in a new direction. Nature,
rather than the occult, was his guide. He had begun to adopt clothes
made of pure white linen or cotton, like the ancient Pythagoreans,
and now added a new prescription to his routine of cold-water washing, fresh air at all times, outdoor exercise and straw beds: inhaling
the scent of newly turned earth was becoming an obsession. "Dig
up the earth in a clean garden," he recommended in the directions
for taking his new medicine, "or rather in a fallow field, common,
or hill-side, lie down with your face in the earth, or in the hole, and
draw the sweet refreshing effluvia for an hour or two at a time, every
day or every other day." He confessed that he had taken to sitting
naked up to his breast in the earth for three hours at a time, two or
three times a week. "This is perfectly safe, and is in effect going to
our mother's womb to be born again and to flourish in the *perpetual
bloom* of youth, personal beauty, and serene *brilliancy* of soul!"

That summer Graham experimented with his first "earthbathing"
patient. Thirty-four-year-old David Robinson was a respectable malt
dealer from Warrington who had been recommended to Graham by
a local JP. By the time Graham met him, after Robinson had made
the usual rounds of orthodox medical practitioners, he had been ill
for six months. His stomach and bowels were vastly swollen, he was
suffering from agonizing constipation, and on the rare occasions he
managed to urinate he passed only blood and foul discharge. Two
months into his treatment, Graham saw little improvement. Lying,
as the Doctor directed, with his face over a newly dug hole for a
few hours each day seemed to revive only Robinson's spirits, without
affecting his constitution. Eventually he became so weak everyone
assumed death was inevitable. "Not knowing what more to do for
him," Graham explained, "I directed him to be stripped totally naked,
and put into a fresh made hole in the earth, and closely covered up
with earth to his chin." August and September were, as usual, very
rainy months in Lancashire. Still Robinson gallantly buried himself

daily for three-hour stretches for nearly eight weeks. By the end of this time, he was "perfectly cured, root and branch".

It took a little while to get the details right. At first Graham and his patients found themselves rather uncomfortable – the holes were too narrowly dug, they were irritated by bits of sharp stone or gravel, or they sat shivering, their head, neck and shoulders exposed to the wind. Eventually the Doctor worked out that three foot wide by five foot long was the best size for their earth baths, with a seat broad enough to support the thighs, and a "place like a child's grave… for your legs and feet to go down". Crossing the arms and resting a hand on each shoulder protected the chest and made breathing easier, and the very weak or reluctant were permitted a few hot bricks buried beneath their feet, or even allowed to keep their clothes on for the first few times – provided they were made of linen or cotton.

> The more that the patient sings or speaks aloud while they are in the earth the better; as the bellows like motion of the breast and bowels, not only keeps alive the natural heat of the body, but also works out disease, and sucks in health and vitality more powerfully and more abundantly from the Earth… the surface of our body and limbs is a mere sponge or mass of dry sand, drinking in with ease and avidity whatever is applied to it: Nature, at every pore of the body and limbs, eats and drinks, like a glutton.

Earthworms were good. As Graham later pointed out, they were to be found in the best earth. But he preferred to avoid soil that had been too much manured, or was "full of grubbs and other troublesome insects". And a good brown or reddish loam, or "light sandy, crumbly, mellow and marrowy Earth" was preferable to very black, blue, yellow, white or clayey soil. Above all it should have that "strong-sweet-refreshing-breast-opening smell".

By January 1786 Graham was ready to take his new medical philosophy to London. After a single somewhat inaudible lecture in the Saloon at the Lyceum debating chambers, Graham took a smart ground-floor room at no. 6 Panton Street, near the Haymarket. He was back in show business. The Doctor imagined that the "Heart of every Lady and every Gentleman, of Education and of Taste" who came to hear him would exclaim "Ah! What are all the Plays, Operas, Concerts, Masquerades, Exhibitions of Paintings or Prints, idle Phusicons, Trial Books, Magazines, or even the celebrated

Pall-Mall Lecture itself which ran on almost every Night for three Years to the Tune of about Ten Thousand pounds, when compared to the truly *natural* Philosophy, and celestial Touchings!" The therapy may have changed, but Graham had returned to his original passion, "Animal Love and Propagation". He had composed "an entirely new and complete Cyprian System of that most profound, most sublime, all-taming, and all-renewing Mystery… that most wondrous Law, Appetite, Passion, mysterious Act or whatever else it should… be called". Yes, his "whims and foibles" had been "many and expensive", but he remained true to his original and best intentions: never to take pecuniary advantage of the public, but devote all his energy to promoting the health and happiness of his fellow creatures. (How could he be driven by financial motivations, he argued, when he was by then even poorer than he had been when he first entered penniless into "public service" twenty-five years previously?)

By spring, he was putting on public exhibitions of earth-bathing at Panton Street, reportedly with the help of one of his daughters. On Good Friday he staged a daringly suggestive "Coffin Scene and Lecture": "at Nine the trumpet will sound, and it is hoped a glorious and happy resurrection will take place." A satirical letter in *The Rambler's Magazine*, which had joyfully serialized Graham's new lecture earlier that year, described earth-bathing as "a new method of promoting longevity" which considered "mankind as so many cabbages or cauliflowers that cannot live without being planted in the earth". Linnaean jokes about planting male and female plants in the same bed drew on a now well-established format of constructing erotica from the latest botanical theories.

An engraving shows the Doctor at work in a grand room, complete with oval mirrors, three sash windows and intrigued spectators peering in from the pavement. On a pile of earth stands a fashionably dressed Dr Graham, tall and handsome as ever, a spade-bearing assistant beside him. In the foreground a half-dressed lady has discarded her upper petticoat to reveal an artificial "derrière", and another such device lies on the floor. Three naked women, one sporting a rather magnificent wide-brimmed hat, are standing or sitting in rectangular pits on the floor. These were probably the remains of the medicinal baths of another alternative practitioner, Dr Dominiceti. He had steamed and sweated and fumigated his patients while issuing Grahamesque challenges to the medical establishment since the mid-1760s in Bristol and then Chelsea, finally setting up his son to extend his work in Panton Street in the summer of 1781.

When fencing master Henry Angelo went to one of Graham's evening lectures, the audience was crowded with ladies as well as men. "In the centre of the room was a pile of earth, in the middle of which was a pit, where a stool was placed: we waited some time, when much impatience was manifested, and after repeated calls, 'Doctor, Doctor!' he actually made his appearance *en chemise*. After making his bow, he seated himself on the stool; when two men with shovels began to place the mould in the cavity; as it approached to the pit of his stomach he kept lifting up his shirt, and at last he took it entirely off, the earth being up to his chin, and the Doctor being left *in puris naturalibus*." His lecture seems to have been earthy in every way. "Whether it was that the men felt for the chastity of the female audience, or they had had quite enough of his imposing information, which lasted above an hour, either the hearers got tired, or some wags wished to make themselves merry at the Doctor's expense, and there was a cry of 'Doctor, a song, a song!'" Nodding and hemming, Graham embarked on a popular number from a long-running stage comedy called *How to Keep Him*. It offered advice more conservative than that espoused in *The Blazing Star*, but still very much in keeping with the Doctor's conjugal philosophy:

> Use the man that you wed like your favourite guitar
> Though there's music in both, they are both apt to jar.
> They should never be used but with delicate touch,
> Not be handled too roughly, nor play'd on too much.

The Panton Street earth baths were a relatively short-lived affair, but Graham did not put away his shovel. The new treatment would be the main weapon in his medical artillery for the rest of his life. In May he was in Paris, advising the relative of a fellow traveller on earth-bathing treatments for his gammy leg, and in August he announced plans to spend some months in Newcastle. That winter he returned once more to Edinburgh, where he continued to practise, prescribing continence and moderation, and painful-sounding alcohol rubs, particularly for the genitalia. He also planned to brush up his medical training. But the professors he had once held up as "living ornaments" were now a disappointment.

During the early 1760s Joseph Black – the thermodynamics pioneer who had first discovered carbon dioxide, or "fixed air" as he called it – had been teaching in Glasgow. Graham was appalled to find that Black, now one of Edinburgh's star professors, conducted "his most noxious processes and experiments" in an airless, lead-lined room crammed with two or three hundred students, every door and window tightly shut. He reported witnessing "the celebrated Professor of chemistry... emaciated, coughing, pale and puling, drinking warm or hot foreign tea", gnawing at a piece of liquorice root as he held forth. The early-morning classes in Medical Practice given by William Cullen, who "when *out* of the college, was one of the pleasantest, politest, and most Courtier-like behaved men in the world", distressed Graham even more. The "very god of medicine" arrived "covered from top to toe, with snuff, horses hair, sheep's wool, and calves skins, coughing incessantly, and incessantly trembling with both hands, like aspen-leaves, while the gawkey and glum Gowks, in the gloomy gallery of the Lecture-room keep glowering and gaping down upon him, in senseless admiration of his long-winded spasmodic doctrines, and of his NICE *nosology,* as he calls it". Graham found the students equally repulsive, and recoiled at "their cadaverous breath". Many of them were up "very late at the vile drinking houses and brothels, many of them diseased and dying... eight or ten of the medical students actually died and were buried, that winter, in the course of a few months."

As Graham's fastidiousness grew, so too did his abhorrence of death in every arena. A few years earlier he had made confident predictions about his own longevity: "I have every reason to expect, (speaking with humble submission to the will of heaven!) that I shall live in uninterrupted health, till I fall like ripe fruit, a hundred years hence, upon the bounteous and ever-teeming lap of her from whom I sprung." Now Graham was becoming fixated on the goal of achieving a Methuselah-length lifespan. The Evangelical strain that had intermittently erupted in his performances and published work began to dominate his life. He had already staged numberless self-resurrections from a succession of earthy theatrical graves. He was now also well on the way to being spiritually reborn.

True to form, Graham's version of evangelism remained rooted in politics. From Panton Street, he had already addressed a passionate anti-war manifesto called *The principal grounds, basis, argument or Soul! of the New Celestial Curtain, (or reprehensory) Lecture!* to Catherine the Great, George III, Louis XVI, Joseph II of Germany – in fact, to "all CROWNED HEADS! GREAT PERSONAGES! And others, whom it may concern." Summoning anthems of freedom and peace in its soul-saving mission, it argued that "the greatest Prince, or King, or Emperor! That ever lived, has no more *right*, in the sight of God, of nature, or of humanity, to make *offensive war* against his own species, than the meanest chimney-sweeper or beggar-man has". Grinding taxation and the curse of colonization were presented in dramatic terms as the forerunners of collapsing kingdoms and empires. Graham signed himself "Formerly a Physician, but now a Christian Philosopher, and loving Follower of Nature".

Dr Graham was born again in late summer, on the Isle of Man. Had it been an event of the kind described in a number of contemporary conversion memoirs, caused by the sudden divine inspiration of a particularly meaningful sermon perhaps, some providentially striking text – or had it triggered the kind of agonizing birth pangs that sometimes left whole congregations in tears or laughter, groaning, weeping, sweating and shaking – the former doctor would undoubtedly have described the occasion in every detail. One charismatic preacher called William Huntington had experienced a vision of brilliant light while pruning a pear tree; his fervent prayers were followed by Christ's appearance "in a most glorious manner, with his body all stained with blood". William Blake first saw an angel on Peckham Rye. But when Graham found Jesus he seems to have been struck by a complex idea rather than an epiphanic vision. Being a man who seemed to live most deeply through his relationship with the public, he felt immediately compelled to communicate his plans to the world. Graham's divine inspiration struck in July 1788: "on the rising in [his] heart of that Bright and Morning Star! Which is the glorious harbinger of the blissful everlasting day", he put to paper his *Proposals for the establishment of a New and True Christian Church.*

He had got it all wrong, he confessed. "I feel my nature, my apprehensions, my views, and my desires, totally altered and even reversed. Selfishness and the world are now to me comparatively dead, and disappear. Humility, love, and childlike teachableness, reign; and to use a modern phrase in a proper sense, I am become a Gentleman." (He had clearly been inspired by all the Adam-like delving he had been doing. He spent much of that summer literally testing the ground in the north of England, beginning work on a book on earth-bathing while living on Blackstone Edge, in Yorkshire, between Halifax and Rochdale.)

Graham heartily denounced the self-interest and pride that had formerly motivated him, making him speak and write "with harsh, unbecoming, and ungentleman-like virulence, against every one who in [his] vain and foolish imagination affronted, opposed, or dishonoured" him. Before he was "born again", he admitted, the dissolute and unchristian lives and conversation of so many officials of the established churches in the world had provoked in him an extreme prejudice, "even a bitter enmity" against all clergymen. He used to delight "on every occasion to asperse and to dishonour them". He did not think he had altogether dug out that "root of bitterness", but, for the sake of their Maker if not their own worthiness, he had at least learnt to pity, respect and even honour them.

Given the complexity of Christian controversies, and the high feelings roused by them during the eighteenth century, Graham's *Proposals* seem in many respects both moderate and, by his own standards, lucid. He entered the fray, he claimed, as a mediator, "to moderate intemperate zeal on the one hand, and to rouse languid affections on the other", hoping that the "sweet light of truth and christianity" might appear from this "collision". Of course it was hardly that simple, as Graham well knew. Heterodoxy seemed to be engulfing Hanoverian Britain. The scientific scepticism that had dominated intellectual thought for the past century allowed freethinkers to move towards atheism. Voltaire famously declared that religion began when the first rogue met the first fool, while Diderot, the French encyclopedist, suggested liberty would come when "the last king is strangled with the entrails of the last priest". Reason applied to religion made deism the "natural" theology for many believers: they rejected scriptural revelation, miracles and superstition. Meanwhile the dioceses of the established Church of England were often both divided along party lines and waging war on evangelism – the "revealed" religion of Methodists and other awakened souls who emphasized the doctrine of justification by faith. Intricate distinctions caused internal rifts within virtually every creed and denomination – Anglican, Dissenting, Baptist, Antinomian, Unitarian, Trinitarian, Arminian, Socinian, Antipaedobaptist, Calvinist, Moravian and so on.

Graham was horrified by the rise of Unitarianism and Deism alike, those "societies... formed for the lamentable purpose of degrading the ever-blessed Jesus". He couldn't resist a ringing call to arms, for all his conciliatory mouthings: "Let us, my brethren, boldly march up to the camp and head quarters of the enemy, in London, Paris, Edinburgh, &c. and by public advertisements call together some of the most zealous friends and followers of our dear Lord!" But this was just a passing thought. His real purpose was to propose a complementary church. He wanted to set up places of worship that would be free, unlocked and open every day simply for the reading of the Bible, basic prayers and the singing of catchy, melodious "soul-touching" hymns. No other Christian sect or denomination could possibly have any objection to coming to the "True Church" as well as their own, for it would teach no particular doctrine, subscribe to no creed, and use no ceremonies. Jews, heathens and even infidels "all, all may assemble peaceably here".

Inspired by the True Church of the Book of Revelation, Graham envisaged his ideal church built in the shape of a perfect square or circle, light and bright. The colours would be white and virgin blue, and there would be huge windows all around, and a domed skylight in the roof. With fresh air pouring in every day, congregations would suffer none of the stinking deadly vapours endured in most dark and gloomy Scottish churches, where "dead corpses …are rotting… under their pews". (An Edinburgh historian had recently bemoaned the "nauseous" scenes and smells in Greyfriars' churchyard, where sextons could not bury a fresh corpse without disturbing an old one "not fit to be touched".) Neither would there be any grasping vergers or doorkeepers watching and rattling with their locks and keys.

The sublime separation of soul from body offered by the Celestial Bed experience shifted to the space of the True Church, or Treasury. Here Graham could enact his long-expressed desire for fewer sermons and "more of that soul-melting, – of that sweetly agonising, – of that true psalm-singing, in which, while we intensely brood over the spiritual sense of the words, our soul is abstracted from earth, snatched up into heaven, and with wonder and delight ineffable sees itself surrounded with innumerable myriads of angels and blessed spirits".

Graham's rebirth as a natural philosopher was as complete as his spiritual renaissance. Declaring himself "the worm" to Priestley's "giant", Graham nevertheless attacked his former hero on scientific as well as theological grounds. (He hadn't actually read much Priestley recently – who indeed could keep up with his prodigious output? – but he had heard him preach in Birmingham a few years earlier and had discussed his writings in "accidental conversation with some literary gentlemen.") Graham's opening gambit must have amazed his old fans and enemies:

How tormenting, how very fatal, ha[ve] Doctor Priestley's books, recommending the application of electrical fire, and of artificially produced airs, to the human body for the cure of diseases, proved to mankind?

Graham continued to admire electricity as part of God's creation. But to "increase and augment that principle" in human bodies was presumptuous and dangerous, even sinful and depraved. A few years later he had convinced himself that his electrical experiments had been the Devil's work. Although in 1788 he still owned his electrical temple, and still described it as magnificent, he had completely given up medical electricity, and hoped all mankind would follow his example.

No longer in command of nature, Graham now declared himself, through God, under nature's command. "Yes, Nature's electrical machines are, walking, frictions, brisk winds, or sea water among rocks, &c. violently dashed and agitated by high winds and tides into a milky white soapy froth; or living rain or spring water rushing down mountains or hills, natural or artificial cataracts... in snowy-white torrents, in which the latent fire of nature is, in her own way, most powerfully excited, and tempered by the grand mediator water." Graham did not abandon the rational vocabulary of science, but put it to new metaphorical use to describe newly clarified religious beliefs. Jesus Christ became "the Prime Conductor" to the Father of Eternal Life, Light, and Felicity". Satan, "the arch-deceiver and destroyer" was said to "to contract and to freeze the minds of mankind, by evaporating, with the diabolical heat of their zeal, the sweet evangelical radical heat of their souls". (Later Graham would write of Jehovah's incorruptible Spirit "operating in the centre of even every atom, as well as of every complete body and system".)

The language of science remained, but the Doctor's conversion experience seems to have swept away his reason. In Whitehaven, a Cumberland ship-building port, he was showing such "signs of insanity" on 19th August that he had to be secured and sent back to Edinburgh in the custody of two constables. A less than reliable but often quoted account of Graham, presumably referring to this period of his life, described him as "wholly an enthusiast", who "would madden himself with ether, run out into the streets, and strip himself to clothe the first beggar whom he met".

To call someone an "enthusiast" in those days was rarely a compliment. It was an accusation often levelled by orthodox Christians at John Wesley's growing band of Methodists. Unregulated enthusiasm implied a particular kind of religious delusion: suffered by individuals, like Graham, who bypassed doctrine and discovered God in themselves and the world about them. Those transported by it saw their intensity of passion as testimony to God's dominion.

Their critics distrusted such uncontrolled responses, and recalled with alarm the "enthusiasms" of the previous century's civil war, and their disastrous, king-killing consequences. So political radicalism, and the dangerous power of the mob, were implicitly entwined in the term.

The man who labelled Graham an "enthusiast" was Robert Southey, future Poet Laureate and nascent establishment Tory. He was writing about Graham in the guise of a bigoted Spaniard, Don Manuel Alvarez Espriella, in his *Letters from England*. Southey gathered the material for this semi-fictional production from a number of friends: Walter Scott may well have supplied him with information about Graham. By 1807, when the *Letters* were published, Southey had turned his back on the youthful radical idealism he had shared with the poet Coleridge. The regicide and Terror of the French Revolution had made zealotry and quackery altogether too menacing in his eyes. A few years earlier Southey declared that a "worse danger than the spread of [m]ethodism can scarcely be apprehended for England". In his *Life of Wesley* he depicted enthusiasm as mental disease, implicitly infectious.

Graham's faith had certainly tipped into religious mania. Whether this was fuelled by ether, the Holy Spirit or a devastating combination of the two is impossible to judge. He was still prescribing ether as an ingredient in a massage tonic in January 1788, and used his own Nervous Aetherial Balsam throughout his life. When he renounced electricity in his *Proposals* in July, he also repudiated "artificially produced airs from certain chemical admixtures". Perhaps he had as much difficulty giving up these addictive narcotics as he did in relinquishing the "scenes of public life".

Back in Scotland, the former physician tried to insert advertisements implying that he was the new messiah in the Edinburgh newspapers:

JAMES GRAHAM the Servant of the Lord! is commissioned to proclaim Glory to God in the highest, and on Earth peace, good will towards Men; and that the Great Shepherd is now come the second time on the Earth, to gather in his Sheep into his Fold...

Neither Graham's money nor his earnest pleas touched the hearts of the city's three newspaper printers. Undaunted, Graham issued free handbills, pressing them onto reluctant passers-by with manic fervour, urging them to reproduce them as often as they wished. The leaflets announced that his New Jerusalem Church was now established "on Earth as it is in Heaven", at his home in Lochend's Close, about halfway down the Canongate. He begged forgiveness of anyone he may have offended or injured in the past, and promised to make amends as fast as his "Loving, Loving, Loving and Wondrous, Wondrous, Wondrous Lord" would allow. He invented a new calendar beginning in January 1788, and he described himself as "James Graham, O.W.L!" This stood for "Oh Wonderful Love".

After just ten days, Graham published *A Very Short History* of his new church, and "of its poor-rich Minister". These must have been difficult times for long-suffering Mary Graham, as well as her son and two daughters. As usual, the Doctor reveals remarkably little about his own family life. But at this point, Mrs Graham seems to have done her utmost to contain her intermittently deranged husband. "Notwithstanding the Minister's Angel of a Wife used all her feet and hands, running to, and standing in all the gaps, and brandishing and turning every way her Flaming Sword... to keep still barred the way", five men did manage to get through their tenement door the first evening the "church" was open. Four appeared to be University students in search of diversion, their leader sitting "in the Chair of the Scorner". One respectful but nameless young man was ready to become Graham's first acolyte, and that was enough for the self-ordained minister.

The following evening, according to his account, about twenty turned up, but as far as Graham was concerned only he and the earnest young man from the previous night formed a true and worthy congregation. But then one of those glorious meteorological moments in which Edinburgh specializes took place, confirming for Graham that his new church was truly blessed: just before sunset the black clouds dispersed, a golden-red sun shone on the rugged hills opposite, and a rainbow appeared, so perfect that the minister and his little flock rushed to the window to admire it.

The next morning was a Sunday. Rising at dawn and kneeling as usual to pray at his open window, Graham held household prayers, ate breakfast, and then, to the competing sounds of different church bells, he set off with his family to Lady Glenorchy's chapel, halfway between the Old Town and the New Town. One of Lady Glenorchy's early forays into the field of church-founding, in the very chapel in Niddry's Wynd where Graham was banned from lecturing in 1783, had been on ambitiously ecumenical principles. Lady Glenorchy herself had died in 1786, and the chapel that still bore her name was becoming a bastion of evangelical Presbyterianism. Here, Graham had a reserved seat, paid for, as was the custom, by a year's advance rent.

As he strode up the Canongate, Graham carried a little white linen bag, containing a Bible, "Mr Craig's Spiritual Poems" and a very small but as yet unread extract from Emmanuel Swedenborg's *Doctrine of the New Jerusalem Church*. He was met at the door of Lady Glenorchy's chapel by the elders, clothed in black. They tried to persuade him that the church was full, then simply said that Graham could not come in. "J.G." related that he remonstrated, accusing them of breaking the laws of the land and of God by preventing a peaceable person from entering during the hours of public worship on the Lord's Day. "He commanded them, in the name of his dear Lord Jesus Christ, to admit him to hear the Word!" When this didn't work, he sent his family inside and then went round to another door, where he was repelled with "equal, or rather with unequal" rudeness.

Eventually, as he stood sheltered from the public gaze in the church porch, he was seized by four soldiers, dragged away "like a thief or a murderer" and locked up in the Guard House with no explanation of what crime he had committed. At this prison, "a long, low, ugly building", which Scott imagined as "a long black snail crawling up the middle of the High Street and deforming its beautiful esplanade", Graham was abandoned for the rest of the day, his requests to see the city's Provost disregarded. "In the dark night, several persons were sent out to spy, to pump, and at length to entreat J.G. to go out of the prison, but he told them, that he would not be threated, coaxed, or smuggled out..." He was waiting to leave in broad daylight, "and in sight of the Sun and people".

When Graham came home on Monday, exhausted and hungry, but ready to officiate at his New True Church, he found that in his absence his house had been broken into. He returned to Lochend's Close to an empty room. His papers were gone, there were now thick iron bars at the windows, and a straw bed was made up on the floor. His own room had been transformed into a prison – or an asylum. Graham collapsed and slept for sixteen hours.

The next morning when he woke and called for breakfast, he was greeted by two or three guards ("or madmen keepers") who continued to confine him – along with "the truth and the light that they expected would rush from the pen &c. of James Graham". The following Sunday, he tried once more to leave his house to attend "Public Worship" and three town guardsmen emerged from his own kitchen, set upon him, and "kept him a prisoner in his house all day". On Monday he somehow committed his tale to a new handbill.

It is all too easy to imagine these scenes, Graham sleeplessly ranting all the while about punishment, delusion and tyranny. It is harder to disentangle the substance of the events from the paranoid narrative printed subsequently by Graham himself. Clearly the powers-that-be were trying to keep the peace and prevent a public disturbance. Mary Graham must surely have been colluding with the city officials as the only way to protect her husband and children from his own worst excesses. Her desperation is understandable.

There is no record of how long this domestic confinement lasted, but Mrs Graham does seem to have kept her husband out of the madhouse. Whatever his affliction was, it appears to have been episodic. On his recovery Graham embarked undaunted on a whole new chapter of renewed travels, writing and public performances, and soon returned to his medical career. The Doctor's resilience was extraordinary, but he continued to wrestle with his soul and his sanity. An undated handbill, probably from this period, addresses God in an effusive outpouring, which disintegrates into those lists of Grahamesque epithets so familiar from his earlier writings on sex. "Be a Wall of Pure and Holy Fire around me and mine through which no Evil can penetrate," he begged. "O be the External, the Internal and the Eternal Sun and Shield of our Soul; and most graciously Ordain, that we may bask in Security and in Peace, Ineffible and Eternal, under the most Genial and Brilliant, yet most Mild, and most Necessary Shadow of the ALMIGHTY Wings of *Thine* Holy Spirit! the White-Wing'd, The Celestial LIGHT! *The Eternal Dove!* The *Holy Ghost*!" In March 1789, a Quaker friend living near Carlisle, who may have been involved in the Whitehaven incident the previous year, wrote an extremely long and affectionate letter to Graham, obviously the continuation of an intense discussion between the two men about inward spirit, electricity and resurrection. "The new Jerusalem is not a place or sect, but a state," consoled Benjamin Dockray. "Then we do not take other men's words and say them… but [use forms of prayer and sermons]… such as the Spirit begotteth in us, and bringeth forth…"

But Graham was not in Edinburgh to receive the letter. By November 1788, he was in Liverpool again, where he heard the alarming news of another attack of madness, one of immense national significance. Graham had managed to escape the confines of his Edinburgh home-asylum, but his sovereign on earth was talking to oak trees, resisting straitjackets and mooning at his pages. In this first bout of insanity (retrospectively but not conclusively diagnosed in the twentieth century as porphyria) fifty-year-old King George III was so ill that misinformed rumours of his death rapidly traumatized the whole country. While the Regency Crisis began to play itself out in London, Graham got instantly to work. He attached a prayer to his wall, sat down to write, and nine uninterrupted hours later was ready to "fly", post-haste, to Windsor. He managed to deliver a letter to the Prince of Wales, explaining that he had established the probable cause and best cure for the King, and suggesting some scriptural consolation for his eldest son. Graham sped on to Hampstead, in order to survey the metropolis from its lofty heights and add a national diagnosis to his opinions on the royal malady. But by the time he was ready to publish the work, the King, now closeted at Kew, was on the mend, and "the Hemorrhagy of the national Heart" had stopped.

Undaunted and cash-strapped, Graham still tried to find subscribers for this new "eccentric" work, informing the nobility and gentry that a full guinea's subscription would be rewarded with a copy bound in his trademark white linen. Surely, he suggested to no less than Sir Joseph Banks, President of the Royal Society, his thoughts on this awkward subject would still be valuable in "arranging, comforting, and assuring – deranging, agonizing, and Horror and Panic-struck Minds, – or, in other Words, dissipating the Clouds and stilling the Storms of intellectual Darkness, Destraction, and Despair, and sweetly and serenely shining, as a Summer's Sun in a Blue Sky, on sunk and shrivelled Souls"? (Indeed cheering them on till they could "bask in Blessedness under the Eternal Meridian of JEHOVAH's Day!")

While he waited hopelessly for subscribers in London, Graham was apparently glimpsed at Newgate. On 1st July 1789, he was said to have stood outside the prison gates, among the crowds attending the hanging of his old accomplice Thomas Denton, the designer of the Celestial Bed. Denton was cast by the press as a genius whose misapplied talents led to his downfall. His skills had taken him into counterfeiting and, to public horror, he died a professed infidel, wishing only that he'd taken the advice of his wife, "the best of mothers, and the best of women". Two weeks later the whole country's attention was taken up by events at another prison, in Paris. The Bastille fell, the French Revolution began and, as Mary Wollstonecraft put it, "all the passions and prejudices of Europe were instantly set afloat".

In print at least, Graham never referred directly to events across the channel. Managing his own professional rehabilitation must have taken up most of his energies at this time. He must also have been preoccupied with the health of one of his daughters, who eventually died of consumption in the early 1790s. Returning to Bath, the scene of his earliest triumphs, Dr Graham published in 1789 a treatise on the *True Nature and Uses of the Bath Waters*, which recycled material from his early days in the city. It was "plain" and "rational" enough to win him some respect and it marked the beginning of yet another comeback, and another national tour. For the next three years, crowds turned out in Newcastle, South Shields, Sunderland, Sheffield, Nottingham, Exeter, Bristol and Bath to watch him and his patients earth-bathing.

Southey's semi-fictional travelogue reports a friend who paid a shilling to see half a dozen of Graham's patients buried up to the chin "in fresh mould... The operation lasted four hours; they suffered, as might be seen in their countenances, intensely from cold for the first two, during the third they grew warmer, and in the last perspired profusely, so that when they were taken out of the mould reeked like a new dunghill..." At this point the demonstrators wolfed down huge quantities of mutton "to prove that when they rose from the grave they were as devouring as the grave itself". This version of events shows Graham enduring his share of hecklers. "The doctor used sometimes to be buried himself for the sake of keeping his patients company: one day, when he was in this condition, a farmer emptied a watering-pot upon his head to make him grow. When J. saw him he was sitting up to the neck in a bath of warm mud, with his hair powdered and in full dress. As he was haranguing upon the excellent state of health which he enjoyed from the practice of earth bathing, as he called it, J. asked him Why then, if there was nothing the matter with him, he sate in the mud? The question puzzled him. – Why, he said, – why – it was – it was – it was to show people that it did no harm, – that it was quite innocent, – that it was very agreeable: and then brightening his countenance with a smile at the happiness of the thought, he added, 'It gives me, sir, a skin as soft as the feathers of Venus's dove.'"

This last part of the account is unlikely, since Graham seems rarely to have been lost for words. He always had a host of explanations for his bizarre behaviour, and seemed to welcome persecution like a good messiah. In one advertisement he evoked the Creation in describing pure virgin soil as "the true Adamic Earth" and "First

Matter". In another, for "Cold Earth and Warm Mud-Bathing" at a public house in Bath, he promised to be ever present to explain his methods fully and satisfactorily to "intelligent" ladies and gentlemen. "Men may despise simple remedies that cost nothing, and esteem dear-bought, scarce, far-fetched, tediously prepared, and dangerous medicines," declared the former apothecary. "'THINGS WHICH ARE DESPISED HATH GOD CHOSEN.'"

Just as he continued to use images drawn from natural philosophy, Graham never turned his back entirely on scientific debate. Hard though it was to reconcile with "Divine Revelation", he confessed he was tempted to set the age of the earth at sixty million years, in line with the emerging discoveries of geologists. James Hutton, the leader in this field, had recently pioneered the idea of "reading" rocks to discover the history of the earth; the Edinburgh artist John Kay portrayed him hammer in hand, scrutinizing the very human features of a rock face. Graham meanwhile compared the Earth to a vast living animal, the mountain ranges its backbone, volcanoes like Etna and Vesuvius its lungs. More than a century before the theory of continental drift was formulated, the doctor delighted in the notion that Europe and America had once been joined.

By 1792 Graham had been successful enough through much of England to persuade himself that the "prejudices" against which he had struggled for most of his life were now "totally removed". At last he felt accepted again by "the genteeler and the more sensible parts of the inhabitants" of Bath as "a regular bred tho' eccentric Physician", whose mobility gave him practical advantages over "other more stationary medical Gentlemen". As usual, he carefully distanced himself from "the numerous herd of Quacks" and "those persons who prowl about England, calling themselves Doctors", whose unprincipled ignorance had, in his view, tainted his own work.

For all Graham's efforts to appear "regular", the effect was undermined by his own eccentric excursions into print. *A clear, full and faithful portraiture*, or *...ardent recommendation of a certain most beautiful and spotless Virgin Princess... to a ...youthful Heir Apparent*, Graham's belatedly published contribution to the Regency Crisis, finally appeared in 1792. It was the only section of his proposed work on the King's "late maladies" ever to reach the booksellers. Ignoring the constitutional wrangling tormenting Whigs and Tories alike, he focused his energies on the worrying prospect of a Britain ruled by a man who had yet to show any sign at all of living up to his God-given authority. It is often hard to tell whether Graham is writing tongue-in-cheek. He had claimed a few years earlier that this work was designed to spare from torture all those *"European* Fair Ones" anxiously hoping for a marriage proposal from England's dissolute heir. Graham argued that the only suitable consort for the Prince was one not just of imperial but of celestial birth – it was high time the Prince began to woo "Wisdom... the Virgin Daughter of the Great *King of Kings!"* Here the Doctor was acting as a pander not for Enlightenment rationality, but "Evangelical Wisdom". Only by walking in the paths of righteousness could the future George IV expect to have his Royal head "permanently crowned with wise, virtuous and truly honourable grey-hairs".

Graham followed an ecstatic paraphrase of the Song of Songs from the Book of Solomon with some "words of advice" to his "Fellow-Creatures and Countrymen". He believed that they were living in the ominous calm before the storm. Graham's anxieties had an apocalyptic ring, and were rooted in political specifics. His arguments about "the often unjust and ruinous administration of the laws" in Britain were punchy. Perhaps he was remembering Denton when he wrote that one person could be hanged, or transported to a life worse than death, "for stealing a few shillings on the highway, or for killing one person, whilst another person is enobled or made a lord of this *Christian* land, for robbing, starving, and murdering millions". Starting with the "rotten root and constitution", Graham condemned the organization of parliamentary representation, and even the fact that both Houses met in the darkness of night rather than the "light of the sun". The cruelties and consequences of boxing, horseracing, window taxes, gambling and revenue-raising from health-injurious tea, coffee, tobacco and snuff were all highlighted in his manifesto.

Graham pre-empted the twentieth-century natural farming movement in his approach to food commodities: he was disgusted by the adulterated bread of the bakers, the "putrid and disease-inoculated meat" of the butchers and the habit of eating vegetables bruised, too quickly washed, and too long out of the soil that had nourished them. Man-midwifery, with its unnatural promotion of forceps and generally corrupting tendencies, criminal justice, as well as the barbarous cruelty suffered by thousands of horses tortured in mail- and stagecoaches were all grouped as national sins, "a disgrace to a Christian nation". Beyond Britain's shores, "the catalogue of our foreign sins and enormities" was "too long and too black to be introduced here". Still, Graham did not neglect to condemn the "slavery, devastation, horror, and carnage" inflicted by Europe on the "once peaceful and happy natives of both the Indies, and of the African and American shores".

Graham raised these issues in the context of prophecy rather than political reform. Any moment now, the country should expect "the angel of equity and retribution" to avenge both individual and national sins at home, and Britain's "more horrid transgressions" in most of the rest of the world. His instincts if not his arguments were close to the radicals Thomas Paine, William Godwin and Richard Price, but his solutions had more in common with the preaching of messianic prophets of the 1790s like Richard Brothers or Joanna Southcott. The answer was simply to abandon wickedness and live "in Jesus Christ… our only possible Saviour".

In the autumn of 1792, at Weymouth, where George III had taken to being "ordinary" each summer, the Doctor managed to achieve his long-desired royal meeting. He placed into the King's own hand his rules of health. It is unlikely they were read. There were far too many other matters of more pressing concern. Trade slumps and harvest failures had brought a national outbreak of rioting, the King and Queen of France were now in prison, and Citizen Tom Paine had begun to burn in effigy across England.

Barely had Graham delivered his advice to George III, than the self-appointed Royal Doctor was on his way to Portugal. He may have been well enough to practice, preach and write, but his behaviour in public was still distinctly peculiar. Graham had been convinced by a vision that he should restore the mental health of another ailing monarch, fast becoming known as Maria the Mad. The Queen, previously Maria the Pious, had descended into melancholia two years earlier, tipped partly by the French Revolution. Her mania revolved around sex and religion. By 1792 her son was beginning to take over public affairs, and Dr Francis Willis, the English doctor who had treated George III, was summoned. Dr Graham embarked for Lisbon.

He was observed on board ship by another medic, William Withering, famous for introducing digitalis to the profession. (He was so admired by Graham's brother-in-law Thomas Arnold that he named one of his sons after him.) A party of travellers in the mess diverted themselves on the voyage by trying to draw Graham into conversation. Dr Withering, who tended to take himself rather seriously, refused to join in, finding his presence "spoiled the sport". He described Graham as "either madly or hypocritically religious, some are of one opinion, some of the other, but as I did not choose to be acquainted with him could not form an opinion myself. He lives upon vegetables, Milk, Honey & Water, & reads from the bible from Morning to night."

On New Year's Eve, 1792, Graham started to fast. By then, he claimed, he had buried himself naked in earth, sand and mud, over three hundred times, usually up to his lips, sometimes right over his head. He found even after six or twelve hours underground, he felt no pangs of thirst or hunger. Now it was time to discover "how to live for weeks, months or years, without eating any thing whatever". Earth-bathing was already practised by seamen in the East and West Indies as a cure for scurvy. In a world where war and famine were continual threats, Graham advocated his refined practice as a life-saving measure for any besieged town or garrison.

Graham was now working in the Plymouth area, doctoring by day and lecturing most nights for two-hour stretches. Instead of food, he applied large, fresh and usually rain-soaked pieces of turf to his body, "bleeding grass roots" to his skin. Each time he put one on, he "had a flood-tide of strength and good spirits, and felt no want of any thing, but as refreshed and strengthened" as if he'd eaten a hearty dinner. Nights were clearly difficult – ten- or twenty-pound sods strapped to the torso made for an uncomfortable and disturbed sleep. As the tall, ageing doctor became progressively thinner, he appeared to swell. His pure white clothing was bulked out by turfs, held on at first by a strong under-waistcoat and three silk handkerchiefs, later by a specially made girth, like that for a horse's saddle, attached by leather straps. When Graham came to London, the Lord Mayor witnessed his experiment under oath amidst the grandeur of Mansion House, on 3rd April 1793. At this point the Doctor took to feeding himself by putting raw red meat on, but not in, his stomach. Otherwise, he only allowed himself pure water, for a full fifteen days.

This episode was not staged, argued Graham, to make himself "singular and admired in the world". These were accusations that clearly still stung. "I live not but to communicate and to do all the good that God... may enable me to do, to the bodies and souls of my fellow-creatures," he protested in his account of the occasion, arguing somewhat disingenuously that his "constant disregard for money" was the proof of his altruism. He claimed to have had the opportunity to amass great wealth in America, Edinburgh, the Adelphi and Pall Mall, forgetting perhaps that what he did make he quickly spent. It is impossible not to smile at Graham's wonderfully boastful expressions of his own selflessness, but equally impossible not to applaud the fundamental good-heartedness of his views on so many aspects of life: war, slavery, colonialism, religious tolerance, women's position in society and of course pleasure itself.

Now the Doctor just wanted to show the nutritious power of simple earth, and the truth of "the repeated assurances of Jehovah... that we were originally formed of the earth, and... are best nourished... by its simplest productions". Roots, fruits, herbs and seeds were all that a healthy body required. To complicate one's diet was to "debauch... the integrity of Nature":

> Lusting after other mistresses, we go a whoring continually after our own inventions – the ARTS of cookery, stimulation, repetition, crudities and excess... We do not eat to satisfy hunger, but luxury and ambition; we are dead while we are alive, and our houses are so much our tombs, that a man might write our epitaph on our very doors; we are poisoned in the very pleasures of luxury, and betrayed to a thousand diseases, pains, and horrors, by indulging our palate.

After his fasting experiences, the doctor seemed to be feeling his age. "Alas, the hoary winter of life has now, or is fast coming on – sensual love is for ever fled," he mourned revealingly in an appendix to his last published work, *Pathetic remonstrances... to old men*. This was a final diatribe against masturbation which still celebrated the "seminal principle". Written as a postscript to his explanation of *How to live for many weeks, months, or years, without eating anything whatever*, Graham's advice interpreted post-coital *tristesse* as nature's sadness for the loss of the luminous balsam.

The last few years of the doctor's life were relatively silent ones, spent in Edinburgh with his family, neither seeking nor attracting attention. His conduct towards his parents was said to be exemplary, even when he was in his "high and palmy state". Graham had once predicted he would die like a ripe fruit falling to the ground. In the event, he was not far off the truth. A brain haemorrhage apparently felled him instantly, at home in Buccleuch Street, on his birthday, 23rd June 1794. Although the newspapers found it hilarious that the one-time celebrity who had so publicly planned to live for a hundred and fifty years was dead at forty-nine, Graham himself was prepared for such an eventuality. In the *Infallible Guide to eternal Blessedness* that he had appended to his marriage advice to the Prince, he had recommended his pamphlet readers, whoever they might be, to

"Retire as much as possible, and more and more from the noise and nonsense, and delusions of the world, of the flesh, and of the devil. Reckon that this day or this night may be your last, and that some day or some night soon must, and inevitably will, be your last." He seemed fairly certain, as he wrote those words, that his own "naked, quivering, and astonished soul" would be received by the angels rather than the devils.

There is no monument to the indefatigable doctor, and unmarked green turf now covers the spot where he was buried in the churchyard at Greyfriars. The public exaltation anticipated by Graham when he long ago imagined his final interment has yet to take place: "When the gentle, unerring, and ever-working hand of Nature is taking my body to pieces in my last and long earth-bath, and disposing each constituent part to the great mass of matter or element from which she took it, and re-animating and preparing the whole to be wrought up and organized a-fresh into new forms of vegetable, or the lower animal, or of human life – thousands of weak, sick, and lame persons, will arise up in health, strength, and happiness, and call me blessed."

Afterword

They did not, of course. Graham never received the recognition he longed for. But sometimes it seems his heirs are everywhere. As my bus draws up at the Elephant and Castle in south London one afternoon, a few streets from where Lord Gordon gathered protestors for his march on Parliament in 1780, the passionate voice of a black pavement preacher drifts heavenwards: "You'll never correct Nature, because Nature belongs to God." His loudspeaker crackles and I catch the words "God made Adam and Eve so that they could have children". Half an hour earlier, a free newspaper had been thrust into my hand by today's equivalent of Gog and Magog. No Kevenhuller hats, but a luminous logo-ed waistcoat. Opening the tabloid, I read about hay-bathing in the Dolomites, or closer to home in a Soho spa.

A few weeks previously, a respectable broadsheet had positively recommended bottled herbal moor water from some unspecified but apparently medicinal lowland. The article promised ravishingly radiant skin at vast expense. Should you find the smell of sewage off-putting, try the freeze-dried capsules instead. "Because you need it," purred the heading. In the United States, thousands of members of the Calorie Restriction Society are convinced that their extreme regimens will slow down their ageing, allowing them to live to be skinny centenarians, hungry but alive. At home, I check my spam filter and find a hundred emails offering sperm enhancement pills, and different versions of Viagra. "Don't be inadequate any more…" reads one. "Increase your Cum By 5-times more," suggests another.

Of course these modern echoes make misleading parallels. The contemporary conviction that medical ethics are invariably incompatible with commerce muddies the waters when it comes to assessing eighteenth-century entrepreneurs. I don't want to relegate Graham once again to mere master of the sales pitch, religious maniac, or even classy fraud. He has already been confined to the context of quackery for so long that he has become somehow flattened. The passing of time now makes it possible to see the doctor of love in better relief. But it would be no more appropriate to promote him as the misunderstood genius he believed himself to be. Graham was a modern man of the Enlightenment, for whom everything that was new and exciting about the world was material ripe to be refashioned – and usually sold, sometimes literally, sometimes metaphorically.

Many of his medical treatments have perfectly respectable adherents today: electro-convulsive therapy continues to be recommended by psychiatrists, magnetic beds are still on sale, and thalassotherapy is a reputable practice. The therapeutic benefits of music are well recognized. His predominantly vegetable diet and regimen of regular exercise are promoted by government agencies. Many of the Doctor's liberal beliefs about women, slavery and colonialism are enshrined in international law. As for sex therapy, it is in endless demand. It was invented by Graham.

Notes

Prologue

p. 3, ...*of every Englishman*: Charles Frederick Nordenskjöld writing to Charles Bernard Wadström in Stockholm, Jan. 1784, *Bryn Athyn, Academy of the New Church: Academy Collection of Swedenborg Documents*, no. 1664.31 (ACSD), quoted in Marsha Keith Schuchard, *Why Mrs Blake Cried: William Blake and the Sexual Basis of Spiritual Vision* (London: Century, 2006), p. 185 [Schuchard, *Why Mrs Blake Cried*].

p. 3, ...*newly published guide to symbolism*: George Richardson, *Iconology, or, A Collection of Emblematical Figures*, 2 vols., 1779. Richardson had been Robert Adam's companion and draftsman on an acrimonious Grand Tour in 1760 and this English version of the Italian Cesare Ripa's 1593 *Iconologia* would have been familiar to many of Graham's visitors, allowing them to "read" his furnishings without much difficulty.

p. 4, ...*an Entertainment for Angels, rather than for Men*: Benjamin Martin, *The young gentleman and lady's philosophy* [1755] (London: 1781), p. 319.

p. 4, ...*the venereal act itself... electrical processes*: James Graham, *A Lecture on the Generation, Increase, and Improvement of the Human Species!* (Nov. 1783), p. 22 [*A Lecture*].

p. 5, ...*medico... Celestial Bed*: *A Lecture*, p. 19.

p. 6, *Miss Harriet Jones... distended parts*: *Harris's List of Covent Garden Ladies*, facsimile edn. (New York and London: Garland Publishing, 1986), p. 27.

p. 6, ...*a cold, glowing, full... infallible barometer*: *A Lecture*, p. 34.

p. 7, ...*his whole Soul*: *Morning Herald*, 18th July, 1783.

p. 8, *Wordsworth, Imitation of Juvenal*: William Wordsworth *Early Poems and Fragments, 1785–1797*, eds. Carol Landon & Jared Curtis (Ithaca, New York and London: Cornell University Press, 1997), p. 800.

Chapter One

p. 9, ...*profession of medicine:* James Graham, *A Sketch, or Short Description of Dr Graham's medical apparatus* (1780), p. 30 [*A Sketch*].

p. 9, *Und[a]unted firmness of resolution... pain and torture*: Edward Foster, *An Essay on Hospitals* (Dublin: W.G. Jones, 1768), p. 61, quoted in Guenter Risse, *Hospital Life in Enlightenment Scotland* (Cambridge: Cambridge University Press, 1986), p. 65.

p. 9, *I have seen several... a cupping glass*: James Gregory, *Additional Memorial to the Managers of the Royal Infirmary* (Edinburgh: 1803), quoted in Risse, p. 66.

p. 10, *The mamma... too shocking to look at*: Quoted in Lisa Rosner, *Medical Education in the Age of Improvement* (Edinburgh: Edinburgh University Press, 1991), p. 42 [Rosner, *Medical Education*].

p. 10, ...*exemplary municipal enterprise*: Hugh Arnot, *The History of Edinburgh* (Edinburgh: 1779), p. 546 [Arnot, *History*].

p. 10 ...*grandfather a lawyer*: Manuscript biography of Graham by Charles Kirkpatrick Sharpe, in his own handwriting. In National Library of Scotland copy of *An Eccentric Lecture... printed for A. Roger, G. Lister and other booksellers* [Sharpe MS].

p. 10, *morning smells*: Robert Fergusson, 'Auld Reikie, A Poem' (1773).

p. 11, ...*a glover, and a blacksmith*: *A Directory of Edinburgh in 1752*, compiled by J. Gilhooley (Edinburgh: Edinburgh University Press, 1988).

p. 11, ...*in Old Parish Records*: Bothkenner OPR 473/1; Falkirk OPR 479/3; Edinburgh, St Cuthberts OPR 685/2/7; Edinburgh OPR 685/1/28; OPR 685/1/29. John Kay, *A Series of Original Portraits... with Biographical Sketches* (Edinburgh: Hugh Paton, 1842), p. 30ff [Kay, *A Series of Original Portraits*].

p. 11, ...*of Graham's Eccentric Lecture*: Sharpe MS. It was pillaged, unsourced, by Robert Thin in the *Book of the Old Edinburgh Club*, vol. 22 (1938) pp. 150–59.

p. 11, ...*old-fashioned... of the strictest kind*: Kay, *A Series of Original Portraits*, p. 36.

p. 12, ...*survived to adulthood*: Paterson allots Graham three sisters and one brother, all of whom are traceable in parish archives. The doctor did claim at one point to have twenty-five living siblings, but he wrote this at a stage when he had every expectation of living "in uninterrupted health, till I fall like ripe fruit, a hundred years hence, upon the bounteous and ever-teeming lap of her from whom I sprung." (*A Lecture*, p. 16). It may have been the ether speaking.

p. 12, *The fatal day... deadly preparation*: Walter Scott, *The Heart of Midlothian* (1818), ch. 2.

pp. 12–13 *I should not have gone... not at the arm*: Basil Cozens-Hardy, ed., *The Diary of Sylas Neville, 1767–1788* (1950), entry for 15th Sept. 1773, p. 205 [*Diary of Sylas Neville*].

p. 13, ...*familiar through long use*: John Bell complained in his *Letters on the Education of a Surgeon* (1810), p. 579, that "[i]n Dr Monro's class, unless there be a fortunate succession of bloody murders, not three subjects are dissected in the year. On the remains of a subject fished up from the bottom of a tub of spirits, are demonstrated those delicate nerves, which are to be avoided or divided in our operations; and these are demonstrated once at the distance of one hundred feet! nerves and arteries which the surgeon has to dissect, at the peril of his patient's life."

p. 13, ...*a smattering of Greek*: Robert Kerr, ed., *Memoirs of William Smellie*, with new introduction by Richard B. Sher. [Reprint of 1811 edition], (Bristol: Thoemmes Press, 1996), p. 18 [*Memoirs of William Smellie*].

p. 14, ...*Russians and Danes*: A. Logan Turner, *Story of a Great Hospital: The Royal Infirmary of Edinburgh, 1729–1929* (Edinburgh: Oliver and Boyd, 1937), p. 152 [Logan Turner, *Story of a Great Hospital*]. See also the letter from Thomas Ismay, student of medicine at Edinburgh in 1771, to his father. 23rd Nov. 1771, *University of Edinburgh Journal*, vol. 8, 1936–37, pp. 57–60.

p. 14, *already rivals... Physic in Europe*: John Morgan, quoted in Rosner, *Medical Education*, p. 24.

p. 14, *1st the Fine Gentleman... ought to associate*: Rosner, *Medical Education*, p. 25. Jones was writing to his brother in 1776.

p. 14, *A College Life... may be long continued*: Letter from Thomas Arnold to Richard Pulteney, Edinburgh, 26th Dec. 1762, Pulteney MSS, The Linnaean Society.

p. 15, *I am well happy... out of my mind*: Letter from Timothy Bentley to Richard Pulteney, 20th Mar. 1762, Pulteney MSS.

p. 15, *regularly bred to Physic and Surgery*: James Graham, *Thoughts on the present state of practice and disorders of the eye and ear* (1775), p. 6 [*Thoughts*].

p. 15, *May Prick nor Purse ne'er fail you*: Letter from Sylas Neville to Mr Baker, Yarmouth, Aug. 1772 (Norfolk Record Office, MC7/1) "The Beggar's Benison is in good health, at least one part of it (I suppose you remember both parts of the Toast). – I shall defer saying anything of the Inoculation, till I see you..."

p. 15, *...apothecary at this point*: Sharpe MS.

p. 15, *...nineteenth-century Royal Commission*: Rosner, *Medical Education*, p. 107.

p. 16, *What should I have been... delightful thought*: 10th Nov. 1805, Box 11, Folder 73, Alexander [Lesassier] Hamilton Collection, Royal College of Physicians of Edinburgh, quoted in Lisa Rosner, *The Most Beautiful Man in Existence* (Philadelphia, PA: University of Pennsylvania Press, 1999), p. 29.

p. 16, *continually haunted... in that Language*: Arnold to Pulteney, Edinburgh, 26th Dec. 1762, Pulteney MSS. His friend Bentley, on the other hand, implored his former master not to think him "pedantick" because he wrote a bit of Latin in a letter: "'tis not because I w'd show my Learning since it requires no great head to make it out & the young Gentlemen here often make use of that Language which is most expressive, among themselves without thinking it pedantry." Letter to Pulteney, Edinburgh, 4th Dec. 1761, Pulteney MSS.

p. 16, *...St Andrews none at all*: The French revolutionary Jean-Paul Marat acquired his MD from the University of St Andrews in 1775, for example.

p. 17, *When I consider... conducive to my Health*: Thomas Ismay, 'Letter from Thomas Ismay, Student of Medicine at Edinburgh, 1771, to his father', *University of Edinburgh Journal*, 8 (1936–37), p. 59 [Ismay letter].

p. 17, *The Professors... by Dr. Rutherford*: *The Edinburgh Evening Courant* and *The Caledonian Mercury*, Wednesday 7th Oct. 1761.

p. 17, *golden age of physic*: According to Irvine Loudon, 'The Nature of Provincial Medical Practice in Eighteenth-Century England', *Medical History* (1985), vol. 29, p. 24.

p. 17, *I think I would not fail... live for ever*: Whitfield Bell, Jr, 'Philadelphia Medical Students in Europe, 1750–1800', *Pennsylvania Magazine of History and Biography* (Jan. 1943), vol. 67, no. 1, pp. 1–29, 14.

p. 17, *Scotch Hippocrates*: Rosner, *Medical Education*, p. 51.

p. 17, *Dr Cullen the inimatable... from any before*: Whitfield J. Bell Jr, 'Thomas Parke's Student Life in England and Scotland, 1771–73', *Pennsylvania Magazine of History and Biography*, vol. 75, no. 3, July 1951, p. 249 [Bell, 'Thomas Parke's Student Life'].

pp. 17–18, *it must certainly... distinctly heard*: Whitfield J. Bell Jr, 'Some American Students of "That Shining Oracle of Physic," Dr William Cullen of

Edinburgh, 1755–1766', *Proceedings of the American Philosophical Society* vol. 94, no. 3, (June 1950), pp. 275–81. Cullen's generosity was as legendary as his learning. He lowered his fees for impoverished patients, and gave free class tickets to a number of students who would have otherwise struggled to afford a medical education. "Dr Cullen lately presented me with a ticket without any solicitation." *Memoirs of William Smellie*, p. 235.

p. 18, *the learned and sagacious Dr Whytt*: James Graham, *Travels and Voyages in Scotland, England, and Ireland* (1783), p. 38 [*Travels and Voyages*].

p. 18, *perfectly the Master... Notice of the Students*: Arnold to Pulteney, 26th Dec. 1762, Pulteney MSS.

p. 18, *His energy and eloquence... art or effort*: Matthew Kaufman, *Medical Teaching in Edinburgh during the 18th and 19th centuries* (Edinburgh: Royal College of Surgeons in Edinburgh, 2003), p. 29.

p. 19, *the seat of the medical muses*: *Memoirs of William Smellie*, p. 238.

p. 19, *Such clouds of dust... thick Obscure*: Letter from Arnold to Pulteney, Edinburgh, 26 Dec. 1762, Pulteney MSS. Fierce public priority disputes with Monro, mainly concerning the lymphatic system, were documented in Hunter's *Medical Commentaries* (1762) and its supplement (1764). See also Alexander Monro, *An Expostulatory Epistle to William Hunter, MD* (1762).

p. 19, *...finished off Ismay*: He would rise "about 7, read till 9, then go to Dr. Cullen's Class, come back at 10, then breakfast and transcribe the Notes which I have taken at his Lecture. From 12 to 1 I walk in Infirmary, from 1 to 3 attend Dr Monro. Then come and dine, and as you may suppose I am very hungry. From 4 to 5 attend Dr Young, from 5 to 6 transcribe the notes I have taken of Dr Young or Dr Monro's Lectures; from 6 to 7 attend Dr Innis Private Demonstrations, from 7 to 9 transcribe the Lectures I have borrowed and at 9 get Supper; from 10–12 write Lectures besides every Tuesday and Thursday from 5 to 6 o'clock I attend the Clinical Lectures." Ismay letter, p. 60.

p. 19, *I have also begun to attend the Hospital*: Diary of Sylas Neville, 16th Nov. 1772, p. 189.

p. 19, *...with formal clinical lectures*: Logan Turner, *Story of a Great Hospital*, p. 133.

p. 19, *I shall give you... vary my prescriptions*: Quoted in Risse, p. 243, from an unpublished manuscript of Dr Rutherford's clinical lectures delivered in 1758, owned and quoted by Logan Turner in *Story of a Great Hospital*, p. 133.

p. 20, *knowing the dangerous... blood-letting in some cases*: Diary of Sylas Neville, 15th July 1772, p. 170.

pp. 20–21, *sent for the best Surgeon... a Dose of Salts*: Bentley to Pulteney, 26th Dec. 1762, Pulteney MSS.

p. 21, *exciting, promoting... in the human body*: Risse, p. 182, quoting James Gregory, *Additional Memorial to the Managers of the Royal Infirmary* (Edinburgh: 1803), pp. 412–413. This disputatious professor achieved a good century of popular posterity thanks to his invention of the celebrated Gregory's powder or Gregory's mixture. This was made of powdered Turkestan rhubarb roots, ginger, and magnesium oxide and acted as an antacid, stomachic, and cathartic.

p. 21, *to place... in the train*: Risse, p. 181.

p. 22, *to stroll... clerk or patients*: *History and Statutes of the Royal Infirmary*, (1778), quoted by D.M. Lyon, 'A Student of 1765–70: A Glimpse of Eighteenth Century Medicine', *Edinburgh Medical Journal* (1941), pp. 185–208.

p. 22, *I take notes... blowing noses*: Bentley to Pulteney, Edinburgh 20th Mar. 1762, Pulteney MSS.

p. 22, *We meet every Saturday... write in Latin*: Letter from Thomas Arnold to Richard Pulteney, Edinburgh, 26th Dec. 1762, Pulteney MSS.

p. 23, *...much lower than in the south*: Loudon, *Medical History*, p. 26.

p. 23, *Nothing is of greater service... in their profession*: Letter to John Ramsay, Yarmouth, Norfolk, written from Inner Temple, 21st Oct. 1776. Norfolk Record Office.

p. 23, *became his patron... into England*: Sharpe MS.

p. 24, *a gentleman who placed... of the young institution*: Henry Thompson, *A History of Ackworth School* (1879), p. 18.

p. 24, *I was highly entertained... turned into a woman*: *Memoirs of William Smellie*, p. 234. Buchan wrote this to his friend William Smellie, in one of a number of letters from which any serious medical or salacious content was removed by the printer's censorious memorializer, Robert Kerr, who destroyed much of what he chose not to publish.

p. 24, *...£60 for five years*: See P.J. and R.V. Wallis, *Eighteenth Century Medics (subscriptions, licences, apprenticeships)*, 2nd improved and enlarged edition (Newcastle: PHIBB, 1988) for examples of medical apprentice fees throughout the century. "The Sums given with Lads, going Apprentices to this Business, are from 20l. to 300l. according to the Reputation and Station the Masters are in", according to *A General Description of Trades, Digested in Alphabetical Order* (London: 1747), p. 2.

p. 24, *...early version of Domestic Medicine*: C.J. Lawrence, 'William Buchan: Medicine Laid Open', *Medical History* (1975), vol. 19, pp. 20–35, p. 22.

pp. 24–25, *Full of anecdote... money from his pocket*: William Buchan (1729–1805), physician, by G.T. Bettany, *DNB* (1886).

p. 25, *he absolutely refuses... jump at such an opportunity*: *Memoirs of William Smellie*, pp. 228–29.

p. 25, *Any booby... most humble servant*: *Memoirs of William Smellie*, p. 250.

p. 25, *...at the end of 1763*: A/FH/01/16/1, London Metropolitan Archives.

p. 25, *WANTED... of Ackworth*: *York Courant*, Tuesday 11th Oct. 1763 and subsequent issues until 1st Nov.

p. 26, *...on 3rd November*: In fact, the Marquis was prevented from attending this meeting by the gangrene in his foot caused by a festering toenail. *York Courant*, 1st Nov. 1763.

p. 26, *recommend a proper Person*: A/FH/D/O1/2/2/1, London Metropolitan Archives, Foundling Hospital, Correspondence to London 1763. Letter from Mr Collinwood, 27th Oct. 1763.

p. 26, *...with an established practitioner*: *York Courant*, 22nd Nov. 1763.

p. 26, *...also getting on in years*: John Tomlinson, *Doncaster from the Roman Occupation to the present time* (1887), p. 333; Pamela Lindley, *Freemen of the Borough of Doncaster 1558–1974*, vols. 1 and 2 (Doncaster and District Family History Society, 1998).

p. 26, *[a] JOURNEYMAN... in the Country*: *York Courant*, 3rd July, 1764.

p. 26, *a young girl with some beauty*: Sharpe MS.

p. 27, *fifty five pounds a year... her own fortune*: Letter from James Graham to Lady Spencer, 24th Mar. 1784, BL Add. 75708, vol. 408, Gore-Gwy – petitions for charity.

p. 27, *...Doncaster apothecary shop*: Sharpe MS.

p. 27, *vie with any town... of small fortune*: Edward Miller, *The History and Antiquities of Doncaster and its Vicinity with Anecdotes of Eminent Men* (Doncaster: 1804), p. 8.

p. 27, *...free-for-all for medical men*: For a full explanation see S.W.F. Holloway, 'The Apothecaries' Act, 1815: A Reinterpretation', *Medical History* (1966), vol. 10, pp. 107–236.

p. 27, *in tatter'd weeds... culling of simples*: *Romeo and Juliet*, Act v, Sc. 1, ll. 37–48.

p. 27, *...bust of Galen*: *The Quacks* (British Museum, no. 6325; Wellcome Library, no. 20790i).

p. 28, *...more lucrative field of general medical practice*: As the regulatory reforms of the Apothecaries' Act of 1815 finally recognized.

p. 28, *...round to the backdoor*: E.M. Sigsworth and P. Swan, 'An Eighteenth-century surgeon and apothecary: William Elmhirst (1721–1773)', *Medical History* (1982), vol. 26, p. 193.

p. 28, *This is a very genteel Business... eminent in their Way*: *A General Description of all Trades* (1747), pp. 1–2.

p. 28, *there is no business... thus turn Apothecary*: *Free Thoughts on Apothecaries and empirics...* (London: 1773), pp. 29–30.

p. 28, *...a good set of patients*: *A General Description of all Trades* (1747), p. 3.

p. 28, *knockt up by Midwifery*: Undated letter from Bentley to Pulteney (no. 7), Pulteney MSS.

p. 29, *Pharmacopoeia Universalis; or, a new universal English dispensatory*: The *Pharmacopoeia Universalis* was by Robert James of James's Fever Powder fame, an outrageous old Lichfield friend of Samuel Johnson.

p. 29, *no set hours for Business*: *A General Directory of Trades* (1747), pp. 2–3.

p. 29, *...their position could secure*: Unlike physicians, apothecaries could only make money from the sale of medicines, and were forbidden to charge a fee for attending a patient. Their drugs charges were notorious, their profits "a bye-word, denoting something uncommonly extravagant", as Adam Smith observed in *An Inquiry into the Nature and Causes of the Wealth of Nations*, vol. 1 (1776; London: Methuen & Co., 1904), p. 113. But even the best-employed apothecary in a sizeable market town could not expect to sell drugs actually worth more than thirty or forty pounds in a year. Without attendance fees, argued Adam Smith, it was perfectly reasonable for him to sell these drugs for as much as a thousand times what they cost.

p. 30, *quietly as lambs*: A late seventeenth-century French traveller quoted by John R. Gillis in *For Better, For Worse: British Marriages, 1600 to the Present* (Oxford: Oxford University Press, 1985), p. 136.

p. 31, *...generalized horror of depopulation*: Andrea Rusnock, *Vital Accounts:*

Quantifying Health and Population in Eighteenth-Century England and France (Cambridge: Cambridge University Press, 2002), p. 181.

p. 31, *Count, measure, compare*: Jean Jacques Rousseau, *The Social Contract*, ed. Maurice Cranston (Harmondsworth, Middlesex: Penguin Classics, 1968), p. 130.

p. 31, *make the Nation… and hardier*: Thomas Short, *A Comparative History of the Increase and Decrease of MANKIND in* England*, and Several Countries Abroad, According to the different soils, situations, Business of Life, Use of the NON-NATURALS, &c. faithfully collected from, and attested by, above Three Hundred Vouchers, and many of them for a long Course of Years, in two different Periods* (1767), p. 25.

p. 31, *of Children, or aged… should they have any*: Short, *A Comparative History*, p. 22.

p. 31, *…Yorkshire newspaper in 1763*: York Courant, 25th Jan., 1763.

p. 32, *– Better thy Heat assuage… a vig'rous Strain*: Claude Quillet, *Advice to new-married persons: or, The art of having beautiful children. In four books*, tr. Nicholas Rowe (1754), p. 18 [Quillet, *Advice*].

p. 32, *William Pickering Graham*: Exact d.o.b. unrecorded, but William Pickering Graham died of consumption on 9th Oct. 1768 aged three years and four months and was buried in Ackworth 11th Oct. 1768. Ackworth Parish registers, West Yorkshire Archives, WDP77/3.

p. 32, *…have not been preserved*: Unfortunately the original Doncaster St George Parish Registers were damaged in a fire and only incomplete transcripts survive, so it is impossible to be conclusive on this matter.

p. 32, *…and bore six children*: The only available information about her date and place of birth is the 1841 Census, which records Mary Stirling (as she became on her marriage in 1796), then living in the Edinburgh parish of Newington, as aged seventy, and born in England. Since census officers were required to round down adults' ages to the nearest five years, this suggests Mary Ann Graham was born at some point between June 1766 and 1771. She was said to be "a very accomplished lady". Kay, *A Series of Original Portraits*, p. 3.

p. 32, *a weakly Offspring*: Quillet, *Advice*, p. 10.

p. 32, *…during the 1760s*: *The New-York Gazette or the Weekly Post-Boy*, 20th Aug. 1770, and elsewhere.

p. 33, *…other than to his own advancement*: See Toby Gelfand, '"Invite the philosopher, as well as the charitable": hospital teaching as private enterprise in Hunterian London', W.F. Bynum and Roy Porter eds., *William Hunter and the Eighteenth-Century Medical World* (Cambridge: Cambridge University Press, 1985), pp. 129–51; Susan C. Lawrence, 'Entrepreneurs and private enterprise: the development of medical lecturing in London, 1775–1820', *Bulletin of the History of Medicine* (1988), 62, pp. 171–192.

p. 33, *I firmly believe… reward in this world*: William Hunter, *Two Introductory Lectures* (London: 1784), pp. 102–103.

Chapter Two

p. 35, *America… with intellectual light*: A Lecture, p. 18.

p. 35, *the spirit of emigration… North Britain*: Patrick M'Robert's *Tour*

Through Part of the North Provinces of America, 1774–5, ed. Carl Bridenbaugh, offprint from *The Pennsylvania Magazine of History and Biography,* Apr. 1935, p. ix [M'Robert, *Tour*].

p. 35, *[I]t was the best country... on an agreeable footing:* M'Robert, *Tour,* p. ix.

p. 36, *for men in this particular... as from a bad:* M'Robert, *Tour,* pp. ix–x.

p. 36, *indulging in those extravagances... return home again:* Sharpe MS.

p. 37, *to be flying... desirable progress there:* Diary of Sylas Neville, 3rd Nov. 1768, p. 49.

p. 38, *...from side to side:* Janet Schaw, *Journal of a Lady of Quality... 1774 to 1776,* eds. Evangeline W. Andrews and Charles M. Andrews (New Haven, CT: 1921), pp. 45–55.

p. 38, *They might as well fall... coarse food and clothing:* Bailyn, *Voyagers to the West: Emigration from Britain to America on the Eve of the Revolution* (London: Tauris, 1987), p. 324, 'Extract of a letter from an officer in the 64th regiment, Boston, 5th Aug. 1773, to his father in Dublin', *Lloyd's Evening Post,* 4th–6th Oct. 1773; *Etherington's York Chronicle,* 27th Jan. 1775.

p. 38, *...referred to them all as his "children":* Bailyn, *Voyagers,* p. 325.

p. 39, *...to which their owners were sunk in debt:* Carl Bridenbaugh, *Myths and Realities of the Colonial South* (1952; Westport, CT: Greenwood Press, 1981), pp. 6–18.

p. 39, *they seldom show... of the human species:* Andrew Burnaby, *Travels through the Middle Settlements in North-America. In the Years 1759 and 1760. With observations on the state of the colonies,* 2nd edn. (London: T. Payne, 1775), pp. 31–32 [Burnaby, *Travels*].

p. 39, *a small neat town... imaginable:* The Maryland Gazette, 25th Jan. 1770; Burnaby, *Travels,* p. 65.

p. 39, *Doctor Graham... several parts of Europe:* The New-York Gazette or the Weekly Post-Boy, 20th Aug. 1770.

p. 39, *...any truly reputable medic:* Thomas Parke to Owen Biddle, Edinburgh, 13th Jan. 1772, Friends Historical Library, Swarthmore College, cited in Bell, 'Thomas Parke's Student Life', p. 246.

p. 40, *'Tis truth... nothing new:* Apostrophe to "The Newspaper", published by John Holt in the *New York Journal,* quoted by Carl Bridenbaugh, *Cities in Revolt: Urban Life in America, 1743–1776* (New York: Alfred A. Knopf, 1955), p. 389 [Bridenbaugh, *Cities in Revolt*].

p. 40, *tenderness and moderation... incurable by other Practitioners:* The New-York Gazette or the Weekly Post-Boy, 20th Aug. 1770.

p. 40, *recommended to some Share... from pretended Knowledge:* The New-York Gazette or the Weekly Post-Boy, 20th Aug. 1770.

p. 41, *flock'd... every day of his exhibition:* New York Journal, 29th Aug. 1771.

p. 41, *...seventh son of a seventh son:* Peter Benes, 'Itinerant Physicians, Healers, and Surgeon-Dentists in New England and New York, 1720–1825', *Medicine and Healing: The Dublin Seminar for New England Folklife Annual Proceedings* (Boston University, 1990), p. 97.

p. 41, *Few physicians... in Egypt:* William Smith, *The history of the province of New-York* (1757; London: 1776).

p. 41, *..."promiscuously" styled doctors:* Helen Brock, 'North American

Medicine' in *The Medical Enlightenment of the Eighteenth Century*, eds. A. Cunningham and R. French (Cambridge: Cambridge University Press, 1990), p. 202, citing Adam Thomson, *A Discourse on the Preparation of the Body for the Smallpox and the Manner of Receiving the Infection* (Philadelphia, PA: 1750).

p. 41, ...*several different newspapers at once*: The New-York Journal; or, the General Advertiser; The New-York Gazette; and the Weekly Mercury and The New-York Gazette or the Weekly Post-Boy.

p. 41, *rather hurts an Europian eye... yearly here*: M'Robert, *Tour*, p. 3.

p. 42, ...*as well as "FEMALE COMPLAINTS in general"*: Repeated in all New York advertisements.

p. 42, *The means of conveying knowledge... thirst for knowledge*: Bridenbaugh, *Rebels and Gentlemen: Philadelphia in the Age of Franklin* (New York: Reynal and Hitchcock, 1942) p. 335 [Bridenbaugh, *Rebels and Gentlemen*]. Thomson was a man whose name was well known to be synonymous with truth, who was one of the two first signatories on the first handwritten draft of the American Declaration of Independence.

p. 43, ...*it remains to this day*: Whitfield J. Bell, Jr, 'The Old Library of the Pennsylvania Hospital', *Bull. Med. Libr. Assoc.*, vol. 60, Issue 4 (Oct. 1972), pp. 543–550, p. 543 [Bell, 'The Old Library'].

p. 43, *elegant Anatomical... as well as the curious*: Newspaper advertisement quoted in *Medical Collectors Association Newsletter*, no. 37 (Aug. 2000), p. 8.

p. 43, ...*his dissecting theatre*: John F. Watson, *Annals of Philadelphia and Pennsylvania* (1857), vol. 2, ch. 17.

p. 43, ...*instrument to play music*: William Barton, *Memoirs of the Life of David Rittenhouse* (Philadelphia, PA: 1813), pp. 202–203.

p. 43, *There wond'ring... maze unfold*: Joel Barlow, *The Vision of Columbus* (1787).

p. 44, *who are daily making Collections*: Bridenbaugh, *Rebels and Gentlemen*, p. 354.

p. 44, *hydraulics... fortification*: Bridenbaugh, *Rebels and Gentlemen*, p. 351.

p. 44, *[t]o those Gentlemen who enquire... many foreign nations*: *Travels and Voyages*, pp. 36–37.

p. 44, *obscure mechanicks... mathematics*: Bridenbaugh, *Cities in Revolt*, p. 383.

p. 44, ...*physicians and their students*: Bell, 'The Old Library'.

p. 44, *made the common Tradesmen... other Countries*: *The Autobiography of Benjamin Franklin*, ed. Leonard W. Labaree (New Haven, CT, and London: Yale University Press, 1964), p. 131.

p. 45, *person of distinction and fortune*: Librarian Revd Jacob Duché, quoted in Bridenbaugh, *Cities in Revolt*, p. 383.

p. 45, ...*once in a session*: Gary Nash, *First City: Philadelphia and the Forging of Historical Memory* (Philadelphia, PA: University of Pennsylvania Press, 2002), p. 17.

p. 45, *[T]he great prince... prince of politicians*: *A Lecture*, p. 18.

p. 45, *the writings of an American... and to general practice*: *Travels and Voyages*, p. 37. Much the same material is also found in Graham, *A Short*

Inquiry into the Present State of Medical Practice (1776), p. 8 [*A Short Inquiry*].

p. 45, ...*with wise Minerva*: 'Au Génie de Franklin', engraving by Jean Honoré Fragonard. See *Journal de Paris*, 15th Nov. 1778, for account.

p. 46, *As this may... in electrical experiments*: Collinson to Colden, 30th Mar. 1745, *The Letters and Papers of Cadwallader Colden*, vol. 3, 1743–1747 (Collections of the New-York Historical Society, 1919), p. 110, quoted in I. Bernard Cohen, *Benjamin Franklin's Science* (Cambridge, Mass: Harvard University Press, 1990), p. 62 [Cohen, *Science*].

p. 46, *[P]rinces were willing... some other circumstances*: 'An Historical Account of the wonderful discoveries, made in Germany, &c. concerning Electricity', *Gentleman's Magazine*, xv (Apr. 1745), pp. 193–97.

p. 47, *was continually full... new wonders*: Max Ferrand, ed., *Benjamin Franklin's Memoirs, Parallel Text Edition* (Berkeley and Los Angeles, CA: University of California Press, 1949), p. 380.

p. 47, ...*he had lived eight hundred miles... A strange project*: Labaree, *Papers of BF*, IV, 480 and V, 522 letter to Dr John Lining, quoted in J.A. Leo Lemay, *Ebenezer Kinnersley: Franklin's Friend* (Philadelphia: University of Pennsylvania Press, 1964), pp. 61–62 [Lemay, *Ebenezer Kinnersley*].

p. 47, *What Spirit Such... not of such confusion*: 'A Letter from Ebenezer Kinnersley to his Friend in the Country', Postscript to the *Pennsylvania Gazette*, 15th July 1740.

p. 48, ...*battery of eleven guns*: *Maryland Gazette*, 14th June 1749.

p. 48, *does not, like common Matter... Spark of it*: Lemay, *Ebenezer Kinnersley*, p. 64.

p. 48, ...*containing not only those... lately made in Philadelphia*: *Maryland Gazette*, 10th, 17th and 24th May, 1749, "Notice is hereby given to the Curious..."

p. 48, *master of words... respectable*: Lemay, *Ebenezer Kinnersley*, p. 86.

p. 49, ...*in the Dömjén mould*: Sylas Neville wrote of his fellow student Dennison's passion for electricity in Edinburgh (*Diary of Sylas Neville*, p. 147), and from time to time a Mr Cross gave electricity lectures in York in the late 1760s.

p. 49, *artificial spider... to catch a fly*: Lemay, *Ebenezer Kinnersley*, p. 62.

p. 49, ...*in any well-to-do home*: J.I. Heilbron, *Electricity in the 17th and 18th Centuries: A Study of Early Modern Physics* (Berkeley, CA: University of California Press, 1979), p. 98 [Heilbron, *Electricity in the 17th and 18th Centuries*].

p. 49, *Some Notice may be taken... Money and Pleasure*: 30th Jan. 1761, British Library; Heilbron, *Electricity in the 17th and 18th Centuries*, p. 164.

p. 50, ...*feathers, straw and so on*: Derived from the Greek word for amber, electricity literally means "ambricity". As Kinnersley observed, if the property had first been discovered in glass, which does the same thing considerably better, our terminology would be different today.

p. 50, *the Electric Virtue... Common Mass of Matter*: I. Bernard Cohen, ed., *Benjamin Franklin's Experiments* (Cambridge, MA: Harvard University Press, 1941), p. 411 [Cohen, *Experiments*].

p. 50, ...*in ever more ingenious trials*: Cohen, *Experiments*, p. 411.

p. 52, *...he thought his life was at an end*: *Gentleman's Magazine*, vol. 16 (1746), p. 163. "It was two days before I recovered from the blow and terror... I would not take a second shock for the kingdom of France." This earned Musschenbroek the epithet the "cowardly professor" from Priestley, in contrast to Wilhelm Richmann, who was killed in St Petersburg while performing a version of Franklin's lightning and sentry-box experiment, or the "magnanimous Mr. Boze, who with a truly philosophical heroism, worthy of the renowned Empedocles, said he wished he might die by the electric shock, that the account of his death might furnish an article for the memoirs of the French Academy of Sciences". Joseph Priestley, *The History and Present State of Electricity*, 3rd edn. (1775; New York and London: Johnson Reprint Corporation, 1966), vol. 1, p. 107 [Priestley, *History and Present State of Electricity*]. The Leyden jar was discovered independently by Georg von Kleist of Cammin in October 1745 and by van Musschenbroek of Leiden in the spring of 1746.

p. 52, *...the onlookers' astonished gaze*: The Florence Museum of the History of Science, which boasts a particularly impressive collection of Enlightenment electrical apparatus, has a nineteenth-century version of this gadget on display. The experiment was originally designed by Nollet in the 1740s as part of his effort to prove his two fluid theory of "effluent" (outgoing) and "affluent" electric streams.

p. 52, *rises into bubbles... electrified finger*: *Gentleman's Magazine*, 1745.

p. 53, *a few years since... overthrow a true one*: Cohen, *Experiments*, p. 415.

p. 53, *a spike of iron... enter the ground*: M'Robert, *Tour*, p. 38

p. 53, *seem to be means... safety and protection*: Burnaby, *Travels*, p. 10.

p. 53, *Deum laudo... fulgura frango*: Schiller's poem, *Die Glocke*, quoted in Cohen, *Science*, p. 119.

pp. 53–54, *...to strike the ringers themselves*: The French electrician Abbé Nollet cited a report describing a storm in Brittany in April 1718, when no less than twenty-four churches between Landernau and Saint-Pol-de-Léon had been struck, with one church utterly destroyed and two bell-ringers killed. The silent churches had been spared. Cohen, *Science*, p. 120.

p. 54, *Atheistical presumption*: Lemay, *Ebenezer Kinnersley*, p. 78.

p. 54, *with pointed... Preservation*: *New York Journal*, 19th Aug. 1773.

p. 54, *...from America to Europe*: George Adams (1787), pp. 330–31, Pl. v, fig. 89.

p. 55, *...transform the oculist's life*: Kinnersley advertised a lecture on 26th Dec. 1771, with further appearances the following year on 2nd Jan., 9th Jan., 30th Jan., 6th Feb., 13th Feb., 28th Oct., 4th Nov., 11th Nov. and 18th Nov., with a single lecture in 1773 on 29th Dec. (Christmas always seemed to produce a demonstration). Lemay, *Ebenezer Kinnersley*, appendix ii, p. 117.

p. 55, *...sceptical about electricity's medical benefits*: Letter To Dr John Pringle, 21st Dec. 1757 in *The Papers of Benjamin Franklin*, vol. 7, ed. Leonard W. Labaree (New Haven, CT, and London: Yale University Press), pp. 298–300 (read at the Royal Society 12th Jan. 1758).

p. 55, *Antonius de Haen... have been effectual*: *The Pennsylvania Chronicle and Universal Advertiser*, 24th Dec. to 31st Dec. 1770 [*Pennsylvania Chronicle*].

p. 55, *Thunder and Lightning produced by human Art*: Bridenbaugh, *Cities in Revolt*, p. 416.

p. 55, *draw down... clouds of heaven*: Graham, *The general state of medical and chirurgical practice, exhibited; shewing them to be inadequate, ineffectual, absurd, and ridiculous* (London: 1779), p. 185 [*The General State*].

p. 56, *...sparks a foot long*: W.D. Hackmann, *Catalogue of Pneumatic, Magnetic and Electrical Machines* (Florence: Museo di Storia della Scienza, 1995) [Hackmann, *Catalogue*].

p. 56, *some considerable addition... coated with tinfoil*: *Dunlap's Penn Packet*, 27th Dec. 1773.

p. 56, *dart towards a little Lady... affected by it*: Lemay, *Ebenezer Kinnersley*, p. 142.

p. 56, *...beautiful electric stars*: *Dunlap's Penn Packet*, 27th Dec. 1773.

p. 56, *illuminated... celestial Brilliance*: *Sketch of the Plan, etc of the Temple of Health*, one-penny handbill (1780).

p. 56, *We have no discoveries... of North America*: Benjamin Rush, *An oration, delivered February 4, 1774, before the American Philosophical Society, held at Philadelphia* (1774), p. 60.

p. 57, *...reached 77 tons in 1770*: Helen Brock, *Medical Enlightenment*, p. 213.

p. 57, *...discover their medical secrets*: *Travels and Voyages*, p. 37.

p. 57, *...extracting such information*: Henry Tufts, *The Autobiography of a Criminal*, edited, with an introduction, by Edmund Pearson (London: Jarrolds, 1931), p. 68.

p. 57, *lower Canada... intoxicating potion*: Tufts, *Autobiography*, p. 254.

p. 57, *Gadding about quack-like*: Tufts, *Autobiography*, title of Chapter II, Book III, pp. 248–54.

p. 58, *suddenly struck... concocted fire*: *A Lecture*, p. 18.

p. 58, *that principle... the sexes meet*: John Cleland, *Memoirs of a Woman of Pleasure* (London: Penguin Classics, 1985), p. 211.

p. 58, *let one of the nicest Ladies... from her Eyes*: *Electrical Eel* (c.1770), p.19.

p. 58, *...disproved the hypothesis*: Joseph-Aignan Sigaud de la Fond, *Précis historique et experimental des phénomènes électriques*, 2nd edn. (Paris: 1785), pp. 230–33, cited in Arthur Elsenaar and Remko Scha, 'Electric Body Manipulation as Performance Art: A Historical Perspective', *Leonardo Music Journal*, vol. 12 (2002), pp. 17–28.

p. 59, *...bruising with its shocks*: W.D. Hackmann, *Electricity from Glass: The History of the Frictional Electrical Machine 1600–1850* (Alphen aan den Rijn: Sijthoff & Noordhoff, 1978) [Hackmann, *Electricity from Glass*].

p. 60, *The first patient... and happily pregnant*: *A Lecture*, p. 18.

p. 60, *They all found... more durable*: *A Lecture*, p. 18.

p. 60, *[A]fter a few months... critical HOUR*: *A Lecture*, p. 18.

p. 61, *I call it an atmosphere... acid smell*: *Gentleman's Magazine*, vol. 15 (1745), p. 197.

p. 61, *...particularly arousing*: Good examples can be found in editions of *The Rambler's Magazine; or, the annals of Gallantry, Glee, Pleasure and the Bon Ton: Calculated for the entertainment of the Polite World; and to furnish the Man of Pleasure with a most delicious banquet of Amorous,*

Bacchanalian, Whimsical, Humorous, theatrical and polite entertainment… (1783–90).

p. 62, *the influence… sweet pleasures*: A Lecture, p. 19.

p. 62, *Wonderful, oftentimes… celestial bed*: A Lecture, p. 18.

p. 62, *that wise… city*: A Lecture, p. 18.

p. 62, *at a Mrs Dugdale's… the ears, &c.*: Pennsylvania Chronicle, 14th–21st Oct. 1771.

p. 63, *How noble… Almighty God*: Front page and first article in *Pennsylvania Chronicle*, 23rd–30th Mar. 1772.

p. 63, *the thundering of Coaches… assaill our Ears*: Bridenbaugh, *Cities in Revolt*, p. 224.

p. 64, *Since his arrival… probably be effected*: Pennsylvania Chronicle, 23rd–30th Mar. 1772.

p. 64, *so curiously fixed… its healthy state*: Pennsylvania Chronicle, 3rd, 12th and 19th Oct. 1772.

p. 64, *Rational and Pleasing Entertainment*: Pennsylvania Chronicle, 8th Mar. 1773.

p. 66, *…of the eyebrows alone*: Nicolas Andry de Boisregard, *Orthopaedia* (1743), Book II, pp. 28–43.

p. 66, *…sight and desire*: "Where does Love enter?" asks a man of his female companion in *Love's Catechism: Compiled… for the Use and Benefit of All Young Batchelors, Maids and Widows* (1707). "Into the eyes," comes her reply.

p. 66, *for they have the Art… Eyes and Actions*: Thomas Stretzer, *New Description of Merryland* (1741), p. 38.

p. 66, *those bewitching… or emanations*: A Lecture, p. 22.

Chapter Three

p. 69, *…and may excentric medical geniuses arise*: Thoughts, p. 2.

pp. 69–70, *the Pennsylvanians are… on [his] Pate*: 27th Nov., 1773, Broadsheet addressed *To the Delaware Pilots [and] Capt Ayres* (Library of Congress, Rare Books and Special Collections Division).

p. 70, *I returned to England… oceans to seek for*: A Lecture, p. 18.

p. 71, *…her monumental History of England*: Catharine Macaulay, *The History of England from the Accession of James I to that of the Brunswick Line*, 8 vols. (London: 1763–83).

pp. 71–72, *She is one of the sights… to see*: W.S. Lewis, ed., *The Yale Edition of Horace Walpole's Correspondence*, vol. 23, p. 92, letter of 1769 [*Walpole's Correspondence*].

pp. 72, *contends for laurels… for flowers*: Letter from Mary Wollstonecraft to Catharine Macaulay, 30th Dec. 1790 (New York Public Library), accompanying a copy of Wollstonecraft's newly published *Vindication of the Rights of Man*. Her *Vindication of the Rights of Woman* was published early in 1792.

p. 72, *very prodigy*: According to Lord Lyttelton. Bridget Hill, *The Republican Virago: The Life and Times of Catharine Macaulay, Historian* (Oxford: Clarendon Press, 1992), p. 23 [Hill, *Republican Virago*].

p. 72, *Above all, beware... any of them back*: Works of Augustus Toplady (1853), p. 855.

p. 72, *...Thomas Wilson*: For example by Lucy Donnelly, in a pamphlet reprinted from her article 'The Celebrated Mrs Macaulay' in *The William and Mary Quarterly*, 3rd ser, vol. 6, no. 2 (Apr. 1949) and Hill, *Republican Virago*.

p. 73, *...large curls of his hair*: Letter of 24th May 1781 from A.J. Lexall to J.A. Euler, quoted in J.T. Alexander, 'A Russian Reflection of Dr James Graham's "Strange Establishment"', *Study Group on Eighteenth-Century Russia Newsletter*, vol. 20 (1992), pp. 178–79 [Alexander, 'Russian Reflection'].

p. 73, *his hair most marvellously... Parnassus*: Walter Scott's marginalia in his copy of Francis Grose's satire, *A guide to health, beauty, riches, and honour* (1785), Abbotsford Library (Faculty of Advocates, Edinburgh).

p. 73, *...in early spring*: Since Graham only began to advertise his practice in England in Bristol in May 1774, the possibility that he could have been the subject of this letter has not previously been given serious consideration. But his last advertisement in the colonies appeared in mid-December the previous year. Transatlantic voyages could by then take little more than four weeks – the tea ship *Polly* had finally been turned back from the Delaware River on Christmas Day 1773, and was safely sailing up the Thames barely a month later. Graham could have moved just as quickly.

p. 73, *a System of Tyranny... every day*: John Adams to Catharine Macaulay, 19th Apr. 1773, Gilder Lehrman Collection, Pierpont Morgan Library.

p. 73, *acquired not a little... MACAULAY: The General State*, p. i.

pp. 74–75: *so far superior... science and men: Thoughts*, pp. 1–3.

p. 75, *pecuniary harvest: Thoughts*, p. 13.

p. 75, *...for the past two months: Bath Journal*, 2nd Jan. 1775.

p. 75, *that great metropolis: Bath Journal*, 16th Jan. 1775.

p. 76, *Vivid pictures... came under Dr. Graham's care: Thoughts*, p. 20.

p. 76, *...describing him as an "apothecary"*: He wrote to the Comtesse de Viry, around 2nd Apr. 1776: "*En un mot, la goutte m'a mis à la torture depuis quatre mois; or, je ne sais comment cela se fait, mais les douleurs excessives ne me rapellent jamais rien d'agréable. Comment s'attendre donc que les angoisses, l'apothicaire Graham, les flanelles, et une chaise longue pussent rappeler à ma mémoire, l'esprit, la vivacité, la bonne humeur et la gaîté?*" [In a word, gout has been torturing me for four months now; yet I don't know how this happens, but the excessive pains usually do not remind me of anything pleasant. How was I then to expect that the anxieties, Graham the apothecary, the flannels and a chaise longue could conjure up to my mind, wit, vivacity, good humour and cheerfulness?], *Walpole's Correspondence*, vol. 41, p. 343.

p. 76, *sweet-flowing... notes*: L.E. Troide, ed., *The Early Journals and Letters of Fanny Burney*, 3 vols. (Oxford: Clarendon, 1988–94) .

p. 76–77, *inimitable sweetness... literary composition*: James Graham, *A Sketch, or Short Description of Dr Graham's medical apparatus* (1780), p. 53 [*A Sketch*].

p. 77, *the humble pious Heart... of Divine Love*: Graham, *The Christian's Universal Prayer*, 3rd edn. (1776), Preface.

p. 77, *On publishing... very well understand*: A Sketch, p. 58.

p. 78, *a person in Russia... study of magnetism*: A Short Inquiry, p. 8.

p. 78, *... in the popular Gentleman's Magazine*: Aepinus, *An Attempt at a Theory of Electricity and Magnetism* (1759), *Gentleman's Magazine*, vol. 28 (1758), pp. 617–19. See also Joseph Priestley, *History and Present State of Electricity* (1767), p. 243.

p. 78, *...as a masterpiece*: Heilbron, *Electricity in the 17th and 18th Centuries*, pp. 401, 426. In 1776, Lichtenberg, professor of pure and applied mathematics at the University of Göttingen, believed that the non-mathematical experimenter had had his day: electricity, he said, "has more to expect from mathematics than from apothecaries".

p. 78, *...in the Gulf of Finland*: Travels and Voyages, p. 216.

p. 78, *...after this trip*: A Short Inquiry, p. 11.

p. 79, *the highest... capable of enjoying*: A Short Inquiry, p. 8.

p. 79, *Consumptions... nervous Weakness*: A Short Inquiry, p. 9.

pp. 79–80, *My method of cure... Divine restorative*: A Short Inquiry, pp. 11–12.

p. 80, *effluvia... celestial*: Bath Chronicle, 28th Nov. 1776.

p. 80, *elegancies... by enchantment*: Stebbing Shaw, *A Tour to the West of England in 1788* (London: 1789), p. 295.

p. 80, *a huge cistern... hot water*: Shaw, A Tour, p. 68.

p. 80, *their Scorbutick carcasses... Stygian Lake*: Ned Ward, *The reformer. Exposing the vices of the age in several characters. ...* (1701), p. 157.

p. 80, *...regularly updated guidebooks*: For example, *The Bath and Bristol Guide: Or the Tradesman's and Traveller's Companion* (Bath: 1753); Philip Thicknesse, *The New Prose Bath Guide, for the year 1778*; George Ellis, *Bath, Its Beauties and Amusements* (1776).

p. 80, *when proper walks... with one another*: John Wood, *A Description of Bath* (1742–43; 2nd edn. 1749; repr. 1765; Bath, Kingsmead Reprints: 1969), p. 411.

p. 81, *Knowing no other... nobles of the land*: Tobias Smollett, *Humphry Clinker* (1771; Harmondsworth: Penguin, 1983), p. 66 [*Humphrey Clinker*].

p. 81, *...extremely diverted... excite my laughter*: Humphrey Clinker, pp. 78–79.

pp. 81–82, *The morning after... minds engagements*: Elizabeth Montagu to the Duchess of Portland, Bath, 27th Dec. 1740, *The Letters of Mrs Elizabeth Montagu*, ed. M. Montagu, 3rd edn., 4 vols., vol. 1, pp. 72–73 [*Letters of Elizabeth Montagu*].

p. 82, *that giddy vortex*: The General State (1778), p. 14.

p. 82, *putrid gums... sal volatile*: Humphrey Clinker, pp. 75, 96.

p. 82, *It is a melancholy assertion... women of fashion*: The General State (1778), p. 14.

p. 82, *temple of sociability*: Peter Borsay, *The Image of Georgian Bath, 1700–2000* (Oxford: Oxford University Press, 2000), p. 27.

p. 83, *...heroes of eighteenth-century republicanism*: He symbolized for republicans the popular liberties lost when Anglo-Saxon England was crushed by the "Norman Yoke". See Hill, *Republican Virago*, p. 32.

p. 83, *...library and his wealth*: That they felt able to do so with any propriety is perhaps surprising. Macaulay's scholarly rival, David Hume, laid a false trail for subsequent historians with a grammatically ambiguous piece of gossip in a letter to a fellow academic. He described Macaulay as "if not a more illustrious, yet a more fortunate Historian, than either of us. There is one Dr. Wilson, a man zealous for Liberty, who has made her a free and full Present of a house of £2,000 Value, has adopted her Daughter by all the Rites of Roman Jurisprudence, and intends to leave her all his Fortune, which is considerable". *The Letters of Hume*, ed. J.Y.T. Greig, 2 vols. (Oxford: Clarendon Press, 1932), vol. 2, p. 321. It was actually Mrs rather than Miss Macaulay whom Wilson had actually adopted, putting his money where his mouth was, as he explained in an effusive letter to their mutual friends, the Northcotes: "...from a high esteem and regard I have for that dear and amiable lady, I have made her perfectly easy, not only while I live, but after my death, by adopting her as *my daughter...* she will have such a share of my fortune, as, with her own, will set her above the world; and I can assure you that no words can express the joy I feel in having it in my power to remove all anxieties from a breast which ought never to have been ruffled. This ought to have been done long ago by persons of opulent fortune, who in words expressed their high veneration for her exalted character as an historian; but Providence reserved that honour for me." John Feltham, *A Tour Through the Island of Man*, 1798, quoting letter from Dr Wilson to Mr Northcote of Honiton, Devonshire, written from Clifton, 16th July 1777.

p. 83, *made herself the centre... constitutional history*: Revd Joseph Hunter, *The Connection of Bath with the Literature and Science of England* (1853), pp. 56–57.

p. 83, *Alas!... tenth Muse*: *Walpole's Correspondence*, Letter to Lady Aylesbury, 1775 (vol. 5, p. 189n.; vol. 10, p. 233; vol. 24, p. 197; vol. 32, p. 196; or vol. 39, pp. 240–41).

p. 83, *...during their grand tour*: The urn itself had been elevated into "Tully's vase". This was on the whim that it might once have belonged to Marcus Tullius ("Tully") Cicero, the Roman statesman who had kept a country seat in Tusculum (by then Frascati) where it had been found.

p. 84, *Lady Miller is a round... very inelegant*: Quoted in Ruth Avaline Hesselgrave, *Mrs Miller and the Batheaston Literary Circle* (New Haven, CT, and London: Yale University Press, 1927), p. 10 [Hesselgrave, *Mrs Miller*].

p. 84, *above fifty carriages... four duchesses*: This is from an account by the Revd Richard Graves of Claverton, who was also a regular visitor to Alfred House. Hesselgrave, *Mrs Miller*, p. 7.

p. 85, *...supposed to have been written*: *Bath Chronicle*, 20th Feb. 1777, advertises the publication of *A Short Inquiry... to which is added, a Letter from the celebrated Historian Mrs. Catharine Macaulay*. The letter itself is dated 15th Mar. 1777.

p. 85, *In January... skill and success*: Letters of Jan. 1778 and Apr. 1777, printed, among other places, in *Travels and Voyages*, pp. 75–76.

p. 85, *...popular Spring Gardens*: *Bath Chronicle*, 3rd Oct. 1776 and 24th Oct. 1776.

p. 85, *a much greater... peculiar art*: *Bath Chronicle*, 6th Mar. 1777.

p. 86, *for throwing... their action upon*: *A Sketch*, p. 11.

p. 86, ...*through the entire body*: Edward Nairne, *The Description and Use of Nairne's Patent Electrical Machine*, 8th edn. (London: 1796).

pp. 86–87, *The prime conductor... or diseased parts*: A *Sketch*, pp. 10–11.

p. 87, *It is well known... bristle of a boar*: A *Lecture*, p. 22.

pp. 87–88, *What may not... perform*: *The General State*, p. 10.

p. 88, ...*composition of air*: He may also have been familiar with the work of Daniel Rutherford, John Rutherford's son, who worked with Joseph Black in Edinburgh on carbon dioxide and in 1772 isolated nitrogen, which he called noxious air or phlogisticated air.

p. 88, *Who can tell... privilege of breathing it*: Joseph Priestley, *Experiments and observations of different kinds of air*, 2nd edn. (1776), p. 45.

p. 88, *the air which... as we deserve*: Joseph Priestley, *The Discovery of Oxygen* (1775; Edinburgh: E&S Livingstone, 1961), pp. 51–54, quoted in Joe Jackson, *A World on Fire* (New York: Viking, 2005), pp. 172–73.

p. 89, ...*the Egyptian haschish*: Henry Bigelow, *Insensibility during surgical operations produced by inhalation* (1846).

p. 89, *immediate relief... memorable*: According to Edmund Rack.

p. 89, ...*particles of air*: W.D. Hackmann, 'The Researches of Dr Martinus Van Marum (1750–1837) on the influence of electricity on animals and plants', *Medical History* (Jan. 1972), vol. 16, p. 12 [Hackmann, 'Researches'].

p. 89, *My neck is now broiling... and brimstones*: Letter from Mary Way to Eliza Way Champlain, 6th Dec. 1818, *Way-Champlain correspondence*, American Antiquarian Society. Mary Way was a painter of miniature portraits who was being treated for advancing blindness with "the usual routine of bleeding, blistering, &c.".

p. 90, ...*the absent rector*: *Gentleman's Magazine*, 47 (1777), p. 458.

p. 90, ...*from death's jaws*: This marble "testimony of the high Esteem" which Wilson claimed to bear "to the distinguished Merit of his Friend" was later reported to have scandalized the devout, astonished the learned and disgusted the Royalists in his congregation. The outrage it caused when erected in September 1777 is well documented, and it did not remain at St Stephen's long. The statue is now in the entrance hall of Warrington Museum and Library. See Hill, *The Republican Virago*, pp. 99–102.

p. 90, *our little Tusculum... frequent this place*: C.L.S. Linnell, ed., *The Diaries of Thomas Wilson* (London: Society for Promoting Christian Knowledge, 1964), p. 6 [*Diaries of Thomas Wilson*].

p. 90, *Wilson's reputation... hunter of a mitre*: *Town and Country Magazine*, 3 (1771), p. 681; *Diaries of Thomas Wilson*, p. 10; *Letters of Elizabeth Montagu*, vol. 4, p. 356, in a letter to Elizabeth Carter; *Walpole's Correspondence*, vol. 28, p. 372. See Hill, *Republican Virago*, pp. 81–82.

p. 91, *numerous and brilliant company*: *Six Odes* (Bath: Cruttwell, 1777), pp. vi-vii.

p. 91, *The morning was ushered in... present times*: *Bath Chronicle*, 3rd Apr. 1777.

p. 91, *contemptible vanity*: *The Works of Augustus Toplady*, p. 877.

p. 91, *Surely nothing ever equalled... firebrand of party*: Revd Montagu Pennington, ed., *Letters from Mrs Elizabeth Carter to Mrs. Montagu*, 3 vols. (London: F.C. and J. Rivington, 1817), vol. 3, p. 98. It is not clear whether by then Richard Samuel had completed his painting of *The Nine Living Muses of Great Britain*, in which Carter and Montagu appeared in neo-classical robes alongside their fellow bluestocking Macaulay. The painting, now in the National Portrait Gallery, was exhibited at the Royal Academy in 1779, but its circulation in print form was advertised in November 1777. See Elizabeth Eger, 'Representing culture: "The Nine Living Muses"' in E. Eger, C. Grant, C. O'Gallchoir and P. Warburton, eds. *Women, Writing and the Public Sphere, 1700–1830* (Cambridge: Cambridge University Press, 2001), pp. 104–132.

p.   91, ...*to affect the former*: The controversialist Philip Thicknesse, an infamously quarrelsome man known by his many enemies as Dr Viper, lifted wholesale a vicious account of the toadying odes from the *Monthly Review* for use in his own book, *The New Prose Bath Guide, for the year 1778*, pp. 68–69.

p.   92, *the pious, learned... Cure of Diseases: Six Odes*, pp. 36–37.

p.   92, *They then dispersed... pine-apples: Six Odes*, p. viii.

p.   92, *The pleasures of Bath... without reason*: Richard Graves, *The Spiritual Quixote* (1773). Graves was the man who had counted Mrs Miller's duchesses, and was described by Edmund Rack as possessing "much *wit* and *humour*, and a great knowledge of mankind; but *wit* and *humour* have seldom resided in a form more unfavourable in its appearance." (Edmund Rack, *A Disultory Journal of Events &c at Bath*, unpublished typescript in Bath Central Library, R691/12675, pp. 42–43 [Rack, *A Disultory Journal*]).

p.   93, *It is the most light... same Effect*: Matthew Turner, *An Account of the Extraordinary Medicinal Fluid, called Aether* (Liverpool, 1761), p. 4 [Turner, *An Account*]. The language employed by Graham also suggests a familiarity with a less successful work on medicinal ether by Richard Lovett, *The subtil medium prov'd, or, That... power... call'd sometimes aether, but oftener elementary fire, verify'd* (1756).

p.   93, *chemical essences... Applications*: Advertisement in *Bath Chronicle*, 26th Dec. 1777.

p.   93, *To apply it Externally... of his Hand*: Turner, *An Account*, pp. 12–13.

p.   94, *Josiah Wedgewood... showroom there: Bath Chronicle*, 1st May 1777.

p.   94, ...*portraitist in the city*: In fact, Dr Wilson had commissioned a painting of himself with his newly adopted granddaughter Catharine Sophia Macaulay from Wright the previous year. (William Bemrose, *Life and Works of Joseph Wright* (1885), p. 45.)

p.   94, ...*of the medical profession: Bath Chronicle*, 24th Apr. 1777.

p.   94, ...*in spring 1779: Travels and Voyages*, pp. 134–35, reprinting a letter in the *Newcastle Journal* of 19th Mar. 1779.

p.   94, *The ingenious... invaluable treasure: Bath Chronicle*, 24th Apr. 1777.

p.   95, *It is not only... topic of conversation*: Letter of 12th Jan. 1778 in *Letters, from the year 1774 to the Year 1796, of John Wilkes, Esq. Addressed to his daughter, the late Miss Wilkes*, 4 vols. (London: 1804), vol. 1, p. 76 [Wilkes, *Letters*].

p.   95, ...*recycling habit*: In the course of just a few years an almost identical poem appeared in newspapers in Bristol, Bath, Newcastle and London, all regretting the Doctor's imminent departure from the relevant city, all supposedly by different patients: "Will GRAHAM go? – who, born to bless mankind, / Gives health of body, firmness to the mind..."*Bath Chronicle*, 8th May 1777.

p. 95, *On his fair front... trembling sounds*: Bath Chronicle, 15th May 1777.

pp. 95–96, *to the south of France... her health*: Mary Hays, *Female Biography, or Memoirs of Illustrious and Celebrated Women...* 6 vols. (London: 1803), vol. 5, p. 294 [Hays, *Female Biography*]. Mary Hays was one of the last of the original bluestockings, and a close friend of Mary Wollstonecraft.

p. 96, *...met her in Paris*: *Walpole's Correspondence*, vol. 7, p. 261 and vol. 6, p. 497. Letter From Madame du Deffand, 5 Dec. 1777.

p. 96, *persons of... eminence*: Hays, *Female Biography*, p. 297.

p. 96, *I saw her yesterday... and ghostly*: Wilkes, *Letters*, 4th Jan. 1778, p. 61.

p. 96, *The rage of politics... worse daily*: Wilkes, *Letters*, 7th Jan. 1778, p. 69.

p. 96, *...hard to determine*: Wilkes, *Letters*, 28th Apr. 1778, p. 93.

p. 96, *...called there by business*: Bath Chronicle, 26th Feb. 1778.

pp. 96–97, *I do assure your Lordship... sink to the grave*: Catharine Macaulay to the Earl of Buchan, Alfred House, Bath, 23rd Feb. 1778, Misc. MSS Macaulay, Catharine, New York Historical Society.

p. 97, *...in his own publications*: See his advertisement, *Edinburgh Advertiser*, 24th July 1777.

p. 97, *own worthy father and mother*: *Travels and Voyages*, pp. 104–7.

p. 97, *...accusations of quackery from Philip Thicknesse*: Thicknesse, *New Prose Bath Guide*, pp. 116–17.

p. 97, *The celebrated Dr Graham... used it with skill*: Walter Scott's marginalia in his copy of Francis Grose's satire, *A guide to health, beauty, riches, and honour* (1785), Abbotsford Library (Faculty of Advocates, Edinburgh).

p. 97, *[T]here was so much suspicion... according to medicine*: H.J.C. Grierson, ed., *The Letters of Sir Walter Scott, 1828–1831* (London: Constable & Co., 1936), vol. 11, pp. 401–2. Letter dated 31st Oct. 1830.

p. 97, *...patron of the architect Robert Adam*: John Fleming, *Robert Adam and His Circle in Edinburgh and Rome* (London: John Murray, 1962).

p. 98, *Sure am I... French fops*: Letters of Sir Walter Scott, p. 402. Walter Scott maintained his interest in Graham throughout his life, and in 1825 bought an extensive collection of his tracts and some manuscripts at a sale in Edinburgh held by bookseller John Stevenson. The volume remains in Scott's Abbotsford Library.

p. 98, *As from previous engagements... younger brother*: Taken from a scurrilous pseudo-biography of Charles James Fox called *The Amours of Carlo Khan* (London: 1789), p. 93.

p. 98, *...opportunities to set up practice*: Alexander Lesassier, a near contemporary at Edinburgh of William Graham, considered there was "little profit to be gained" from being a navy surgeon and bemoaned the "poor plight one's character is in when one wishes to settle in the world". Rosner, *Medical Education*, p. 21.

pp. 98–99, *To the great surprise... are the mighty fallen*: Diaries of Thomas Wilson, p. 19.

p. 99, *...praising Arnold's gentle approach*: For example in *Travels and Voyages*, p. 44, and elsewhere.

p. 99, *Mrs Montagu thought… by the senses*: Elizabeth Montagu's letters to Hester Thrale, Manchester University, John Rylands Library, Eng. MSS 551, quoted in Hill, *Republican Virago*, p. 118 and *Walpole's Correspondence*, vol. 33, p. 84–85.

p. 99, *Poor Mrs. Macaulay!… thou are fallen*: Revd R. Polwhele, *Traditions and Recollections*, 2 vols. (1826), vol. 1, pp. 122–23. Polwhele later wrote a poem called 'The Unsex'd Females' (1798) attacking Wollstonecraft and other eighteenth-century proto-feminists. It delighted reactionary reviewers.

p. 99, *…attached to a corpse*: "Il semblait voir un enfant attaché à un cadavre." J.-P. Brissot, *Mémoires* (1754–1793), ed. C. Perroud (Paris: Librairie Alphonse Picard & Fils, 1912), vol. 1, pp. 347, 350 [Brissot, *Mémoires*].

p. 99, *tumbled from a greater height*: *Walpole's Correspondence*, vol. 33, pp. 84–85.

p. 100, *By a sweet… lovely sixteen*: Bath Chronicle, 7th Jan. 1779.

p. 100, *she could not resist… Dr. Graham's brother*: St James's Chronicle, 1st Dec. 1778 (written from Bath, 28th Nov.).

p. 100, *…a Haymarket farce*: The Female Patriot (1779), probably by R.P. Jodrell; A Remarkable Moving Letter (1779); A Bridal Ode on the Marriage of Catherine and Petruchio (1779); Richard Paul Jodrell, A Widow – No Widow (1780), staged at the Haymarket in July 1779.

p. 100, *carrying an electrical conducting tube*: 'The auspicious marriage', Town and Country Magazine, 10 (Dec. 1778), p. 623.

p. 101, *I was [at Alfred House]… declared favourite*: Wilkes, Letters, p. 130.

p. 101, *to write… Friends were alarmed*: Rack, A Disultory Journal, 12th Jan. 1780, p. 21.

p. 102, *…by "a maid, Betty"*: Wilkes, Letters, p. 165.

p. 102, *an Arbitrator… expect anything*: Rack, A Disultory Journal, pp. 21–22.

p. 102, *frequent and powerful… entrails*: Wilkes, Letters, pp. 224–25.

p. 102, *…put into Chancery*: Diaries of Thomas Wilson, p. 24.

p. 102, *…with the Russian empress*: Dedications to The General State.

p. 103, *To be Sold… fair Valuation*: St James's Chronicle, 26th Nov. 1778.

Chapter Four

All Graham quotations describing the house in this chapter are from
A Sketch, unless otherwise indicated.

p. 105, *Deign… in thine*: An ACROSTIC, supposedly "By a Gentleman restored to perfect health, from the last stage of a Consumption, after having been given over by the principal Physicians in Scotland, and in the North of England", first printed in *Dr Graham is now preparing the largest and most elegant medico-electrical-aerial and magnetic apparatus…* (1779) [*Dr Graham is now preparing…*].

p. 105, *…London's river frontage*: Old and New London, vol. 3 (1878), pp. 100–10.

p. 106, *…Both barely survived*: Only the foundations and embankments had been finished when the Scottish workmen, realizing that they were being underpaid and overworked compared with London bricklayers, revolted en masse. They indignantly cast off what they termed "the curse of Adam" to seek more remunerative if less melodious work elsewhere in the capital. The problem was solved by shipping in a new workforce of Irish labourers, whose low pay and lack of accompaniment inevitably led to grim jokes about the replacement of the bagpipe with "the fiddle". At the point at which shovels had begun to sound in 1768, the Adams had also been rashly casual about securing written agreements with the owners of their building site. This was an eighteenth-century equivalent of failing to apply for planning permission on a very grand scale. Only after work had begun did they manage to sign a lease with the freeholder of the land, the financially beset Duke of St Albans, a year before he was imprisoned for debt in Brussels. In 1771, the brothers belatedly applied for authority to reclaim the land from the river, only to meet with furious indignation from the City. Occupying the tidal banks, foul as they were, was seen as a cavalier appropriation of common land. The Corporation of London lawyer sneered "that Messrs. Adams were very able and experienced architects; but although he admired the elegance of their buildings, he never could allow from thence alone arose a right of building on that land". (*Survey of London*, vol. 18, p. 100.)

p. 106, *Paperwealth*: *London Magazine*, 1777, p. 469, quoted by Paul Langford, *A Polite and Commercial People: England 1727–1783* (Oxford: Clarendon Press, 1989), p. 568 [Langford, *A Polite and Commercial People*].

p. 106, *...Mess. Richardson and Goodluck*: See for example *The Public Advertiser*, 12th Nov. 1779.

pp. 106–107, *Whate'er the wretched... Speculation*: Christopher Anstey, *Speculation, or a Defence of Mankind*, 1780 [Anstey, *Speculation*].

p. 107, *...of visiting tourists*: *Sophie in London 1786, Being the Diary of Sophie v. la Roche* (London: Jonathan Cape, 1933), p. 161 [*Sophie in London*].

p. 107, *The extreme depth... of the skilful*: Thomas Malton, *Picturesque Tour through London and Westminster, 1792*, p. 43 [Malton, *Picturesque Tour*].

p. 107, *[E]very spectator... deserves the preference*: Malton, *Picturesque Tour*, p. 42.

p. 108, *...fit to Entertain princes*: Anonymous diary of an Irish clergyman, 26th Aug. 1772, BL Add. MSS. 27951, quoted in David G.C. Allan, *The Adelphi Past and Present: A History and a Guide* (London: Calder Walker, Assoc., 2001), p. 41 [Allan, *Adelphi Past and Present*]; *A Sketch*, p. 3.

p. 108, *...row of houses*: Simon Bradley and Nikolaus Pevsner, *The Buildings of England: London 6: Westminster* (New Haven, CT, and London: Yale University Press, 2003), p. 326.

p. 109, *...national calamity*: 'The British Theatre', *London Magazine* (1776), pp. 230–31, quoted in Langford, *A Polite and Commercial People*, p. 309.

p. 109, *as a prince... actor*: According to V&A exhibit label.

p. 109, *seldom heard... decorum*: R. Brimley Johnson, *The Letters of Hannah More* (London: John Lane, 1925), p. 30.

p. 109, *My dear Adelphi... people in England*: Allan, *Adelphi Past and Present*, p. 38.

p. 110, *...water closets galore*: Robert Adam collection at Sir John Soane's Museum Archive, No. 42/60–67.

p. 110, *to which the subterranean... sublimity*: Malton, *Picturesque Tour*, p. 42.

p. 111, *...new ceilings*: Soane Archive, *Ceilings* III, vol. 13/21–40. See *Survey of London*, vol. 18: plate 78 has photograph of ceiling, and plate 79 shows the mantelpieces of the first floor front (sphinxes) and back rooms.

p. 111, *he has made me... glimpse of them*: Quoted in Christopher Simon Sykes, *Private Palaces* (London: Chatto & Windus, 1985), p. 199.

p. 112, *...to other treatments*: *Dr Graham is now preparing...*, p. 12.

pp. 112–13, *...cross-breeds of all kinds*: For example, Christian Clauss's Guitar Forte Piano, advertised in the *Morning Herald*, 5th July 1783.

p. 113, *as if all the instruments... listen to it daily*: *Sophie in London* (1786), pp. 139–40.

p. 113, *...inexplicably moving*: *Music for the Glass Harmonica*, Bloch et al, (Naxos).

p. 113, *incomparably sweet... of any other*: Benjamin Franklin, *Experiments and Observations on Electricity* (1769), pp. 427–33.

p. 113, *...disappointed in love*: 'The Glassharmonica' by Thomas Bloch, translated by Michelle Vadon, www.finkenbeiner.com/gh.html.

p. 114, *Can there be... acute complaints*: *The General State*, p. 58.

p. 114, *THE SALUTARY POWER... nervous system*: *The General State*, p. 59.

p. 114, *...in Edinburgh in his youth*: Christopher Lawrence, 'The Nervous System and Society in the Scottish Enlightenment', *Natural Order: Historical Studies of Scottish Culture*, eds. Barry Barnes and Steven Shapin (Beverly Hills, CA, and London: Sage Publications, 1779), pp. 19–40, p. 33.

p. 114, *just a smith's... intense fervour*: *The General State*, p. 66.

pp. 114–15, *the universal living fire... his other works*: Graham, *The guardian goddess of health: or, the whole art of preventing and curing diseases; and of enjoying peace and happiness of body and of mind to...* (1780), pp. 19–20. In a footnote, Graham categorically refuses to argue about whether or not the soul is immaterial, since it is not a point "essential to happiness".

p. 116, *always disposed... guarantee of success*: Benjamin Wilson, 'New experiments and observations on the nature and use of conductors', *Philosophical Transactions of the Royal Society*, 68, pp. 245–313, p. 247.

p. 116, *have a scene... Purfleet by nature*: Benjamin Wilson, *An Account of Experiments Made at the Pantheon, on the Nature and Use of Conductors* (1778), p. 3.

p. 116, *...while I can literally... NEVER GOETH OUT*: *A Sketch*, p. 29.

p. 117, *...extravagant experiment*: Illustration and description in Benjamin Wilson, *An Account of Experiments* (1778).

p. 117, *that it brought to his mind... on fairy ground*: *Gazetteer and New Daily Advertiser*, 29th Jan. 1772. From: 'The Pantheon', *Survey of London*, vols. 31 and 32: 'St James Westminster', Part 2 (1963), pp. 268–83.

p. 117, *in prosecuting discoveries... apparatus, &c.*: *The General State* (1778), p. 35.

p. 118, *producing either positive... at one time*: *A Sketch*, p. 18.

p. 118, *As to poor Mrs Garrick... any body in*: Quoted by Austin Brereton, *The Literary History of the Adelphi and Its Neighbourhood* (London: T. Fisher Unwin, 1908), p. 159.

p. 118, *...plainest green bottles*: *The Picture of Newcastle upon Tyne* (Newcastle: 1807).

p. 118, *...and other luxuries*: Catherine Ross, 'The Flint Glass Houses on the Rivers Tyne and Wear during the Eighteenth Century', *The Glass Circle*, no. 5 (1986), pp. 75–85.

p. 119, *the largest... Apparatus in the world*: *Dr Graham is now preparing...*

p. 119, *...and candelabra*: See Geoffrey Beard, *Craftsmen and Interior Decoration in England, 1660–1820* (Edinburgh: John Bartholomew and Son, 1981), pp. 32–33 [Beard, *Craftsmen*].

p. 119, *...was known in France*: Hackmann, *Electricity from Glass*, p. 114.

p. 120, *...could command £2,000*: Heilbron, *Electricity in the 17th and 18th Centuries*, p. 152.

p. 120, *it breathes health... principle of all things*: *A Sketch*, pp. 17–18.

p. 120, *...transparent or coloured*: See C.R.S. Sheppard & J.P. Smith, *Glass from the Restoration to the Regency* (London: Mallett and Sheppard and Cooper, 1990).

p. 121, *most elegant and SUPERB... exquisite workmanship*: *A Sketch*, pp. 6–7.

p. 121, *a massy pillar... of the rainbow*: *A Sketch*, p. 19.

pp. 121–22, *no less than twelve... richest harmony*: *A Sketch*, pp. 19–20.

p. 122, *superb brilliant... highest polish*: *A Sketch*, p. 24. Graham did not neglect to plug their manufacturer: "These, and some of the most curious and beautiful pieces of my cut glass work, were executed by Messrs. Polhill and Blades, the celebrated Glass Manufacturers, No. 5, Ludgate Hill." Newcastle glassworks often sent their most elaborate pieces to be finished off by experts in London.

p. 122, *[N]o man could be... liberty*: W. Hone, 'Biographical sketch', in J. Murray, *Sermons to Asses* (1819), p. iv.

p. 123, *the lucrative emoluments... opinion of the public*: *Travels and Voyages*, p. 127.

p. 123, *earnest request*: *Dr. Graham is now preparing...*, pp. 2–3; *Travels and Voyages*, p. 128.

p. 123, *On hearing that Dr. GRAHAM... 8th of April*: *Travels and Voyages*, pp. 137–38.

p. 125, *to low methods... little sphere*: Letter to the printer of the *Newcastle Journal*, 9th Mar. 1779, *Travels and Voyages*, p. 134.

p. 125, *...very early in life... drove me mad*: *A Sketch*, p. 30.

p. 125, *the boasted advances... application of it*: *The General State*, pp. 13–14.

p. 126, *friendly powerfulness*: *Dr Graham is now preparing...*, p. 10.

p. 126, *the electric fluid... vital principles*: *Travels and Voyages*, pp. 52–53.

pp. 126–27, *arguments... please her imagination*: William Smellie, *A Treatise on the Theory and Practice of Midwifery*, 3 vols. (1752–64), vol. 1, p. 137.

p. 127, *perfectly convinced... hears them or not*: *A Sketch*, p. 50.

p. 127, *the various faculties... comprehension we stop*: *A Sketch*, p. 12

Chapter Five
Quotations from Graham's works in this chapter are taken from *Travel and Voyages* or *The General State*, unless otherwise specified.

p. 129, *Goodness... & death*: Letter from James Graham to Lady Spencer, Spa, 13th Aug. 1779, BL Add. MSS. 75708.

p. 129, *...and Foote would suggest*: Anne F. Woodhouse, 'Eighteenth-Century English Visitors to France in Fiction and Fact', *Modern Language Studies*, vol. 6, no. 1 (Spring 1976), pp. 37–41.

p. 129, *...cause of neoclassicism*: Beard, *Craftsmen*, p. xxiii.

p. 130, *...do the same trick*: Hackmann, *Catalogue*, p. 150.

p. 130, *...batter[ies] of philosophical cannon... loud and tremendous*: *A Sketch*, p. 25.

p. 130, *...caricature of the Doctor*: *The Quacks* (British Museum no. 6325, Wellcome Library, no. 20790i).

p. 131, *...two feet long*: Equivalent to about 300,000 volts.

p. 132, *...four copyists simultaneously*: Heilbron, *Electricity in the 17th and 18th Centuries*, p. 313.

p. 132, *...some sort of crocodile*: Petrus Camper, 'Conjectures Relative to the Petrifactions Sound in St. Peter's Mountain, Near Maestricht', *Philosophical Transactions of the Royal Society of London*, vol. 76 (1786), pp. 443–56.

p. 132, *..."crime" of the act*: Samuel Tissot, *Onanism: or, a treatise upon the disorders produced by masturbation: or, the dangerous effects of secret and excessive venery*, 3rd edn. (London: 1767), p. vii [Tissot, *Onanism*].

p. 132, *Hoffman has seen... blows of a cudgel*: Tissot, *Onanism*, p. 9.

p. 133, *...in that direction himself*: Roy Porter, '"I think ye both quacks": The Controversy between Dr Theodor Myersbach and Dr John Coakley Lettsom', in William F. Bynum and Roy Porter, eds., *Medical Fringe and Medical Orthodoxy, 1759–1850* (London: Croom Helm, 1987).

p. 133, *I am a long way... seems to work best*: Mauduyt, *Extraits des journaux tenus pour quatre-vingt-deux malades qui on été électrilisés...* (Paris: 1779), p. 38 [Mauduyt, *Extraits*]. His name is also written Maduit, Mauduyt or Mauduit. Graham probably read his 'Sur le traitement électrique, administré à quatre-vingt-deux malades', *Histoire et Mémoires de la Société Royale de Médecine*, 1777–1778, II, pp. 199–432 and 'Sur les effets généraux, la nature et l'usage de fluide électrique, considéré comme médicament', ibid., pp. 432–55.

p. 134, *...out of women's clothes*: These measures would minimize the dangers of losing the electrical field through accidentally earthing the patient, or concentrating the charge so much that sparks might be created.

p. 134, *is to get patients... are afraid*: Mauduyt, *Extraits*, p. 39.

p. 134, *...confused results*: Hackmann, 'Researches', p. 19.

p. 134, *a sensation... spider's web*: Mauduyt, *Mémoire sur les différentes manières d'administrer l'électricité...* (Paris, 1784), p. 6 [Mauduyt, *Mémoire*].

p. 134, *...size of her head*: Mauduyt, *Mémoire*, p. 152, fig. 16.

p. 135, *...presumed dead from drowning*: James Delbourgo, 'Electrical Humanitarianism in North America: Dr T. Gale's *Electricity, or Ethereal*

Fire, considered (1802) in Historical Context', *Electric Bodies: Episodes in the History of Medical Electricity*, eds. Paula Bertucci and Giuliano Pancaldi, *Bologna Studies in History of Science*, 9 (2001), pp. 117–156; pp. 140–141 [Delbourgo, 'Electrical Humanitarianism'].

p. 135, ...*targets of its practitioners*: Criticizing the hostility of so many conventional medics in his radical lay textbook *Primitive Physick, or an Easy and Natural Method of Curing Most Diseases* (1747), John Wesley, the founder of English Methodism, came up with another explanation for this attitude toward electrical therapy. It was probably as well founded as it was cynical: "They must not disoblige their good friends, the apothecaries. Neither can it consist with their own interest to make (although not every man) so many men their own physicians." Quoted in Delbourgo, 'Electrical Humanitarianism', p. 143.

p. 135, *when he would point... to the ground*: Mesmer, *Schreiben über die Magnetkur* (1776), Appendix, p. 36, quoted in Adam Crabtree, *From Mesmer to Freud: Magnetic Sleep and the Roots of Psychological Healing* (New Haven, CT, and London: Yale University Press, 1993), p. 8.

p. 136, ...*or somnambulism*: See Patricia Fara, *Sympathetic Attractions: Magnetic Practices, Beliefs and Symbolism in Eighteenth-Century England* (Princeton, NJ: Princeton University Press, 1996), p. 196 [Fara, *Sympathetic Attractions*].

p. 136, ...*blindness and deafness*: *Mesmer's tub; or a faithful representation of the operations of animal magnetism*, Henri Thiriat (Wellcome Library no. 11826i).

pp. 136–37, *My initial urge... lost patience with them*: *The Memoirs of Elisabeth Vigée-le Brun*, translated from the French by Sian Evans (London: Camden Press, 1989), p. 338.

p. 137, ...*denouncing the practice*: Mesmer, *Mémoire sur la découverte du magnétisme animal* (1779).

p. 138, ...*in the Hanoverian British world*: Peter Clark, *British Clubs and Societies 1580–1800: The Origins of an Associational World* (Oxford: Clarendon Press, 2000), p. 325.

p. 138, ...*far from a secret society*: Harry Carr, ed., *The Early Masonic Catechisms* (London: Quatuor Coronati Lodge, 1975).

p. 138, ...*too sparse to be certain*: *Premier Grand Lodge Membership Register, 1768–1813*, CD ROM, p. 59; Revd Arnold Whitaker, *No. 4: An Introduction to the History of the Royal Somerset House and Inverness Lodge* (London: Bernard Quartich, 1928). Schuchard states in *Why Mrs Blake Cried* that Graham was a member of the Ancient Lodge, no. 38.

p. 139, ...*putative family arms*: *A Sketch*, p. 42.

p. 140, ...*called "Le Musée de Paris"*: Nicholas Hans, 'UNESCO of the Eighteenth Century. La Loge des Neuf Sœurs and Its Venerable Master, Benjamin Franklin', *Proceedings of the American Philosophical Society*, vol. 97, no. 5 (30th Oct. 1953), pp. 513–524.

p. 140, *No-one was more fashionable... famous man*: *The Memoirs of Elisabeth Vigée-Lebrun*, p. 319.

p. 140, *I was walking... fixed on him*: Brissot, *Mémoires*, p. 350.

p. 140, ...*vegetarians were known at the time*: The same Pythagoras familiar to every child for his right-angled triangle theorem founded a community of mystical mathematicians in the 6th century BC in Croton, Calabria, Italy. Pythagoras's adherents refused to eat animals on the basis that they had a right to live in common with mankind.

p. 140, *...of the "cap of liberty"*: Pigott was probably the "gentleman in Geneva" so convinced by Graham's dietary theories that he helped save his mentor from poverty with an annuity of £50 a year in "his latter years." Kay, *A Series of Original Portraits*, p. 35.

pp. 140–41, *Graham was poor... divert attention*: Brissot, *Mémoires*, p. 351.

p. 141, *[W]hile I from... firmest resolutions*: BL Add. MSS 75911, Althorp papers, vol. 611 (1769–82), 10th Nov. 1782.

p. 141, *If no objects... fly away*: BL Add. MSS 75911, Althorp papers, vol. 611, (1769–82), 21st Aug. 1781.

p. 141, *the mere association... ensure success*: Amanda Foreman, 'Cavendish, Georgiana, duchess of Devonshire (1757–1806)', *Oxford Dictionary of National Biography* (Oxford University Press, Sept. 2004).

p. 142, *as I never hear... or an arm*: Lady Clermont to Lady Spencer, Dublin, 12th Aug. 1780, British Library, Althorp papers.

p. 142, *It is curious to see... through the grass*: Devonshire MSS, Chatsworth, 5th Duke's Group, *Journals of Georgiana, Countess Spencer*, 2014.10–102, 30th June 1779.

p. 142, *in so putrid a state... on his crutches*: BL Add. MSS 75708 1/1, reprinted with some variations in *The General State*, 1779.

p. 143, *thirty sovereigns... resident physicians*: Edwin Lee, *The Principal Baths of Rhenish Prussia* (London: 1870), p. 81.

p. 143, *the custom at Spa... change every dance*: Elizabeth and Florence Amson, eds., *Mary Hamilton, at Court and at Home from Letters and Diaries, 1756–1816* (London: John Murray, 1925), pp. 43, 47.

pp. 143–44, *horrid news... highest Pitch*: Devonshire MSS, 26th June 1779.

p. 144, *Method... hobby-horse*: The Earl of Bessborough, ed., *Lady Bessborough and Her Family Circle* (London: John Murray, 1940), p. 2.

p. 144, *...of which Graham never approved*: *Walpole's Correspondence*, vol. 9, p. 27, Letter to Montagu, Thurs 5th June 1746; Karl H. Wegert, review of *The Hessian Mercenary State: Ideas, Institutions, and Reform under Frederick II, 1760–1785*, by Charles W. Ingrao, in *The Journal of Modern History*, 1989, pp. 384–85. "And great the folly and expence is / Of hiring aid from foreign princes": Anstey, *Speculation*.

p. 144, *I am making my debut... to that end*: Quoted in Robert Darnton, 'How Historians play God', *Chromohs*, 11 (2006), www.cromohs.unifi.it/11_2006/darnton_historians.html.

p. 145, *I have enquir'd... write next*: BL Add. MSS 75694, Letters from Rachel Lloyd to Lady Spencer (1773–1784), Spa, 28th June 1781.

p. 145, *...and other grandees*: Marie François Henri de Franquetot (1737–1821), the Duke de Coigny, held the highest military position in France, and was another intimate of Queen Marie-Antoinette.

p. 146, *Her ladyship will find... Dowager Angel*: BL Add. MSS 75708, vol. 408, Gore-Gwy, Petitions for Charity, 2/8, 25th July 1779.

p. 146, *seen, and certified... humanity of Doctor Graham*: "*vu, certifié, par nous, comme très véritable, & s'etant passé sous nos yeux, dans un intervalle très court, qui fait honneur aux connoissances, au zele, & à l'humanité du Docteur Graham."*

p. 146, *that, he will earnestly... better man*: BL Add. MSS 75708, vol. 408, Gore-Gwy, Petitions for Charity, 6/8, 21st Aug. 1779.

p. 146, *...at the card table*: On 11th May 1780, Rachel Lloyd wrote to Lady Spencer to say she had won sixty-nine guineas at whist, macao and quinze.

pp. 146–47, *I left England... as my Lord Spencer's*: BL Add. MSS 75708, vol. 408, Gore-Gwy, Petitions for Charity, 5/8, Letter from Dr Graham to Lady Spencer, Spa, 13th Aug., 1779.

p. 147, *...in impressive shoals*: A Sketch, p. 15.

p. 148, *...down to the last detail*: BL Add. MSS 300–4, f. 76, Miles to Wilson, 29th Nov. 1750.

p. 148, *a manifest... electricity*: Priestley, *History and Present State of Electricity* (1767), p. 147.

p. 148, *balsam of Peru*: The highly aromatic Myroxylon Pereiræ, not to be confused with Peruvian Bark, or cinchona.

p. 148, *...[I]f thro'... meridian sun*: A Sketch, pp. 80–81.

p. 148, *...effects of inhaling them*: Graham's prose is so dense and allusive, his approach to sex so startling, that until now the doctor's references to this other branch of natural philosophy have been ignored by modern readers.

p. 149, *...breakthroughs in the field*: Priestley's study of airs, 'Observations on different kinds of air', published in the *Philosophical Transactions of the Royal Society* for 1772, was hugely significant. It announced the isolation and identification of nitric oxide and anhydrous hydrochloride acid gases, and introduced eudiometry and photosynthesis. Its descriptions of simple apparatuses and manipulative techniques enabled others to take his work further. The paper won the Royal Society's Copley Medal in 1773.

p. 149, *the great... Dr. PRIESTLEY*: Travels and Voyages, p. 38.

p. 149, *What is the simple... road to conquest*: Gazetteer and New Daily Advertiser, 15th Aug. 1780.

p. 150, *...and burning glasses*: "Upon the table, round the cistern, are placed all sorts of vessels and tubes for producing, combining, containing and conveying to any part of the body, internally or externally, fixable, nitrous, inflammable, phlogisticated, dephlogisticated, phosphoreal, aetherial, and vivifying air; eudiometers for ascertaining (by means of nitrous criterion air) the qualities and degrees of goodness of atmospheric and other air; and lastly, curious vessels out of which my patients inhale various effluvia, or drink medicines impregnated with the electrical fluid, &c. &c." A Sketch, p. 8.

p. 150, *various kinds... culinary fire*: A Sketch, p. 6.

p. 150, *...bigger than the standard*: John Nooth's apparatus, invented in 1774, made it possible to produce "spa water" at home, and it enjoyed brisk sales. Three glass vessels were attached with airtight joints. Carbon dioxide generated in the lowest vessel passed through a valve into water contained in the middle vessel. The top vessel would become filled with any water displaced upwards by the gas. When ether was first used as a general anaesthetic during surgery, it was administered by an adapted form of

Nooth's apparatus. See also J. Priestley, *Directions for impregnating water with fixed air; in order to communicate to it the peculiar spirit and virtues of Pyrmont Water, and other mineral waters of a similar nature* (1772).

p. 151, *A thrilling… pleasures and pains*: Humphry Davy, *Researches, Chemical and Philosophical; chiefly concerning Nitrous Oxide, or dephlogisticated nitrous air, and its respiration* (London: 1800), pp. 487, 496, 513, 521, 525, 534 [Davy, *Researches, Chemical and Philosophical*].

p. 151, *vital air*: Thomas Beddoes and James Watt, *Considerations on the Medicinal Use, and on the production of factitious airs* (1795), p. 60 [Beddoes and Watt, *Considerations*].

p. 151, *[W]e must either… extraordinary gas*: Davy, *Researches, Chemical and Philosophical*, p. 513. This James Thomson combined his outstanding skills in industrial chemistry and visual design to become the "Duke of Wellington of calico printing" in the early nineteenth century.

p. 152, *sensations so delightful… convulsed with laughter*: Davy, *Researches, Chemical and Philosophical*, pp. 521, 525, 496, 487, 534; Beddoes and Watt, *Considerations*, p. 60.

p. 152, *an art in infancy*: Davy, *Researches, Chemical and Philosophical*, p. 558.

p. 152, *…as an anaesthetic*: By a Boston dentist, William Thomas Green Morton. See K. Bryn Thomas, *The Development of Anaesthetic Apparatus* (Oxford: Blackwell Scientific Publications, 1975), p. 5.

p. 152, *The poet Robert Southey… composed of this gas*: Davy, *Researches, Chemical and Philosophical*, p. 507.

p. 152, *printed on royal… richly gilt*: *A Sketch*, p. 25.

p. 152, *Mr. Cox's… itself*: *A Sketch*, p. 48.

p. 153, *…always with fresh… scrupulous exactitude*: M. D'Archenholz, *A Picture of England: containing a description of the laws, customs, and manners of England* (Dublin: T. Byrne, 1791), p. 68 [D'Archenholz, *A Picture of England*]. D'Archenholz was formerly a captain in the service of the King of Prussia. The Swan automaton is now in the Bowes museum.

pp. 153–54, *…completed the effect*: *A descriptive catalogue of the several superb and magnificent pieces of mechanism and jewellry, exhibited in Mr. Cox's Museum, at Spring Gardens, Charing-Cross* (London, 1772) [Cox, *Descriptive Catalogue*].

p. 154, *…for 6–7th October 1779*: Roger Smith, 'James Cox (c.1723–1800): A Revised Biography', *Burlington Magazine*, vol. 142, no. 1167 (June 2000), pp. 353–61.

p. 154, *these Royal portraits… on every side*: Cox, *Descriptive Catalogue*.

pp. 154–55, *a beautiful… most excellent effects*: *A Lecture*, p. 16.

p. 155, *…dependable Dr Warren*: Amanda Foreman, *Georgiana, Duchess of Devonshire* (London: HarperCollins, 1999), p. 71 (quoting Chatsworth 252 Ls to GD, Oct. 1779 – rest of letter destroyed) [Foreman, *Georgiana*]. Warren was the most sought-after society doctor in England, and it was reputed he instinctively transferred a guinea piece from one pocket to another whenever he looked at his own tongue in the morning.

p. 155, *…Duke's late mistress*: Foreman, *Georgiana*, p. 72.

p. 155, *…first-floor balconies*: In the 1770s, "the several exhibitions of Jervais's and the Pearsons' stained glass… dramatized the spectacular possibilities of light flowing through a painted, translucent medium". Richard D. Altick, *The Shows of London* (Cambridge, MA: Harvard University Press, 1978), p. 119 [Altick, *Shows of London*]. *The Public Advertiser*, 30th Sept. 1779 At Drury Lane: 'The Wonders of Derbyshire, or, Harlequin in the Peak, All the Scenery, machinery, &c, designed by Mr. De Loutherbourg, and executed under his Direction'.

p. 155–56, TEMPLUM… *restoring health*: A Sketch, p. 4.

p. 156, …*middle of the floor*: "The Alteration shall be made under the inspection of Messrs Adam…" Letter of 23rd Dec. 1779 from James Graham to John Henderson, in the Jean Kislak Collection of Emma Hamilton.

p. 156, *genteel… Adelphi Temple*: Quoted from *Morning Post* by Kelman Dalgety Frost in 'Charlatan or Prophet? The story of Dr James Graham', *The Scots Magazine*, Mar. 1947, p. 476.

p. 157, …*walking on air*: 'Emma Hart' (as she renamed herself when she took up with Charles Greville, Sir William Hamilton's nephew) 'as the goddess of health', National Maritime Museum, PW4385.

p. 158, *After many years… believe his eyes*: J.W. Goethe, *Italian Journey 1786–1788*, translated by W.H. Auden and E. Mayer (London: Collins, 1962), pp. 199–200.

p. 158, …*over and over again*: Before her marriage Emma was George Romney's best-loved muse, and she was also painted by Joshua Reynolds, Friedrich Rehberg, Angelica Kauffman, William Mineard Bennett and Elisabeth Vigée-Lebrun, among others.

p. 158, …*by the reverend canon*: Quoted in a letter from Sir William Hamilton, His Majesty's Minister at the Court of Naples, to Sir Joseph Banks, President of the Royal Society, 30th Dec. 1781, reprinted in Richard Payne Knight, *Discourse on the Worship of Priapus* (1786), pp. 13–23.

p. 159, *completely insulated… in the world*: A Sketch, p. 47.

p. 159, *prudence… soul of business*: A Sketch, p. 9.

p. 159, *The extended promotional… powers-that-be*: A Sketch, pp. 77–78.

p. 159, *abhorrence or contempt*: A Lecture, p. 5.

pp. 159–60, *I have it… scientific apparatus*: A Sketch, p. 62.

p. 160, …*on a few potatoes*: Brissot, *Mémoires*, p. 351.

p. 160, *the four quarters… to Man*: A Sketch, p. 48.

Chapter Six

p. 161, *I cannot fail… immortal fame*: Travels and Voyages, p. 33.

p. 161, *Here is charming… them as Whitehall*: BL Add. MSS 75694, Letters from Rachel Lloyd to Lady Spencer 1773–1784, 2nd June 1780. The Catholic Relief Act of April 1778 had extended the Protestant right to own and inherit land to English and Welsh Catholics, and allowed Catholic priests to officiate at religious services, and to teach. After rioting in Edinburgh and elsewhere on the issue in the summer of 1779, the Government backed down from introducing an equivalent bill for Scotland.

p. 161, *a time of terror*: "Such a time of terror you have been fortunate in not seeing", Dr Johnson to Mrs Thrale, quoted by Christopher Hibbert,

King Mob: The Story of Lord George Gordon and the Riots of 1780 (Stroud: Sutton Publishing, 2004), p. 8 [Hibbert, *King Mob*].

p. 162, *the choicest... individual*: *General Evening Post*, London, 8th June 1780.

p. 162, *We were surrounded... in our danger*: Hibbert, *King Mob*, p. 90, quoting Lady Anne Erskine writing to the Earl of Buchan.

p. 163, *Many noble... fury of the mob*: *London Chronicle*, 6th June to 8th June 1780.

p. 163, *like a volcano*: Hibbert, *King Mob*, p. 112.

p. 163, *...coming west again*: *Walpole's Correspondence*, vol. 33, pp. 188, 194.

p. 163, *This day is published... Borough of Southwark*: *General Evening Post*, London, 17th June 1780.

p. 164, *You may insert... thousand times*: D'Archenholz, *A Picture of England*, p. 44.

p. 164, *Every thing in London... stand in need of*: D'Archenholz, *A Picture of England*, pp. 231–32.

p. 164, *[T]he object... dealt in mockery*: Andrew Oliver, ed. *The Journal of Samuel Curwen, Loyalist* (Cambridge, MA: Harvard University Press, 1972), vol. 2, p. 656.

p. 165, *...wake of the recent riots*: *Public Advertiser*, Weds 26th July 1780.

p. 165, *...delivered by the porters*: *Morning Chronicle and London Advertiser*, 1st July 1780.

p. 165–66, *The "solemn dedication"... a hundred years*: *Sketch of the Plan, etc of the Temple of Health* (one penny handbill, 1780); *Morning Post*, 8th Feb. 1781.

p. 166, *Garlands... gaiety*: Alexander, 'Russian Reflection', pp. 178–9.

p. 166, *explaining the true nature... human body*: *A Sketch*, p. 47.

p. 167, *he is a most wonderful... hear him, at least*: Miss Rachel Lloyd to Lady Gower, 8th July 1780, London, PRO 30/29/4/7 no. 74.

p. 167, *...Baron Munchausen*: Raspe's later career as an essayist was caricatured by Walter Scott in his novel *The Antiquary* (1816), in which Raspe appears as the dishonest Hermann Dousterswivel. R.E. Raspe, *Singular travels, campaigns and adventures of Baron Munchausen: with an introduction by John Carswell* (1948).

p. 167, *Though there is... Your Excellency's country*: Letter from Rudolph Erich Raspe to Dr Benjamin Franklin, London, 25th July 1780.

p. 168, *The Temple of Health... the morning sun*: *Morning Chronicle*, 22nd July 1780.

p. 168, *all the wonders of art... observation of the curious*: D'Archenholz, *A Picture of England*, p. 69.

p. 169, *...under their upholstery*: Alvar González-Palacios, 'The Prince of Palagonia, Goethe and Glass Furniture', *Burlington Magazine*, 113, no. 821 (Aug. 1971), pp. 456–61, pp. 456–57.

p. 169, *...in the late nineteenth century*: For an in-depth treatment of this see Jane Shadel Spillman, *European Glass Furnishings for Eastern Palaces* (Corning, NY: Corning Museum of Glass, 2006).

p. 170, *...papist principles and politics*: *London Chronicle*, 13th–15th June 1780.

p. 170, *with all the force… on the hottest day*: *The Life and Times of Frederick Reynolds, written by himself*, 2 vols., 2nd edn. (London: Henry Colburn, 1827), pp. 154–55 [*Frederick Reynolds*].

p. 170, *DEAR DOCTOR… you'll put it in*: *Frederick Reynolds*, p. 154.

pp. 170–71, *[T]he present object… fat of nonsense*: *Gazetteer and New Daily Advertiser*, 22nd Aug. 1780.

p. 171, *…he's inspired!… above his line*: *Gazetteer and New Daily Advertiser*, 14th Aug. 1780.

p. 171, *…by a "Caledonian"*: Prejudice against the Scots was rife at this time, and was particularly concentrated on Scottish members of the medical profession. A squib about the Adam brothers' perceived theft of the Thames in *The New Foundling Hospital for Wit* (1771–73) included the lines: "O Scotland! Long it has been said, Thy teeth are sharp for English bread."

p. 171, *…at masquerades*: Masquerade Intelligence, *Morning Chronicle*, 17th Nov. 1780, 7th June 1781.

p. 171, *…to the "Emperor of Quacks"*: *The Quintessence of Quackism* (1780, British Museum no. 5766). This medallion seems to have been well known, for it was also referred to in *The Amours of Carlo Khan*, p. 92: under the care of Dr Graham, Macaulay "received a perfect cure, which she has acknowledged in the body of his work: and for which good offices, like her compeer Catherine of Russia, she liberally rewarded him, besides complimenting him with her miniature picture, which he long afterwards wore in his bosom."

p. 171, *The present Gang… of Rioters*: *Public Advertiser*, 2nd Sept. 1780.

p. 172, *sweetest… wall-flowers*: *A Short Extract from "Medical Transaction"* (1781), p. 3. An extravagant claim, obviously, but at much the same time Benjamin Franklin was discussing (semi-seriously) how to make urine smell of violets with the help of turpentine pills, and joked that finding a way of perfuming flatulence might be more useful to mankind than all the philosophy of Aristotle, Descartes and Newton. 'To the Royal Academy of Brussels' (Passy: printed by Benjamin Franklin after 19th May 1780), www.franklinpapers.org.

p. 172, *Come all ye… my tongue*: *Gazetteer and New Daily Advertiser*, 12th and 14th Aug. 1780. Graham's religious aspirations had been related to his speech. It was even implied that the Doctor's celestial claims made him speak in tongues. One parody in the style of the prayer book had him solemnly committing himself to using and creating every opportunity of "puffing" himself.

p. 173, *And what of… habits and manners*: Sir George Townwood, archetypal country squire retorts to Miss Ogle in Hannah Cowley's *The Belle's Stratagem* (1781), cited by Diana Donald, *The Age of Caricature* (New Haven, CT, and London: Yale University Press, 1996), p. 82.

p. 173, *Dr. Graham kept his… champagne*: Henry Angelo, *The Reminiscences of Henry Angelo* (New York and London: Benjamin Blom, 1969), p. 98.

p. 173, *…soon be felt at the Adelphi*: *Morning Chronicle*, 20th July 1780.

pp. 173–74, *protruded… refused to give him*: George Colman (the younger), *Random Records* (1830), vol. 2, p. 16 [Colman, *Random Records*].

p. 174, *mere entrance… roar of laughter*: Colman, *Random Records*, vol. 2, pp. 17–18. (Both young men were great friends with Henry Angelo, Frederick Reynolds and the artist Thomas Rowlandson, who later also became an Adelphi resident and Graham caricaturist.)

p. 174, *an empyric oration... through the house*: *Morning Post*, 4th Sept. 1780.

p. 174, *an ancient gossip's... end of them*: Quoted in Schuchard, *Why Mrs Blake Cried*, p. 193.

p. 175, *...reviewers adored it*: *The Genius of Nonsense*. By George Colman the elder and Samuel Arnold (composer), an entertainment, afterpiece, unpublished (Huntington Larpent MS no. 532. Advertised as a "Whimsical, Operatical, Pantomimical, Farcical, Electrical, Naval and Military Extravaganza". *Songs* printed for T. Cadell (1780); score printed by Harrison and Co., for the author (1784).

p. 175, *The Nonsense of Genius*: John Adolphus, *Memoirs of John Bannister, Comedian* (London: Richard Bentley, 1838), p. 62.

p. 175, *all spectators... real representation*: *Morning Post*, 4th Sept. 1780.

p. 175, *elegant apartment... parade of electricity*: *The Lady's Magazine; or entertaining companion for the Fair Sex*, vol. 11 (1780), pp. 471–75. The review was reprinted from the *London Evening Post*.

p. 175, *the female voice... Doctor's house*: *London Gazette*, 4th Sept. 1780.

p. 176, *a wooden thing on wires*: *Walpole's Correspondence*, vol. 33, p. 217, letter to Lady Ossory, Weds 23rd Aug. 1780, quoting Lady Wishfort in William Congreve's comedy *The Way of the World*, Act III, Sc. 1. When Walpole's dismissive description of Graham as the dullest "mountebank of his profession" is trotted out, it is never mentioned that he also described the philosopher David Hume as a "superficial mountebank" (vol. 10, p. 176; vol. 16, p. 266; vol. 42, p. 78).

p. 176, *...by a 1760s sea-captain*: Walpole had written a satire on press reports of the Patagonians, as reported by Hon. John Byron, captain of the *Dolphin*, entitled *An Account of the Giants Lately Discovered; in a Letter to a Friend in the Country* (1766).

p. 176, *remarkable for their excellence*: *Morning Herald*, 13th Nov. 1780.

p. 176, *...travelling menagerie*: Altick, *Shows of London*, p. 39.

p. 177, *...at the Gordon Riots*: *A Hit at the Late Riots* was probably directed at crowd psychology and herd behaviour, perhaps drawing parallels between audiences flocking to the Temple and the recently rioting mob. Electricity would have provided a fine image for contagion and conflagration, ideas associated with the Gordon Riots.

p. 177, *clearly see... of the piece*: *Morning Herald*, 13th Nov. 1780.

p. 177, *Does any rich... he was of yore*: *Gazetteer and New Daily Advertiser*, 14th Aug. 1780.

p. 178, *...palenchic, and caprimantic*: *Morning Chronicle*, 7th Apr. 1781.

p. 179, *...well-known actual event*: *Morning Post*, 27th Feb. 1781.

p. 180, *Man was...later that evening*: Ephraim Hardcastle [pseud. W.H. Pyne], *Wine and Walnuts; or, After Dinner Chit-Chat* (London, 1823), vol. 1, pp. 282–298.

p. 180, *...a West End clientele*: 'Pall Mall, South Side, Past Buildings: Nos 80–82 (consec.) Pall Mall: Old Schomberg House', *Survey of London*, vols. 29 and 30: 'St James's Westminster', Part 1 (1960), pp. 368–77. The rent was

£150 a quarter, only £4 less than the Royal Terrace, Adelphi. Westminster Record Office, MF698, vol. D1111, St James's Piccadilly, Parish Records.

p. 180, *Take me... raptur'd proof*: *The Celestial Beds; or, a Review of the Votaries of the Temple of Health, Adelphi, and the Temple of Hymen, Pall-Mall*. London, printed for G. Kearsly, No. 46, in Fleet-Street, 1781, p. 15 [*The Celestial Beds*].

p. 181, *to insure... human species*: *A Lecture*, p. 19.

p. 181, *...Thomas Denton*: C.J.S. Thompson, *Mysteries of History* (London: Faber & Gwyer, 1928), ch. 19.

p. 181, *paid his admission... set about his work*: Andrew Knapp and William Baldwin, *The Newgate Calendar* (London: J. Robins and Co., 1825), vol. 3, p. 150.

p. 182, *...decades of success*: Gaby Wood, *Living Dolls: A Magical History of the Quest for Mechanical Life* (London: Faber & Faber, 2002).

p. 182, *tint of charlatanism... of the masses*: Henri Decremps, *La Magie blanche dévoilée* (Paris: 1784), quoted in *Living Dolls*, p. 77.

p. 182, *forty pillars... electrical fire*: *A Lecture*, p. 20.

p. 184, *About fifteen hundred pounds... and so pleasing*: *A Lecture*, p. 20.

p. 185, *...to a magnet*: Fara, *Sympathetic Attractions*, p. 150.

p. 185, *...into indoor swings*: *Morning Amusement, Merlin's Mechanical Exhibition* (1787–89), pp. 6, 8, 9, 12–13.

p. 185, *he can follow his lady... corpulency*: *A Lecture*, p. 20.

pp. 185–86, *tender dalliances... blissful collusions*: *A Lecture*, p. 20.

p. 186, *...already a buzzword*: D.S. Katz, 'The Occult Bible: Hebraic Millenarianism in Eighteenth-Century England', eds. James Force and Richard Popkin, *Millenarianism and Messianism in Early Modern European Culture*, vol. 3, *The Millenarian Turn* (Dordrecht, Boston, MA and London: Kluwer Academic Publishers, 2001), p. 120.

p. 186, *...the two men's cosmologies*: Schuchard, *Why Mrs Blake Cried*, pp. 172, 185.

p. 186, *for nearly an hour... great success*: This was translated into Russian for the *Moskovskie vedomosti*, 6th Apr. 1784. Quoted in Alexander, 'Russian Reflection', pp. 178–9.

pp. 186–87, *Every man at forty... with the performer*: Frederick Reynolds, p. 155.

p. 188, *...as "Celestial" too*: See, for example, an inscribed print in the Graham collection in McGill University Library, Osler 2810, Item 1.

p. 188, *Alas!... away our vitals*: Graham, *Medical Transactions at the Temple of Health in London* (June 1781), p. 24.

p. 188, *Haste... villain Fate!" The Celestial Beds*.

p. 190, *the personages... nocturnal sports*: *Morning Herald*, 16th Apr. 1781.

p. 191, *Coquette... passions and projects*: *Walpole's Correspondence*, vol. 23, p. 345.

p. 191, *...this kind of publicity*: See Stella Tillyard's *Aristocrats* (London: Vintage, 1995) for a sympathetic portrait of Louisa Lennox.

p. 192, *...solution to the evils of prostitution*: Revd Martin Madan, *Thelyphthora, or a Treatise on Female Ruin, in its Causes, Effects, Consequences, Prevention, and Remedy; considered on the Basis of the Divine*

Law: under the following Heads, viz. Marriage, Whoredom and Fornication, Adultery, Polygamy, Divorce; with any Incidental Matters; particularly including an Examination of... the Marriage Act (London: J. Dodsley, 1780), 2 vols.

p. 192, *Proceed... work of Chance*: Handbill announcing imminent opening of Temple of Hymen, 21st Mar. 1781, NLS MS 9834.

p. 192, *entertaining her visitors... novel*: *Morning Herald*, 28th Apr. 1781.

pp. 192–93: *To't Luxury... pow'rful is the Doctor*: *Songs, Duetts, Trios &c*, in *The Genius of Nonsense*, 2nd edn. (London: 1781). Reference to King Lear's line, in his "let copulation thrive!" speech: "To't luxury, pell-mell..." (Act IV, Sc. 5).

p. 193, *If one may judge... extraordinary indeed*: *Morning Post*, 18th Apr. 1781.

p. 193, *Hence, ye vulgar herd*: This was the Cumaean Sibyl's cry as Virgil's Aeneas was about to descend to the underworld, to be told of the founding of Rome. In July, the prologue to a new play called *The Baron* mocked manufactured coats of arms, linking courtesans like Robinson with the Marriage Act, polygamy debates, poets, brothels, and inevitably, Graham himself:

> "Let two gilt porters, ranged on either side,
> Support the 'scutcheon with gigantic pride;
> Long mottoes, charg'd with genuine classic fire,
> Bid, with a *shock*, – the vulgar crowd retire."
> (*Morning Post*, 14th July 1781).

p. 193, *deter... polluting the Temple*: Graham, *Dr Graham is oppressed with shame...* (1781), p. 2 [*Dr Graham is oppressed*].

p. 193, *her chaste hand... lovely body*: *Morning Herald*, 30th Apr. 1781.

p. 193, *being a mark... of a bagnio*: *Morning Herald*, 12th May 1781.

p. 193, *...his advertised specialities*: Mercury was a common though lethal cure for venereal disease, by this time loudly rejected by Graham. By October the following year, he was giving public "Lectures on the nature, prevention, and cure of Venereal Diseases... In these new and eccentric Lectures, the dangerous roughness, the provoking tediousness, the horrid filthiness, and the eventual insufficiency of the mercurial and other medicines, recommended and used by Astruc, Sydenham, Turner, Cullen, Falcke, Fordyce, Simmons, Leake Clare, and by the most celebrated practitioners in Europe, regular and empirical, are clearly pointed out; and new, more rational, speedier, and more effectual remedies and methods, both for prevention and cure, are liberally explained, and warmly inculcated, without technical terms, for the real benefit and information of those Gentlemen who are not of the medical profession." *Morning Herald*, 24th Oct. 1782.

p. 193, *Whatever the Doctor's... Thieves and Imposters*: *Morning Post*, 19th Apr. 1781.

p. 194, *...Graham's true allegiances*: *Morning Herald*, 10th July 1781, according to *Il Convito Amoroso*, p. 50.

p. 194, *Great numbers of nuns... St James's Park*: D'Archenholz, *A Picture of England*, pp. 193–194.

p. 194, *The Temple... cuckoldom and adultery*: *Dr Graham is oppressed*, p. 2.

p. 194, *practical knowledge... terrestrial*: *Morning Herald*, 4th June 1781.

Chapter Seven
Unless otherwise stated, all quotations by Graham in this chapter are from the
Lecture or *A Private Advice*.

p. 195, *I must myself… mankind*: Preface to *A Lecture*.

p. 195, *There Venus… plunder*: *Morning Herald*, 7th May 1781.

p. 195, *…Southwark prison buildings*: Joanna Innes, 'The King's Bench Prison
in the Later Eighteenth Century: Law, Authority and Order in a London
Debtors' Prison', John Brewer and John Styles, eds., *An Ungovernable People:
The English and their Law in the Seventeenth and Eighteenth Centuries*
(London: Hutchinson, 1980), pp. 250–298.

p. 196, *When they can carry… luxury and riot*: W. Smith, *Mild Punishments
sound Policy* (London: 1778), p. 64.

p. 196, *continue to labour… his Majesty's subjects*: *Morning Herald*, 9th July
1781.

p. 196, *The grand Hymenean Forge… solemnity*: *Morning Herald*, 2nd July 1781.

p. 196, *pretty loudly… amusements within*: *Morning Herald*, 2nd July 1781.

p. 196, *Scarcely has one… apartment is reached*: Unsourced contemporary
account in Harvey Graham, *A Doctor's London* (London: Wingate, 1952),
p. 78.

p. 197, *…after his wife's death*: See British Museum satire no. 5901

p. 197, *…Poll Kennedy turned up*: Kennedy was painted by Reynolds for
Bunbury and was renowned for her avarice.

p. 198, *…causing mayhem*: *Morning Herald*, 30th June 1781.

p. 199, *Britain… race of giants*: Edward Trapp Pilgrim, 'On Dr Graham's
Celebrated Lecture in the Temple of Health', *Poetical Trifles* (London: 1785),
p. 8.

p. 199, *…pointed the finger at war*: Richard Price, *Essay on Population* (1780).

p. 199, *My soul shrinks… conflicts. No*: *Morning Post*, 20th Nov. 1780: "But
as that ingenious gentleman [probably Price] has clearly proved the rapid depopulation of this country, it might be improper to lay any tax at present on
fornication, as it may with the collateral aids of Dr. Madan's Telypthora, and
Dr Graham's electricity, be the means of remedying that alarming evil."

p. 200, *Let us deluge… such enormities*: *A Lecture*, p. 3.

p. 200, *…as well as corporeal powers*: "Luxury impairs the faculties of the
soul, clouds the understanding, renders the will listless and inactive, stupefies
the judgment, blunts the edge of our spirits; in short, for a time, diverts us
of our reason." Samuel Falconer, *An Essay on Modern Luxury* (London:
1765), p. 33.

p. 200, *…of the consumer revolution*: See Maxine Berg and Elizabeth Eger,
eds., *Luxury in the Eighteenth Century: Debates, Desires and Delectable
Goods* (London: Palgrave, 2002).

p. 201, *…had to be abandoned*: On 4th Nov. 1780, Samuel Curwen had attended a meeting of the "Belle Assemblee or Ladys disputing Society", where
the question proposed was "Would it not be prudent and proper, considering
the great demand for public supply, and the difficulty of raising them, to lay
a tax on old bachelors?"

p. 202, *Skipping as it were… Conception may arise*: Lazarus Riverius, *The*

Practice of Physick (1658), quoted in Angus McLaren, *Reproductive Rituals: The Perception of Fertility in England from the Sixteenth to the Nineteenth Century* (London and New York: Methuen, 1984), p. 20 [McLaren, *Reproductive Rituals*].

p. 202, *it is well known... compact children*: This had been spotted also by the influential William Harvey (McLaren, *Reproductive Rituals*, p. 26).

p. 202, *...reproduced since the 1670s*: The ovum was identified by the embryologist Dr Karl Ernest von Baer in 1827. Theodore Kerckring's foetal osteology report for the Royal Society had been frequently recycled. Lisa Forman Cody, *Birthing the Nation: Sex, Science and the Conception of Eighteenth-Century Britons* (Oxford: Oxford University Press, 2005), pp. 102–104 [Cody, *Birthing the Nation*].

p. 203, *the Womb... miscarry*: Quoted and discussed in Cody, *Birthing the Nation*, p. 107.

p. 205, *The many good hints... at least at present*: MS undated, but probably written around 1761. See Norah Smith, 'Sexual Mores in the Eighteenth Century: Robert Wallace's "Of Venery"', *Journal of the History of Ideas*, vol. 39, no. 3 (July–Sept. 1978), pp. 419–33.

pp. 206–207, *O my son... form thee*: John Armstrong, *The Oeconomy of Love: A Poetical Essay* (1736), ll. 101–107.

p. 207, *...immoderate consumer spending*: Thomas W. Laqueur, *Solitary Sex: A Cultural History of Masturbation* (New York: Zone Books, 2004).

p. 209, *Among much... observations*: Norfolk Record Office, MC7/16 395x2.

p. 209, *most men... from year to year*: Robert Willan, *Reports on the Diseases of London* (1801), p. 304.

p. 210–11, *Within a fortnight... species of entertainment*: *Morning Herald*, 17th July 1781.

p. 211, *snowy blooming health... BLESSED*: Advertisement in *Morning Post*, 16th July 1781, and elsewhere.

p. 211, *He uses the plainest... scruple*: Quoted unsourced, Harvey Graham, *A Doctor's London*, p. 78.

p. 211, *Heard the King... to hear him*: Norfolk Record Office, MC7/16 395x2.

p. 212, *...disguised as social concern*: Kevin L. Cope, ed., *Eighteenth Century British Erotica II*, vol. 3, p. 284.

p. 212, *Your Private Advice... body understands*: *The Rambler's Magazine*, Apr. 1783, p. 123.

p. 212, *...sitting on a gentleman's lap*: *A Lecture on Generation* (London: 1780), British Library.

p. 213, *That extraordinary Physician... enrapture the practice*: *Modern Propensities; or, an Essay on the Art of Strangling, &c.* (1791). Reprinted in Rictor Norton, ed., *Eighteenth-Century British Erotica*, vol. 5: 'Sex Doctors and Sex Crimes' (London: Pickering and Chatto, 2002), pp. 255–56. Its author was probably Martin van Butchell, a revolutionary vegetarian healer who sold elastic garters that could be used for erotic purposes as well as for holding up stockings.

p. 214, *...from her son's bedside*: 8th July 1781, BL Add. MSS 75708, 7/8.

p. 214, *I never like the hurry... letter carriage*: BL Add. MSS 75911, Althorp papers vol., 611 1769–82, 25th July 1781.

p. 215, *The Temple... ladies of this kingdom*: *Morning Herald*, 10th Aug. 1781. "Any Chalybeate water, or water fully impregnated with fixed air" is recommended for washing the private parts in *A Private Medical Advice to married Ladies and Gentlemen; to those especially who are not blessed with children*, pirated in *The Rambler's Magazine* (May 1783), p. 161.

p. 215, *...preservation of identity*: *Morning Herald*, 6th Aug. 1781.

p. 215, *A bed that's celestial... top to the toe*: *Morning Herald*, 26th July 1781, reprinted as 'Doctor's Porter' in *Garrick's jests, or the English Roscius, in high glee. Containing all the jokes of the wits of the present age... being... repartees... and the favourite songs sung this season at Vauxhall and the London play-houses* (1785).

p. 216, *An apprehension... understanding orders*: *Morning Herald*, 2nd Aug. 1781.

p. 216, *The Lectures of this worthy Professor... must be considerable*: Robert Jephson, Esq., *The Confessions of James Baptiste Couteau* (Dublin: 1794), pp. 139–45.

pp. 217–18, *"Mary "Perdita" Robinson... Mr. Optic gravely*: Mary Robinson, *Walsingham* (Toronto, ON: Broadview Press, 2003), pp. 227–42.

p. 218, *The Grand Celestial Bed... chain to ditto*: Handwritten note of uncertain origin attached to a copy of *A Lecture*, Library Company of Philadelphia.

p. 219, *The chief object... noble families*: *Dr Graham is oppressed*, p. 2.

p. 219, *so many hundred pounds... in this kingdom*: *Morning Herald*, 19th Sept. 1781.

p. 220, *...in the flesh is ambiguous*: *Morning Chronicle*, 18th Dec. 1781.

p. 220, *Dr Graham's Efforts... CELESTIAL BED*: *Morning Chronicle*, 12th Oct. 1781.

p. 220, *slow dances of half-naked wretches*: Harvey Graham, *A Doctor's London* (London: Wingate, 1952), p. 80.

p. 220, *His Highness... Pall-Mall*: *Morning Herald*, 19th Sept. 1781.

p. 220, *Where can our sailors... war*: *Morning Post*, 19th Sept. 1781.

pp. 220–21, *It is needless to say... [and Hymen]*: *Morning Herald*, 21st May 1782.

p. 221, *the strength... effectually improve*: *Morning Chronicle*, 29th Jan. 1782.

p. 221, *Society in those days... cut and shuffled*: George Otto Trevelyan, *The Early History of Charles James Fox* (London: Longmans, Green & Co, 1880), pp. 88–89.

p. 221, *...cared about losing it*: Gillian Russell, '"Faro's Daughters": Female Gamesters, Politics, and the Discourse of Finance in 1790s Britain', *Eighteenth-Century Studies*, vol. 33, no. 4 (Summer 2000), pp. 481–504.

p. 222, *When this bell... profits of the cheat*: *Morning Herald*, 8th May 1781.

p. 222, *...winnings of £15,000*: *Morning Post*, 12th June 1782. This was probably the Duke of Grafton – one of first members of Brooks's, along with the Duke of Richmond and others. Fox was joined to it by his father at the age of sixteen. *Parliamentary History*, XXIII, p. 110. Byng, MP for Middlesex said on 5th June 1782: "E.O. tables were now to be found in every part of the town... he did not doubt, but shortly the electric bed would be turned into an E.O. table." Eventually, after a six-hour trial, a John Wiltshire was convicted of involvement in "keeping the E.O. tables at Dr Graham's on Pall Mall". *British Magazine and Review* (Dec. 1782), p. 476.

p. 222, *as Lady Chewton... morning is dead*: *Walpole's Correspondence*, letter to Lady Ossory, 13th June 1782, vol. 33, p. 335.

p. 222, *all the windows... destroyed*: *Morning Post*, 13th June 1782.

p. 222, *...as they escaped*: *Morning Post*, 31st July 1782.

p. 222, *...caricature by Gillray*: *Morning Post*, 3rd Aug. 1782; James Gillray, *The W—st—r JUST ASSES a Braying – or – the Downfall of the E.O. Table*, published on 26th Aug. 1782 by W. Humphrey.

p. 223, *...with "decency and decorum"*: *Morning Post*, 28th Sept. 1782.

p. 223, *the Peasant... pleasing scenes*: *Morning Post*, 6th Aug. 1782.

p. 223, *the surprising Irish giant... Goddess Venus*: Wendy Moore, *The Knife Man*, p. 299, cites *Parker's General Advertiser*, 24th Aug. 1782.

p. 223, *...at the Haymarket*: A new comic opera called *Il Convito Amoroso* opened on Tuesday 3rd December 1782 at Sheridan's King's Theatre in the Haymarket, libretto by Antonio Andrei, music by Ferdinand Bertoni.

pp. 223–24, *Adepts Hibernian... and more fat*: *Il Convito Amoroso*, pp. 9–10.

p. 225, *As we decline... disappears*: *Il Convito Amoroso*, p. 89.

p. 225, *the dashes... eighteenth century*: Sharon Harrow, Institute of Historical Research review of Karen Harvey's *Reading Sex in the Eighteenth Century: Bodies and Gender in English Erotic Culture* (Cambridge: Cambridge University Press, 2005), www.history.ac.uk/reviews/paper/harrow.html.

pp. 225–26, *...vessels for procreation*: *Il Convito Amoroso*, pp. 11–12.

p. 226, *...about to be served*: *Il Convito Amoroso*, p. 1.

p. 226, *very merry meetings... institution*: *Morning Chronicle*, 19th Dec. 1782. See *James Graham lecturing from a podium, to a crowd of ladies and gentlemen*. Etching by J. Boyne, 1783 (Wellcome Library no. 544690i). Mary Robinson, Charles James Fox and John Wilkes are among the crowd.

p. 227, *a most ready elocution... some gentlemen*: *Journal of Samuel Curwen*, vol. 2, 19th Feb. 1783, p. 898.

p. 228, *...artificial father*: *Rambler's Magazine*, vol. 1 (1783), p. 123.

p. 228, *...into the wider world*: At this point Graham was employing a rather tragic younger sister of the adored cult actress Sarah Siddons to deliver versions of *The Blazing Star*. Ann Julia Kemble, lame and smallpox-scarred, and far less successful on the stage than her siblings, had discovered herself to be bigamously married. Claiming ill treatment by her theatrical family, she had resorted to the newspapers to advertise her financial distress, seemingly unrelieved by the publication of a volume of poetry that year.

pp. 228–29, *The ladies ought not... portraits*: *The Blazing Star*, 25th Mar. 1783, pp. 12–13. Graham, *Tracts, &c*, printed and MS by James Graham, MD, Abbotsford Library (Faculty of Advocates, Edinburgh).

p. 229, *Gentlemen, ye are born... important matters*: *Blazing Star*, pp. 27–28.

p. 230, *In the course of the Lecture... ineffable bliss*: *Morning Herald*, 9th July 1783.

p. 230, *...must-have accessory*: *Morning Herald*, 15th July 1783.

p. 231, *O delicate... rise and fall*: *A Poetical Epistle to the Very Celebrated Doctor Graham* (Derby: 1783).

p. 231, *a few impures... not without humour*: *Diary of Sylas Neville*, p. 307.

Chapter Eight

p. 233, *Alas!... piteous plight*: Manuscript letter by Dr Graham, NLS MS 9834, undated.

p. 233, *He was very early... in prison*: *Morning Chronicle*, 1783, undated, Collection of Cuttings, Wellcome Library.

p. 233, *...quarter of the Exchange*: *The Edinburgh Advertiser*, 29th Aug.–5th Sept. 1783.

p. 233, *down upon them... rotten cheese*: Walter Scott's marginalia in his copy of Francis Grose's satire, *A guide to health, beauty, riches, and honour* (1785), Abbotsford Library (Faculty of Advocates, Edinburgh), p. 153.

p. 234, *publishing Lascivious... within the city*: Edinburgh Tolbooth Records, HH21/21 f.197v.

p. 234, *A prison is... honest men among*: W.J. Forsythe, ed., *The State of the Prisons in Britain, 1775–1905*, vol. 2 (London: Routledge/Thoemmes Press, 2000), pp. 187–196.

p. 234, *proceedings... INQUISITIONS*: *An Appeal to the Public concerning the case of James Graham, M.D.* (1783), no copies in existence.

p. 235, *...Enlightenment anatomy*: Tristram Stuart believes Graham was heavily influenced by Thomas Tryon, "that seventeenth-century brahminical prophet of prelapsarian purity", *The Bloodless Revolution: Radical Vegetarians and the Discovery of India* (London: HarperPress, 2006), p. 333.

p. 235, *the seeds of horrors... incest*: James Graham, *A Discourse Delivered on Sunday, August 17, 1783, in the Tolbooth of Edinburgh* (1783), pp. 12, 13 [*A Discourse*].

p. 235, *every part and particle... even in Britain*: *A Discourse*, p. 18.

p. 236, *Ark of Separation... strength to build*: *A Discourse*, p. 31.

p. 236, *...layers of clothing*: "I call the venereal act the casting off of the *middle* garment of nature; the outer I take to be the visible body, and the inner garment the invisible life, or spirit; to both of which the middle one adheres so closely, that it cannot be frequently shed or cast off, without shrinking, shrivelling, and debilitating both the others very sensibly." *A Lecture*, p. 8.

p. 236, *He began to write... Irregularities*: Only a unfinished draft in the doctor's handwriting remains of this letter, certified by his nephew John Smith. Manuscript letter by Dr Graham, NLS MS 9834 (undated, approx. 1783)

p. 236, *...made up of men*: Portrait of J. Graham delivering a lecture, John Kay (Wellcome Library, Iconographic Collection no. 1184.1).

p. 236, *...to the lecturing room*: *Edinburgh Advertiser*, 26th Aug., 1783.

pp. 236–37, *There shall come... drive you to despair*: Dr Graham letter, 27th Aug. 1783, Central Library, Edinburgh.

p. 237, *shook... off his feet*: *A Lecture*, p. iv.

p. 237, *vile, gutling... liberality and science*: *A Lecture*, p. i.

p. 238, *eagerly inserted... will make them*: *A Lecture*, p. i.

p. 238, *what play... set of scenery*: *A Lecture*, p. i.

p. 239, *...tub of froth*: Mary Robinson, Dally the Tall and another representative of the Cyprian Corps took the top seats, while Fox and North, attached by a string to their puppet the Duke of Portland, the nominal head of a failing coalition, shared the middle row with a pair of bishops. *The Aerostatick Stage Balloon*, 1783, satirical hand-coloured etching by John Nicholson, 23rd Dec. 1783 (British Museum no. 6284; Science Museum/ Science & Society Picture Library no. 10411052).

p. 239, *...in any kind of luxury*: *A Lecture*, p. 21.

p. 239, *standing for Middlesex*: *Edinburgh Evening Courant*, 12th May 1784. See also *The Rambler's Magazine* (Apr. 1784), p. 136.

p. 240, *God knows!... to promote*: 24th Mar. 1784, British Library.

p. 240, *...remove the Temple's insignia*: Schuchard, *Why Mrs Blake Cried*, p. 186.

p. 241, *dangerous... eternal happiness*: Graham, *Temple of Health, South-bridge Street, Edinburgh*, in *A Collection of handbills, etc., of Graham's works...*, Osler Library, McGill University.

p. 242, *...triangle with Graham and Katterfelto*: British Museum print no. 7545, *Billy's gouty visit, or a peep at Hammersmith*, engraving (coloured), 20th July 1789.

p. 242, *Dig up the earth... brilliancy of soul*: 'A Very Short Account of the Composition and Virtues of this most Admirable Medicine! With Directions for taking it' (undated, post-1784), Graham, *Tracts*.

pp. 242–43, *Not knowing... root and branch*: Graham, *A Short Treatise on the all-cleansing, all-healing, and all-invigorating qualities of the Simple Earth* (Newcastle upon Tyne: 1790), pp. 12–13 [*A Short Treatise*].

p. 243, *The more that the patient... like a glutton*: *A Short Treatise*, pp. 16–17.

p. 243, *full of grubbs... breast-opening smell*: *A Short Treatise*, pp. 15–16.

pp. 243–44, *Heart of every Lady... celestial Touchings*: 'Doctor Graham's entirely new Lecture... in Panton-Street', *Tracts*, p. 2 and *The Rambler's Magazine* (1786), p. 44.

p. 244, *...twenty-five years previously*: *The Rambler's Magazine* (1786), p. 45.

p. 244, *at Nine... resurrection will take place*: *Morning Herald*, 12th Apr. 1786.

p. 244, *a new method... planted in the earth*: *The Rambler's Magazine* (1786), p. 226.

p. 244, *...in the summer of 1781*: *The Critical Review, or, Annals of Literature*, vol. 51 (Jan.–June 1781), pp. 178–185.

p. 245, *...some months in Newcastle*: Letter in Graham collection, Osler Library, McGill University.

p. 245, *...for the genitalia*: Letter of 23rd Jan. 1788, Graham, *Tracts*.

p. 246, *his most noxious... the course of a few months*: *A Short Treatise*, p. 18.

p. 246, *I have every reason... from whom I sprung*: *A Lecture*, footnote, p. 16.

pp. 246–47, *all CROWNED HEADS!... or beggar-man has*: James Graham, *The Principal Grounds, Basis, Argument of Soul! Of the New Celestial Curtain, (or reprehensory Lecture! Most humbly addressed to all crowned heads! Great personages!* (1786), p. 12.

p. 247, *...in every detail*: See Clare Brant, *Eighteenth-Century Letters and British Culture* (London: Palgrave Macmillan, 2006), pp. 325–28 [Brant, *Eighteenth-Century Letters*].

p. 247, *in a most glorious... stained with blood*: Clare Brant, 'Huntington, William (1745–1813)', *Oxford Dictionary of National Biography* (Oxford: Oxford University Press, 2004).

p. 247, *on the rising... everlasting day*: Graham, *Proposals for the Establishment of a new and true Christian Church* (1788), p. 4 [*Proposals*].

p. 247, *...delving he had been doing*:
"When Adam delved and Eve span,
Who was then the gentleman?"
This popular proverb dating from the fourteenth century was the text on which John Ball preached to the rebels at Blackheath at the start of the Peasants' Revolt of 1381.

p. 247, *...and Rochdale*: *A Short Treatise*, p. 18.

p. 248, *to moderate... collision*: *Proposals*, p. 4.

p. 248, *the last king... last priest*: Quoted in David Katz and Richard Popkin, *Messianic Revolution: Radical Religious Politics to the End of the Second Millennium* (New York: Hill and Wang, 1999), p. 107.

p. 248, *societies... our dear Lord*: *Proposals*, p. 10.

p. 249, *dead corpses... pews*: *Proposals*, p. 33.

p. 249, *nauseous... to be touched*: Arnot, *History*, p. 158.

p. 249, *more of that soul-melting... blessed spirits*: *Proposals*, pp. 28–29.

p. 249, *accidental... gentlemen*: *Proposals*, p. 7.

p. 250, *Yes, Nature's... heat of their souls*: *Proposals*, pp. 7, 2.

p. 250, *operating in the centre... body and system*: Graham, *A clear, full, and faithful portraiture... of a certain virgin princess* (Bath: 1792), p. 7 [*A clear, full, and faithful portraiture*].

p. 250, *...custody of two constables*: According to the *Whitehaven Packet*, quoted in *The Caledonian Mercury*, 21st Aug. 1788.

p. 250, *wholly... beggar whom he met*: Robert Southey, *Letters from England: by Don Manuel Alvarez Espriella. Translated from the Spanish*, ed. Jack Simmons (1807; Gloucester: Alan Sutton, 1984), p. 297 [Southey, *Letters from England*].

p. 250, *...rarely a compliment*: The term was in uneasy transition, edging towards its Romantic literary rehabilitation to describe a person experiencing a powerful and poetic effusion of emotion, but at this point more redolent of religious fanaticism.

p. 251, *...implicitly infectious*: Emma Mason, 'Emily Brontë and the Enthusiastic Tradition.' *Romanticism On the Net* 25 (Feb. 2002), users.ox.ac.uk/~scat0385/25mason.html.

p. 251, *...impossible to judge*: Southey was not the only writer to connect Graham with another Great Awakening. Catharine Macaulay's friend and fellow historian in America, Mercy Otis Warren incorporated the Doctor into her 1785 satirical comedy *Sans Souci, Alias Free and Easy*, confident her theatrical audiences would be familiar with the Celestial Bed and its proprietor: "We could blind one half the old women in town, by telling them the celebrated Doctor Graham intended to deliver evening lectures on various subjects – they would at least think him a second Whitfield."

p. 251, *...throughout his life*: Letter written from Edinburgh, 23rd Jan. 1788, Graham, *Tracts*.

p.   251, *artificially... admixtures*: *Proposals*, p. vii.

p.   251, *JAMES GRAHAM... Sheep into his Fold*: James Graham, *A very short History of the New Jerusalem True Church, and of its poor-rich Minister...* (1788) [*A very short History*] Like Priestley and a growing band of millenarian philosemites, Graham was convinced that without the conversion of the Jews, Jesus could not return to earth.

p.   252, *Oh Wonderful Love*: The would-be prophet William Huntington par-odied the DD after the names of doctors of divinity by signing himself with SS, standing for Sinner Saved. Brant, *Eighteenth-Century Letters*, p. 305.

p.   252, *...ambitiously ecumenical principles*: This tolerance was too much for some people, who denounced her for promoting sects. Arnot, *History*, p. 161.

p.   253, *...Swedenborg's Doctrine of the New Jerusalem Church*: *A very short History*, p. 1.

p.   253, *...to see the city's Provost disregarded*: Scott, *The Heart of Midlothian*, ch. 5.

p.   254, *kept him... all day*: *A very short History*, p. 2.

p.   254, *Be a Wall... Holy Ghost*: Unsigned and undated broadsheet handbill, *Tracts*, item 5.

p.   254, *The new Jerusalem... bringeth forth*: Letter to Graham from Benjamin Dockray, 21st Mar. 1789. It was returned to him and sent again to Graham, at Bath, on 6th May 1790. See Graham, *Tracts*.

p.   255, *arranging, comforting... JEHOVAH's Day*: *Proposals for printing (by subscription) a Work... [about] the KING's late severe, dangerous, and most universally and deeply lamented corporeal and mental Maladies* (London: 21st May 1789).

p.   255, *the best... of women*: *The Complete Newgate Calendar*, vol. 4, p. 172.

p.   255, *all the passions... set afloat*: Mary Wollstonecraft, *A Historical and Moral View of the French Revolution,* in *Works*, eds. Janet Todd and Marilyn Butler, vol. 6 (London: 1989), p. 146.

p.   256, *...in the early 1790s*: She may have inherited some of her father's eccentricities, since she was said to have died in the early 1790s in the apartments at the Observatory on Calton Hill in Edinburgh. This would have been as close to living on Arthur's Seat as anyone could have achieved. Kay, *A Series of Original Portraits*, p. 31.

p.   256, *in fresh mould... Venus's dove*: Southey, *Letters from England*, pp. 297–98

p.   257, *Men may despise... HATH GOD CHOSEN*: *Bath Journal*, 4th and 9th Jan. 1792.

p.   257, *...human features of a rock face*: National Portrait Gallery no. D18643 (1787).

p.   257, *...had once been joined*: *A Short Treatise*, p. 2.

p.   257, *prejudices... stationary medical Gentlemen*: Appendix to *Dr Graham has had the honour. . . publication of cures* (approx. 1792), p. 19.

p.   257, *the numerous herd... calling themselves Doctors*: Appendix to *Dr Graham has had the honour. . . publication of cures* (approx. 1792), p. 19.

p.   258, *England's dissolute heir*: *Proposals... for the King's Late Malady* (1789).

p. 258, *permanently crowned… grey-hairs*: A *clear, full and faithful portrai-ture*, p. v.

p. 258, *for stealing… murdering millions*: A *clear, full and faithful portrai-ture*, p. 29.

p. 259, *…his rules of health*: James Graham, A *New and Curious Treatise of the Nature and Effects of Simple Earth, Water and Air… How to Live for many weeks, months or years, without eating anything* (1793), p. 4 [*How to Live*].

pp. 259–60, *either madly… from Morning to night*: W. Withering to the Revd W. Scholefield, 11th Nov. 1792, Osler Bequest MSS, Royal Society of Medicine, London.

p. 261, *the repeated assurances… simplest productions*: *How to Live*, p. 1.

p. 261, *Alas, the hoary winter… for ever fled*: *How to Live*, p. 29.

p. 261, *high and palmy state*: Kay, *A Series of Original Portraits*, p. 35.

p. 261, *…his birthday, 23rd June 1794*: As reported by the *Morning Chronicle*, 30th June 1794, and *Musgrave's Obituary*, vol. 3 (London: 1900), although Edinburgh Old Parish Records state Graham's death as 24th December 1794.

pp. 261–62, *Retire as much as possible… rather than the devils*: Graham, 'The infallible Guide to Eternal Blessedness' in *The guardian of health, long-life, and happiness: or, Doctor Graham's general directions as to regimen, &c. for the cure or alleviation of all …* (Newcastle upon Tyne: 1790), p. 7.

p. 262, *when the gentle… call me blessed*: *How to Live*, p. 4.

Brief Bibliography

James Graham's Main Publications:

Thoughts on the present state of practice in disorders of the eye and ear ... and an Address to the Inhabitants of Great Britain (1775)

A Short Inquiry into the present state of Medical Practice (1776)

The Christian's Universal Prayer (1776)

The General State of Medical and Chirurgical Practice (1778)

Dr Graham is now preparing the largest and most elegant medico-electrical-aerial and magnetic apparatus... (1779)

A Sketch, or Short Description of Dr Graham's medical apparatus (1780)

Advertisement: Dr Graham is oppressed with shame... (1781)

The Guardian Goddess of Health (1781)

Medical Transactions at the Temple of Health in London (June 1781)

Il Convito Amoroso! Or a Serio-comico-philosophical lecture! (1782)

A discourse delivered on Sunday, August 17, 1783, in the Tolbooth of Edinburgh (1783)

Temple of health, South Bridge Street, Edinburgh (1783)

Travels and voyages in Scotland, England and Ireland, France, America, Hungary... 6th edition (1783)

A Lecture on the Generation, Increase, and Improvement of the Human Species! (November 1783) NB This is the edition from which I have quoted, abbreviated to *A Lecture*. Various pirated editions of this text also exist.

The Blazing Star; or, Vestina, the Gigantic, Rosy, Goddess of Health: being a complete defence of the fair sex. Delivered by the High Priestess of the Temple, as written by the Doctor Himself (1783) [Item 18 in Walter Scott's *Tracts*, Abbotsford Library]

Health! Soundness! Strength! And happiness! To the people! (Manchester, 1784)

The Principal Grounds, Basis, Argument of Soul! Of the New Celestial Curtain, (or reprehensory Lecture! Most humbly addressed to all crowned heads! Great personages!) (1786)

A very short History of the New Jerusalem True Church, and of its poor-rich Minister... (1788)

Proposals for the Establishment of a new and true Christian Church (1788)

Proposals for printing (by subscription) a Work... [about] the KING's late severe, dangerous, and most universally and deeply lamented corporeal and mental Maladies (1789)

A New, plain and rational treatise on the true nature and uses of the Bath Waters (1789)

Dr Graham's Address to the diseased, weak and lame...(Newcastle, 1790)

A Short Treatise on the all-cleansing, all-healing, and all-invigorating qualities of the Simple Earth (1790)

The guardian of health, long-life, and happiness: or, Doctor Graham's general directions as to regimen, &c. for the cure or alleviation of all... (1790)

A Clear, Full, and Faithfull Portraiture, or Description... of a... Virgin Princess (1792)

Dr Graham has had the honour of publicly exhibiting... the nature and effects of Earth-Bathing (1792)

A New and Curious Treatise of the Nature and Effects of Simple Earth, water and Air, when applied to the Human Body; How to Live for many weeks, months, or years, Without eating any Thing whatever... (1793)

Newspapers and Magazines:

Bath Chronicle
Bath Journal
Connecticut Courant
General Evening Post
Gentleman's Magazine
Lady's Magazine
London Chronicle
London Courant
Morning Herald
Morning Post
Newport Mercury
New-York Journal; or, the General Advertiser
New-York Gazette; and the Weekly Mercury
New-York Gazette; or the Weekly Post-Boy
Pennsylvania Chronicle and Universal Advertiser
Pennsylvania Packet
Public Advertiser
Rambler's Magazine; or, the annals of Gallantry, Glee, Pleasure and the Bon Ton
St James's Chronicle
Town and Country Magazine
York Courant

Selected Secondary Texts, Organized by Theme:

Chapter 1

A. Cunningham and R. French, eds., *The Medical Enlightenment of the Eighteenth Century* (Cambridge: Cambridge University Press, 1990)
W.F. Bynum and Roy Porter, eds., *William Hunter and the Eighteenth Century Medical World* (Cambridge: Cambridge University Press, 1985)
Helen Dingwall, *A History of Scottish Medicine* (Edinburgh: Edinburgh University Press, 2003)
Irvine Loudon, *Medical Care and the General Practitioner, 1750-1850* (Oxford: Clarendon Press, 1986)
Christopher Lawrence, *Medicine as Culture: Edinburgh and the Scottish Enlightenment*, Ph.D. thesis, University of London, 1984.
Guenter Risse, *Hospital Life in Enlightenment Scotland* (Cambridge: Cambridge University Press, 1986); *New Medical Challenges During the Scottish Enlightenment,* (Amsterdam: Rodopi, 2005)
Lisa Rosner, *Medical Education in the Age of Improvement* (Edinburgh: Edinburgh University Press, 1991)

Chapter 2

Bernard Bailyn, *Voyagers to the West: Emigration from Britain to America on the Eve of the Revolution* (London: Tauris, 1987)
Paola Bertucci and Giuliano Pancaldi, eds., *Electric Bodies: Episodes in the History of Medical Electricity* (Bologna: Dipartimento di Filosofia, Università di Bologna, 2001)
Carl Bridenbaugh, *Rebels and Gentlemen: Philadelphia in the Age of Franklin* (New York: Reynal and Hitchcock, 1942); *Myths and Realities: Societies of the Colonial South* (Baton Rouge: University of Louisiana Press, 1952); *Cities in Revolt: Urban Life in America, 1743-1776* (New York: Alfred A Knopf, 1955)
I. Bernard Cohen, *Benjamin Franklin's Science* (Cambridge, Mass. and London: Harvard University Press, 1990)
Patricia Fara, *An Entertainment for Angels: Electricity in the Enlightenment,* (Cambridge: Icon Books, 2002)
Francisco Guerra, *American Medical Bibliography 1639–1783* (New York: Lathrop C. Harper, 1962)
Nina Reid-Maroney, *Philadelphia's Enlightenment, 1740–1800: Kingdom of Christ, Empire of Reason* (London & Westport, Connecticut: Greenwood Press, 2001)

Michael Schiffer, *Draw the Lightning Down: Benjamin Franklin and Electrical Technology in the Age of Enlightenment* (Berkeley and London: University of California Press, 2003)
J.L. Heilbron, *Electricity in the 17th and 18th Centuries: A Study of Early Modern Physics* (Berkeley and London: University of California Press, 1979)

Chapter 3

Peter Borsay, *The Image of Georgian Bath, 1700–2000* (Oxford: Oxford University Press, 2000)
Penelope Corfield, *Power and the Professions in Britain, 1700-1850* (London & New York: Routledge, 1995)
Trevor Fawcett, *Voices of Eighteenth-Century Bath* (Bath: Ruton, 1995)
Bridget Hill, *The Republican Virago: The Life and Times of Catharine Macaulay* (Oxford: Clarendon Press, 1992)
Sarah Knott and Barbara Taylor, *Women, Gender and Enlightenment* (London: Palgrave Press, 2005)
R.S. Neale, *Bath 1680–1850: a Social History* (London: Routledge & Kegan Paul, 1981)
Michael Neve, *Natural Philosophy, Medicine and the Culture of Science in Provincial England: the Case of Bristol, 1790–1850*, Ph.D. Thesis, University of London, 1984.
Roy Porter, *Health for sale: quackery in England, 1660–1850* (Manchester & New York: Manchester University Press, 1989)

Chapter 4

David Allan, *The Adelphi Past and Present, A History and a Guide* (London: Calder Walker Associates, 2001)
Geoffrey Beard, *Craftsmen and Interior Decoration in England, 1660–1820* (Edinburgh: John Bartholomew, 1981)
Arthur Bolton, *The Architecture of Robert & James Adam* (London: Country Life, 1922)
John Brewer and Roy Porter, eds., *Consumption and the World of Goods* (London: Routledge, 1993)
Eileen Harris, *The Genius of Robert Adam: His interiors* (New Haven and London: Yale University Press, 2001)
Paul Langford, *A Polite and Commercial People: England 1727-1783* (Oxford: Clarendon Press, 1989)
Catherine Ross, 'The Flint Glass Houses on the Rivers Tyne and Wear during the Eighteenth Century', *The Glass Circle*, no. 5, 1986, pp. 75–85

Alistair Rowan, *Vaulting Ambition: The Adam Brothers, Contractors to the Metropolis in the Reign of George III* (Sir John Soane's Museum, 2007)

Jane Shadel Spillman, *European Glass Furnishings for Eastern Palaces* (Corning, New York: The Corning Museum of Glass, 2006)

Survey of London, vols. 18 & 29 (London: LCC, 1937)

Christopher Simon Sykes, *Private Palaces: Life in the Great London Houses* (London: Chatto & Windus, 1985)

Jenny Uglow, *Nature's Engraver: A life of Thomas Bewick* (London: Faber & Faber, 2006)

Chapter 5

Patricia Fara, *Sympathetic Attractions: Magnetic Practices, Beliefs, and Symbolism in Eighteenth-Century England* (Princeton, New Jersey: Princeton University Press, 1996)

W.D. Hackmann, *Electricity from Glass: The History of the Frictional Electrical Machine, 1600–1850* (Alphen aan den Rijn, The Netherlands: Sijthoff & Noordhoff, 1978)

Margaret C. Jacob, *The Radical Enlightenment: Pantheists, Freemasons and Republicans* (London: George Allen & Unwin, 1981)

Thomas W. Laqueur, *Solitary Sex: A Cultural History of Masturbation* (New York: Zone Books, 2004)

Daniel Pick, *Svengali's Web: The Alien Enchanter in Modern Culture* (Yale and London: Yale University Press, 2000)

Kate Williams, *England's Mistress: The Infamous Life of Emma Hamilton* (London: Hutchinson, 2006)

John Joseph Merlin: The Ingenious Mechanick (The Iveagh Bequest, Kenwood, GLC, 1985)

Chapter 6

Richard D. Altick, *The Shows of London* (Cambridge, Mass.: Harvard University Press, 1978)

Maxine Berg and Elizabeth Eger, *Luxury in the Eighteenth Century: Debates, Desires and Delectable Goods* (Basingstoke: Palgrave, 2003)

Paula Byrne, *Perdita: the Life of Mary Robinson* (London: HarperCollins, 2004)

James Chandler and Kevin Gilmartin, eds., *Romantic Metropolis: The Urban Scene of British Culture, 1780–1840* (Cambridge: Cambridge University Press, 2006)

Stella Tillyard, *Aristocrats* (London: Chatto & Windus, 1994)

David Wormersley, *Cultures of Whiggism: New Essays on English*

Literature and Culture in the Long Eighteenth Century (Newark: University of Delaware Press, 2005)

Chapter 7

Lisa Forman Cody, *Birthing the Nation: Sex, Science, and the Conception of Eighteenth-Century Britons,* (Oxford: Oxford University Press, 2005)
Lesley Hall and Roy Porter, *The Facts of Life: the Creation of Sexual Knowledge in Britain, 1650–1950* (New Haven, Yale University Press, 1995)
Karen Harvey, *Reading Sex in the Eighteenth Century: Bodies and Gender in English Erotic Culture* (Cambridge: Cambridge University Press, 2005)
Tim Hitchcock, *English Sexualities, 1700–1800* (Basingstoke: Macmillan, 1997)
Angus McLaren, *Reproductive Rituals The Perception of Fertility in England from the Sixteenth to the Nineteenth Century* (Methuen: London and New York, 1984)
Angus McLaren, *Impotence: a Cultural History* (Chicago, Ill.: University of Chicago Press, 2007)
Julie Peakman, *Lascivious Bodies: A Sexual History of the Eighteenth Century* (London: Atlantic Books, 2004)
G.S. Rousseau and Roy Porter, *Sexual Underworlds of the Enlightenment* (Manchester: Manchester University Press, 1987)
Marsha Keith Schuchard, *Why Mrs Blake Cried: William Blake and the Sexual Basis of Spiritual Vision* (London: Century, 2006)
A. Pettit and P. Spedding, eds., *Eighteenth-Century British Erotica*, Parts I and II (London: Pickering and Chatto, 2004 and 2005)

Chapter 8

Clare Brant, *Eighteenth-Century Letters and British Culture* (London: Palgrave Macmillan, 2006)
J.E. Force and R.H. Popkin, eds., *Millenarianism and Messianism in Early Modern European Culture*, vol. 3, *The Millenarian Turn* (The Netherlands: Kluwer Academic Publishers, 2001)
Ida Macalpine and Richard Hunter, *George III and the Mad-Business* (1969; London: Pimlico, 1991)
Jon Mee, *Romanticism, Enthusiasm, and Regulation: Poetics and the Policing of Culture in the Romantic Period* (Oxford: Oxford University Press, 2003)

Acknowledgements

The jigsaw story of Graham's life was pieced together and set in context with the help of numerous individuals at a variety of institutions: I should particularly like to thank Glenn Adamson and his colleagues at the Victoria and Albert Museum, Stephen Astley and Mike Nicholson at the Sir John Soane Museum, Gail Bardhan at the Corning Museum of Glass, Ray Bates (The British Clockmaker in Vermont), Gina Douglas at the Linnaean Society, John Jenkins and his Sparkmuseum, Phil Lapsansky at the Library Company of Philadelphia, Mark Frazier Lloyd at the University of Pennsylvania, Lindsay Levy and Andrea Longson at the Faculty of Advocates, Edinburgh, Ana Ramirez Luhrs at the Gilder Lehrman collection at the New York Historical Society, Pamela Miller and Lily Szczygiel at McGill University, Montreal, Andrew Pepitt at the Devonshire Archives, Chatsworth, and Cathy Ross at the Museum of London.

I am also indebted to the collections and the helpful staff of the Bath Record Office, Benjamin Franklin House, the British Library, the Central Library of Edinburgh, the Czech Museum of Music, Dr Johnson's House, the Guildhall Library, the Hunterian Museum at the Royal College of Surgeons of England, the Institute and Museum of the History of Science in Florence, the Library and Museum of Freemasonry, London, the London Library, the London Metropolitan Archives, the Old Operating Theatre, the National Library of Scotland, the National Portrait Gallery, the Norfolk Record Office, the Prague Pharmacy Museum, the Royal Academy, the Royal College of Physicians of Edinburgh, the former Theatre Museum (Victoria & Albert), the Wellcome Library, the West Yorkshire Archives and the Westminster Archives.

I wish it had been possible to thank in person Roy Porter, who posthumously introduced me to James Graham. My agent, James Gill, made it possible for a passing thought to become a published book; he is a great rock. Thank you to everyone at Alma for all their hard work. Vital encouragement at early stages came from Antony Wood at the Wellcome Trust, Marybeth Hamilton, Michael Hunter and Daniel Pick at Birkbeck College, London University, as well as Anne Janowitz, Elizabeth Eger and other scholarly friends. Thanks must also go to Diane Baptie and Ian Marson for their genealogical research. John Elmes, Esther Godfrey, Natasha Lehrer, Lea Ouai, Polly Radcliffe and Rosemary Scoular all helped me in important ways. Thank you, Kate Summerscale, for critical insight and library companionship. A lifetime of friendship and support from Andrew Shaw and Clare Brant extended to ongoing discussions and short-notice mercy missions on this book: undertaken by both with characteristic grace and rigour.

My whole family has been heroic, and utterly indispensable: huge thanks to parents and siblings, Lucy Gaster, Nick Deakin, Luke Syson and Antonia Syson. My wonderful children Phoebe, Adam, Rufus and Solomon have endured my obsessions and my absences, physical and mental, with great humour. As for my partner, Martin, this book could not exist without his unshaking faith and practical support. *Doctor of Love* is dedicated to my beloved grandfather, Jack Gaster (1907–2007).

Index

Pennsylvania Gazette: 47
Penn, William: 63
Perdita: see Mary Robinson
Phallus worship: 158
Philadelphia: 14, 17, 38, 41, 42–45, 47,
    48, 49, 50, 53, 55, 62–63, 64, 65, 69,
    74, 87, 138, 147, 154, 156, 182
    Arch Street: 48, 62, 63
    College of Philadelphia: 45, 48, 49
    Fourth Street: 42
    Front Street: 41
    Library Company: 44, 46
    Loganian Library: 44
Phlebotomy: see Bloodletting
Phlogiston (dephlogisticated air): see
    Oxygen
Pickering, Mary: see Graham, Mary
Pigott, Robert: 140
Pills: 15, 29, 126, 147, 171, 172, 189,
    263
    Imperial pills: 147
Pivati, Gianfrancesco: 148
Placebo: 126
Pleasure Gardens: 179
Pneumatic chemistry: 88, 148
Politics: 6, 36, 45, 49, 70, 71, 72, 76,
    83, 96, 98, 102, 109, 122, 140, 142,
    144, 159, 162, 170, 197, 198, 200,
    216, 217, 221, 235, 239, 241, 246,
    251, 258, 259
Polwhele, Rev. Richard: 93
Polygamy: 180, 192, 298
Population: 30–31, 36, 80, 199
Pornography: 61, 212, 213, 228
Preformationism: 201–203
    'ovist': 201, 202
    'spermist': 201, 203
Presbyterianism: 11, 27, 33, 252
Price, Richard: 199
Priestley, Joseph: 55, 59, 86, 88, 94,
    140, 148, 149, 249
Prince of Wales: 190, 255
Pringle, John: 149
Pringle, Mark: 123–25
Prostitution: 6, 41, 105, 108, 157, 189,
    192, 194, 200, 211, 213
Publicity: 7, 9, 25, 26, 31, 38, 39, 40,
    41, 42, 48, 55, 62, 63, 64, 65, 71, 72,

74, 75, 79, 85, 88, 86, 89, 94, 101, 103,
    106, 111, 122, 123, 124, 144, 146, 151,
    153, 154, 155, 156, 158, 162, 163, 164,
    165, 166, 167–68, 171, 172, 176, 177,
    178, 187, 188, 191, 192, 193, 196, 212,
    215, 223, 229, 233, 234, 238, 241, 248,
    251, 256
Puffery: see Publicity
Pulteney, Richard: 14, 15, 28
Puppet theatre: see Patagonian Theatre:
Purfleet, Essex: 116–17
Purging: 79, 89, 124, 142, 190
Pyne, William: 180
Pythagoras: 140, 235, 242

Quackery: 7, 16, 40, 41, 57, 94, 97, 98,
    133, 164, 167, 171–72, 174, 175, 185,
    189, 203, 211, 229, 236, 238, 251, 257,
    263
Quakers, the: 30, 43, 46, 66, 156, 209,
    254
Queen Charlotte: 76, 154, 198

Rack, Edmund: 85, 99, 101, 102, 282
Rambler's Magazine, The: 61, 204, 212,
    227, 228, 239, 244
Ranelagh Gardens, London: see London
Raspe, Rudolph Erich: 167
Ravenscroft, George: 119
Regency crisis: 255, 257
Religion: see Arminianism; Baptist
    Church, the; Catholicism; Dissent;
    enthusiasm; Evangelism; God; Great
    Awakening, the; Methodism; natural
    theology; New True Church; Presby-
    terianism; Quakers, the
Reproduction: see Generation
Republicanism: 36, 72, 83, 91, 99
Reynolds, Frederick: 170, 186
Reynolds, John: 162
Reynolds, Sir Joshua: 24, 109, 179,
    193, 196, 197
Richmond, Duchess of: 198
Richmond, Duke of: 197
Rittenhouse, David: 43
Robinson, Mary (Perdita): 190, 217,
    225, 239

List of Illustrations

1. Illustration of electricity machine and apparatus for electrical experiments in *An introduction to electricity in six sections by James Ferguson*, 1775, Institute and Museum of the History of Science, Florence.

2. *An Experiment with Lightning Conductors*, 1778–1780, by Michelangelo Rooker, Science Museum/Science and Society Picture Library, London.

3. *Mesmer's tub; or a faithful representation of the operations of animal magnetism*, by Henri Thiriat, Wellcome Library, London.

4. *View of Adelphi and the Thames*, by Agostino Brunias, 1770, Guildhall Library, City of London.

5. *Emma Hart afterwards Lady Hamilton as the goddess of health while being exhibited in that character by Dr Graham in Pall Mall*, by Richard Cosway, *c.* 1780–90, © National Maritime Museum, Greenwich, London

6. 'The Celestial Couch or Sofa', Osler Library of the History of Medicine, McGill University, Montreal, Quebec, Canada.

7. *The Quacks, or Two unorthodox medical practitioners, J. Graham and G. Katerfelto battling against each other, each surrounded by objects symbolising his practice*, 1783, Wellcome Library, London.

8. *James Graham lecturing from a podium, to a crowd of ladies and gentlemen*, by John Boyne, 1783, Wellcome Library, London.

9. *The Aerostatick Stage Balloon*, by John Nicholson, 1783, Science Museum/Science and Society Picture Library, London.

10. *James Graham; possibly Miss Dunbar*, by John Kay, etching, 1785, © National Portrait Gallery, London.

11. *Dr Graham's Cold Earth and Warm Mud Bathing Establishment at 26 Fleet Street, London* (pen & ink with w/c over graphite on paper) by Rowlandson, Thomas (1756–1827) Yale Center for British Art, Paul Mellon Collection, USA/The Bridgeman Art Library